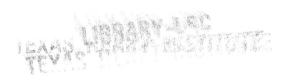

Essential Paediatric Haematology

Essential Paediatric Haematology

Edited by

Owen P Smith, MA, FRCP, FRCPath
Consultant Paediatric Haematologist, Senior Lecturer in
Haematology, Our Lady's Hospital for Sick Children,
St James's Hospital and Trinity College, Dublin, Ireland

and

Ian M Hann, MD, FRCP, FRCPath
Consultant Haematologist, Camelia Botnar Laboratory, Great
Ormond Street, London, UK

MARTIN DUNITZ

© 2002 Martin Dunitz Ltd, a memeber of the Taylor & Francis Group

First published in the United Kingdom in 2002
by Martin Dunitz Ltd, The Livery House, 7–9 Pratt Street, London NW1 0AE

Tel: +44 (0) 20 74822202
Fax: +44 (0) 20 72670159
E-mail: info@dunitz.co.uk
Website: http://www.dunitz.co.uk

Although every effort has been made to ensure that all owners of copyright material have been acknowledged in this publication, we would be glad to acknowledge in subsequent reprints or editions any omissions brought to our attention.

Although every effort has been made to ensure that drug doses and other information are presented accurately in this publication, the ultimate responsibility rests with the prescribing physician. Neither the publishers nor the authors can be held responsible for errors or for any consequences arising from the use of information contained herein. For detailed prescribing information or instructions on the use of any product or procedure discussed herein, please consult the prescribing information or instructional material issued by the manufacturer.

A CIP record for this book is available from the British Library.

ISBN 90-5823-179-8

Distributed in the USA by
Fulfilment Center
Taylor & Francis
7625 Empire Drive
Florence, KY 41042, USA
Toll Free Tel.: +1 800 634 7064
E-mail: cserve@routledge_ny.com

Distributed in Canada by
Taylor & Francis
74 Rolark Drive
Scarborough, Ontario M1R 4G2, Canada
Toll Free Tel.: +1 877 226 2237
E-mail: tal_fran@istar.ca

Distributed in the rest of the world by
ITPS Limited
Cheriton House
North Way
Andover, Hampshire SP10 5BE, UK
Tel.: +44 (0) 1264 332424
E-mail: reception@itps.co.uk

Composition by Wearset Ltd, Boldon, Tyne & Wear

Printed and bound in Spain by Tallers Grafics Soler, SA

Contents

Preface

Paediatric haematology is a rapidly expanding specialty and enormous advances in terms of molecular diagnostic and therapeutic strategies have been seen in the past three decades or so, particularly in the areas of coagulation, blood transfusion, bone marrow failure, white and red cell disorders. One such example is childhood acute lymphoblastic leukaemia, a death sentence in the 1960s that now has cure rates in excess of 80%.

It was our intention from the outset that *Essential Paediatric Haematology* would be a relatively compact book containing concise, practical up-to-date information with detailed tables, and algorithms where appropriate. To this end we have been ably assisted by nine colleagues, each with great expertise in the fields in which they have contributed. The information contained within this book should prove useful for those key members involved in the care of children with blood disorders, namely trainee doctors, nurses, pharmacists, radiotherapists, social workers, psychologists, and laboratory staff, to name a few.

We would like to thank our wives, Jude and Julie, and also Alison Campbell, Clare Lack and Máire Collins from Martin Dunitz Publishers for their forbearance during the time that this book has been prepared.

OPS, *Dublin*
IMH, *London*

Contributors

Erika A de Wynter, PhD
Molecular Medicine Unit
Clinical Sciences Building
St James University Hospital
Leeds LS9 7TF
UK

Helen Enright, MD, FRCPI, FRCPath
Department of Haematology
Adelaide and Meath Hospital Dublin
& National Children's Hospital
Tallaght
Dublin 24
Ireland

Ian M Hann, MD, FRCP, FRCPath
Camelia Botnar Laboratory
Great Ormond Street
London WC1N 3JH
UK

Meriel EM Jenney, MD, MRCP
Department of Paediatric Haematology and
Oncology
Llandough Hospital
Penlan Road
Penarth CF64 2XX
UK

Mark Lawler, PhD, MRCPath
Department of Haematology and
Institute for Molecular Medicine
St James's Hospital and Trinity College
Dublin 8
Ireland

**Michael M Reid, MD, FRCP, FRCPath,
FRCPCH**
Department of Haematology
Newcastle upon Tyne Hospitals
NHS Trust
Newcastle upon Tyne NE1 4LP
UK

Irene Roberts, MD(Hons), FRCP
Department of Haematology
Imperial College Faculty of Medicine
Hammersmith Hospital
Du Cane Road
London W12 0HS
UK

Owen P Smith, MA, FRCP, FRCPath
Department of Haematology and Oncology
Our Lady's Hospital for Sick Children
St James's Hospital and Trinity College
Dublin 8
Ireland

Nydia G Testa, MD, PhD
CRC Experimental Haematology Group
Patterson Institute for Cancer Research
Christie Hospital
Wilmslow Road
Withington
Manchester M20 4BX
UK

George Vassiliou, MRCP
Department of Haematology
Imperial College Faculty of Medicine
Hammersmith Hospital
Du Cane Road
London W12 0HS
UK

David KH Webb, MD, FRCP, FRCPath
Department of Haematology
Great Ormond Street Hospital for
Sick Children NHS Trust
Great Ormond Street
London WC1N 3JH
UK

Dedication

This book is dedicated to our many trainee doctors who have over the years been the source of great inspiration.

1 Normal haemopoiesis

Nydia G Testa and Erika A de Wynter

INTRODUCTION

Haemopoiesis is the process responsible for generating mature blood cells. Mature myeloid cells are condemned to live for only a few hours, as in the case of granulocytes, or a few weeks, as in the case of erythrocytes. This indicates that every day, new cells have to be produced just to replace steady state loss. Normally, of the order of 10^{11} myeloid cells per day are produced in a normal adult. More may be produced in response to increased demand following, for example, blood loss, infection, decreased oxygen availability or abnormal cell destruction. It is known that these cells derive from a common ancestor population, the pluripotential stem cells. The stem cells are relatively few in number, comprising less than 0.001% of the total bone marrow cells, and are defined by characteristic features. These are the ability to produce more stem cells (self-renewal), the capacity to differentiate and generate more development-restricted progenitor cells for all the myeloid and lymphoid lineages, and the potential for extensive proliferation (expressed in their progeny), which ensures enormous amplification in cell numbers.

Our knowledge of the function of the haemopoietic system has progressed enormously due to the variety of experimental assays that allow precise definition of developmental stages. The observation that some bone marrow cells could give rise to clonal colonies containing mature granulocytes and macrophages allowed the development of quantitative assays for the detection of progenitor cells. These assays in turn permitted the discovery of an array of regulatory cytokines, many of which have already been incorporated into clinical practice. In addition, the haemopoietic tissue offers to developmental biologists a system where physiological differentiation, proliferation and senescence can be investigated. Thus, the rapid pace at which we have increased our understanding of the system is expected to continue. In this chapter, we will consider the development and structure of the tissue and the regulation of cell production.

HAEMOPOIETIC TISSUE

Development

In embryogenesis, the first haemopoietic cells are seen in the yolk sac in blood islands. In the fetus, haemopoietic cells are first detected in the aorta–gonad–mesonephros region, from where they migrate to fetal haemopoietic sites and, in time, originate the definitive haemopoiesis. Any contribution of the yolk sac to definitive haemopoiesis is controversial. During early development, after the twelfth week of gestation, the fetal liver is the main site of haemopoiesis, with erythropoiesis starting as dominant, and granulopoiesis developing later. The spleen is also haemopoietic until about the time of birth, although making a smaller contribution than the liver. From week 20 of gestation, the bone marrow becomes increasingly more important and it eventually becomes the main haemopoietic organ. Haemopoietically active marrow is found in all bones for the first 2–3 years of life, but, later, part of this is gradually replaced by inactive fatty marrow. In the adult, active marrow is only found in the epiphyses of long bones and in the trabecular bone in the sternum, ribs, cranium, vertebrae and pelvis. There is no further normal expansion of the tissue after infancy, though there may be a decrease in older people.

The inactive marrow, liver and spleen, however, conserve the capacity to sustain haemopoiesis throughout life. If required (for example, in patients with haemolytic anaemia) the extramedullary sites may be recolonized by stem cells from the bone marrow that have migrated via the circulation. It follows from this that stem cells are found in the peripheral blood, albeit in very low numbers, in normal individuals. It is noteworthy that, at the time of birth, there are still large numbers of primitive cells in the cord blood, with an incidence similar to that in the adult bone marrow. Although the incidence of primitive cells in blood falls rapidly after birth, the administration of cytokines can increase it to a magnitude that makes blood a viable alternative to bone marrow as a source of cells for transplantation.

Structure

Stem cells

The haemopoietic, intestinal and skin systems belong to the hierarchical tissues of the body, where short-lived differentiated end cells are continuously being replaced through processes of proliferation, differentiation and maturation, starting at the level of the stem cells. This is illustrated in Fig. 1.1. Normally, stem cells are quiescent, most residing in the G_0 state of the cell cycle. They are only reluctantly induced to divide, as seen by their relative resistance to cell-cycle-active agents such as 5-fluorouracil. Indeed, even after in vivo cytotoxic injury, about 48 hours are required before primitive populations of quiescent cells are recruited into the cell cycle and enter its S phase. This is, perhaps, not surprising when one considers that, as seen from experimental transplantation, the stem cell compartment has a functional capacity vastly in excess of that required to maintain cell production for a normal lifetime, even if a response to serious and repeated proliferation stress (such as chemotherapy) has taken place. There is an evolutionary argument supporting the difficulty of recruiting stem cells into cycle: up until this century, the prolifera-

tion stress caused by loss of mature cells (for example, by haemorrhage) resulted in compensatory mechanisms that swiftly increased cell production. These mechanisms include expansion of active marrow sites, induction of extramedullary haemopoiesis (reversing the stages of normal development described above), shortening of the intermitotic time in differentiating cells, increase in the proportion of progenitors in active cell cycle and earlier release of cells into the blood. For example, the last of these is seen as increased numbers of reticulocytes in the circulation when there is an increased requirement for production of red cells. All these mechanisms ensure increased mature cell production without necessarily requiring any extra contribution from stem cells. Indeed, it is only in the last century that random stem cell kill by cytotoxic drugs or radiation, or regeneration of haemopoiesis following transplantation, necessitated stress activation of stem cells.

Experimentally, stem cell function is assessed by transplantation. Thus, we may define the marrow repopulating cells (MRC) as those that regenerate haemopoiesis in the long term following transplantation into ablated recipients (Fig. 1.1). Transplant assays for human cells are only possible using xenografts: the most widely used involves immunosuppressed NOD/SCID (non-obese diabetic/severe combined immunodeficient) mice, which, when inoculated with human haemopoietic cells following sublethal irradiation, allow establishment of active human haemopoiesis. Although this assay is being widely used, it is not fully understood: the numbers of human cells required for successful transplantation are about one order of magnitude higher than those of murine cells required to rescue mice from haemopoietic death following ablation. The reasons for this low efficiency are not clear. Furthermore, there is a bias towards B-cell differentiation, and the numbers of human myeloid cells produced may be relatively small.

An alternative in vitro assay that detects a primitive cell population containing MRC (at least in mice) is the long-term culture-initiating cell (LTC-IC) assay. These cells are defined by their capacity to generate clonogenic progenitor cells after at least 5 weeks of

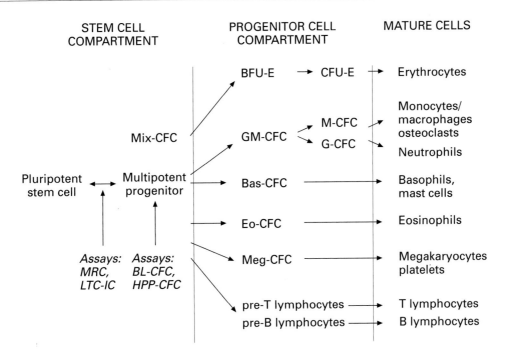

STEM CELL COMPARTMENT **PROGENITOR CELL COMPARTMENT** **MATURE CELLS**

Figure 1.1

Schematic representation of haemopoiesis, showing the three major compartments of haemopoietic populations: BFU-E, burst forming unit erythroid; CFU-E, colony forming unit erythroid; GM-CFC, granulocyte–macrophage colony forming cell; M-CFC, macrophage CFC; G-CFC, granulocyte CFC; Bas-CFC, basophil CFC; Eo-CFC, eosinophil CFC; Meg-CFC, megakaryocyte CFC.

culture in the presence of competent stromal cells (Fig. 1.1). The LTC-IC assay detects a population that partially overlaps with stem cells, at least in mice, but it may also detect primitive progenitor cells.

In conjunction with biological assays, progress has also been made in determining the phenotype of primitive haemopoietic cells (Table 1.1). This allows the purification of discrete cell subpopulations, or even isolation of single cells that may be characterized further in biological assays. At present, the CD34 marker used in cell selection protocols has been applied for clinical use, while most others, such as CD133 (previously known as AC133), CCR1 and CXCR4, remain experimental.

Table 1.1 Phenotypic markers of primitive haemopoietic cells

	Stem cells	Progenitor cells
CD34	+[a]	–
CD38	–	+
CD33	–	+
CD133	+	Some +
Lineage	–	+
HLA-DR	–/+	+
CD71	–	+
Thy-1	–/low	+
CD45RA	low	+
c-Kit	+	–/low
CCR1	+	Some +
CXCR4	+	?
Rhodamine	low	+

[a] A minority are CD34-negative.

Progenitor cells

In the continuum of cell proliferation and differentiation, the progenitor cell population encompasses the immediate progeny of stem cells (which may still conserve some of the stem cell properties) through to committed cells that have not only lost multipotentiality, but also show a more limited capacity for proliferation (Table 1.2).

It is generally agreed that the decision to enter a particular differentiation pathway distinguishes the progenitor from the stem cell populations. The commitment to differentiation appears to be irreversible. This was demonstrated using erythroid progenitors manipulated to express receptors for macrophage colony stimulating factor (M-CSF) which has an important role in macrophage development. When exposed to M-CSF, the erythroid progenitors still develop into erythroid cells. Conversely, macrophage progenitor cells manipulated to express the receptors for erythropoietin (EPO), which has an important role in erythroid development, develop into macrophages and not into erythroid cells in response to EPO stimulation.

However, commitment to differentiation can be manipulated. Although knowledge in this field is very limited, we know that decisions about the choice between self-renewal and differentiation (and which lineage to follow after the latter) can be altered by manipulating either the levels of cytokine that cells are exposed to or the levels of some transcription factors. However, the mechanisms that determine or allow stem cell fate decisions are largely unknown. The genetic programme involving the presumably complex regulatory pathways is only beginning to be elucidated. Phillips et al (2000) have recently published a wide gene expression analysis on putative purified murine stem cells, and found that a significant percentage of the several thousand gene products characterized corresponded to previously unrecognized molecules with properties that suggest regulatory functions.

Progenitor cells were defined following the observation, more than 30 years ago, that clonal colonies containing mature neutrophils and macrophages would develop when haemopoietic cells are cultured in a soft gel matrix containing feeder cells or media conditioned by the growth of some non-haemopoietic cell types. Since then, our knowledge of both the cells giving rise to the colonies (colony forming cells, CFCs) and the

Table 1.2 Developmental changes in primitive haemopoietic cells

Parameters	Stem cells	Early progenitor cells	Late progenitor cells
Incidence in normal bone marrow	$1{:}10^4{-}10^5$	$2{-}5{:}10^5$	$50{-}600{:}10^5$
% of cells in S phase	<10	20–50	50–80
Lineage markers	−	±	++
Self-renewal	++	+	−
Proliferation potential	+++	++	+
Microenvironmental control (matrix molecules, stromal cells, adhesion molecules)	+++	++	±
Humoral control	±	+	++

molecules first described as colony stimulating factors (CSFs) has advanced enormously. Similar advances, which will not be discussed in this chapter, were being made regarding the development of B and T cells (reviewed in Collard and Gearing, 1994).

The progenitor cells are also called CFCs, preceded by a notation that describes their lineage commitment, such as GM (granulocyte–macrophage)-CFC, Eo (eosinophil)-CFC and Meg (megakaryocyte)-CFC. Historically, early erythroid (E) progenitors are called burst forming units (BFU)-erythroid (BFU-E) to describe the appearance of the erythroid colony (burst), with late erythroid progenitors being called colony forming units (CFU-E) (Fig. 1.1).

Within the variety of clonal assays for progenitor cells there are some that almost certainly overlap partially with assays for stem cells. The cells that originate blast cell colonies (Bl-CFCs) are able to originate progenitor cells, which, if replated, will in turn, originate further colonies. The high-proliferative-potential (HPP) CFCs also share with stem cells some phenotypic markers and express high proliferation capacity and multipotentiality. They are also normally quiescent. Thus, these colony assays detect cells placed in the boundary between the stem and the progenitor cell populations (Fig. 1.1). Following in the differentiation–maturation pathway are cells that originate colonies composed of cells belonging to many of the myeloid lineages. These cells are called Mix(ed) CFCs, or GEEMM (granulocytic, eosinophilic, erythroid, macrophage, megakaryocytic) CFCs. They may be classified as early progenitor cells (Table 1.2). Within these large colonies, which may contain up to 10^4 cells, new progenitor cells may also be generated.

The progenitor cells become progressively more limited in their potential for differentiation and proliferation until eventually they are restricted to one lineage and only give rise to colonies of less than 100 cells. Thus, along these processes: (a) the incidence of (late) progenitors increases due to amplification taking place by cell division, (b) the proportion of progenitors in cell cycle also increases and (c) phenotypic changes occur with the acquisition of lineage-specific markers. These changes are illustrated in Table 1.2.

Regulation

Growth Factors

The haemopoietic tissue is able to maintain cell production between the narrow normal values and is also capable of eliciting a response to exceptional requirements for mature cells. The varied functions of the mature blood cells require that the signal for varied levels of cell production may originate outside the bone marrow. For example, a local infection results in enhanced production of factors that will increase granulocyte production and migration to the appropriate site; anoxic conditions will increase production of EPO by the kidney and this will, in turn, stimulate erythropoiesis.

The role of EPO in the stimulation of red cell production was first described at the beginning of the century. However, as mentioned above, only the development of CFC assays in the 1960s allowed first the description and later the purification of CSFs. Later, the use of DNA technology allowed the isolation of the genes coding for diverse cytokines and the production of large amounts of material using appropriate expression systems. Following the recombinant molecules that first became available in the 1980s, more than 30 cytokines are now known to influence haemopoietic cell production (Table 1.3).

It is appropriate here to clarify the varied nomenclature used for haemopoietic regulators, which was developed using descriptive, response-related terminology. One example has already been given: CSFs were defined by their capacity to stimulate in vitro colony growth. The interleukins (ILs) were described as molecules produced by white cells, such as T cells, able to exert their effect on (other) white cells. Later, it became apparent that the effects of interleukins were much wider, and could be targeted on several tissues. For example, receptors for IL-1 are expressed not only on a wide variety of haemopoietic cells, but also on fibroblasts, endothelial and neural cells, indicating that IL-1 has a wide range of effects. There are well-characterized effects of IL-1 on embryo implantation in experimental systems and some described also in humans. From these examples, it is obvious that

Table 1.3 Some growth factors and target colony forming cells		
Growth factor[a]	**Chromosome location**	**Target colony forming cell**[b]
IL-3	5q23–31	Mix-CFC, HPP-CFC, GM-CFC, Eo-CFC, Ba-CFC, Meg-CFC, BFU-E
GM-CSF	5q23–31	HPP-CFC, GM-CFC, Eo-CFC, Meg-CFC, BFU-E
G-CSF	17q21–22	HPP-CFC, Mix-CFC, GM-CFC
M-CSF	5q33	HPP-CFC, GM-CFC
EPO	1q	CFU-E
SCF	12q22–24	Mix-CFC (s), HPP-CFC (s), GM-CFC, BFU-E, Bas-CFC
IL-1α	2q12–21	HPP-CFC (s)
IL-4	5q31	GM-CFC (s), Bas-CFC (s), BFU-E (s)
IL-5	5q23–31	Eo-CFC (s)
IL-6 (IFN-β2)	7q14–21	HPP-CFC (s), GM-CFC (s)
IL-9	5q31.1	BFU-E (s), GM-CFC (s), BFU-E (s)
IL-11	19q13.3–13.4	Meg-CFC (s), GM-CFC (s), BFU-E (s)
TPO	3q23–27	Meg-CFC (s), Other CFC
FLT ligand (Flk-2 ligand)	13q12	Mix-CFC (s), BFU-E (s), GM-CFC (s)
bFGF (FGF-2)	4q25–27	BFU-E (s), GM-CFC (s)
LIF	5q12–13	Meg-CFC (s), BFU-E (s)

[a] IL, interleukin; GM-CSF, granulocyte–macrophage colony stimulating factor; G-CSF, granulocyte CSF; M-CSF, macrophage CSF; EPO, erythropoietin; SCF, stem cell factor; TPO, thrombopoietin; bFGF, basic fibroblast growth factor; LIF, leukaemia inhibitory factor.
[b] CFC, colony forming cell; BFU, burst forming unit; CFU, colony forming unit; Mix, mixed; HPP, high-proliferative potential; GM, granulocyte–macrophage; Eo, eosinophil; Bas, basophil; Meg, megakaryocyte; E, erythroid; (s) synergism with other cytokines.

cytokines (perhaps with the exception of EPO) do not fit the classic definition of hormones (Table 1.4). It also follows that many cytokines have pleiotropic effects, and their variety of actions may overlap to a partial extent. Some examples are shown in Table 1.5. Several general properties are ascribed to cytokines:

- they may be produced by a variety of cells and tend to have a variety of effects on different (or even on the same) target cells;

- different cytokines may have similar actions (Table 1.5);
- they may synergize when acting on the same cells (Table 1.3), and this is observed particularly at the level of the more primitive cells;
- cytokines may modulate the expression of receptors for other cytokines, increasing or decreasing the number of receptors;
- cytokines may increase or decrease signalling by receptors for other cytokines.

Table 1.4 Properties of hormones and cytokines

Classic hormones	Cytokines
Polypeptides, proteins, steroids	Polypeptides, proteins, glycoproteins
Each produced at a specific site	Produced by many cells, tissues
Action not at site of production	Action local or distant
Receptors in one (occasionally two) target cell types (target specificity)	Receptors in several cell types (may also be on producer cells)
Unique actions (no biological redundancy)	Overlapping biological activities (leading to some biological redundancy)
Constitutive production	Constitutive production low (even absent in some cases)

Table 1.5 Examples of overlapping biological profiles of cytokines

Action	Endpoint	Cytokines[a]
Cell proliferation	Stimulation of neutrophilic granulocyte colonies	G-CSF, GM-CSF, M-CSF, IL-3, SCF
Common target cells	CFC (Eo, G, M, GM, E, Meg, Bas) CFC (Meg, E) Platelet formation	IL-3 EPO TPO, IL-6, IL-11
Receptors	Common β-chain subunit Common gp130 subunit	GM-CSF, IL-3, IL-5 LIF, IL-6, IL-11, others

[a] See Table 1.3 for abbreviations.

A group of cytokines originally described by their property of exerting chemotactic effects on cells involved in inflammatory processes are called chemokines (chemotactic cytokines). Not only their known roles but also their number have increased. There are at present about 60 chemokines described, many of which exert effects on the regulation of haemopoietic cell production or function. One of these chemokines, with established and important effects on haemopoiesis, is MIP-1α (macrophage inflammatory protein 1 alpha).

Inhibitors of haemopoiesis need to be postulated as a way of avoiding fluctuations in the number of cells produced and also to stop overproduction once an exceptional need has been satisfied. The two most commonly described are MIP-1α and transforming growth factor β (TGF-β). They fulfil the characteristics of inhibitors: they are not toxic and their actions are reversible. Primitive haemopoietic cells exposed to MIP-1α do not enter the DNA synthesis (S) phase of the cell cycle. Although this effect is seen in primitive cells, MIP-1α may also exert a stimulatory action on some of the more mature subpopulations of CFCs. The inhibitory role of TGF-β on the proliferation of early and late progenitor cells is similar. The tetrapeptide

AcSDKP also has a reversible action and inhibits cell progress into S phase. Tumour necrosis factor (TNF) inhibits colony formation by CFCs, but at low concentrations and, acting in conjunction with GM-CSF and IL-3, it has a stimulatory effect. Other molecules such as prostaglandins, interferon-inducible protein, lactoferrins and isoferritins have also been described as inhibitors of haemopoiesis, but their effect may be indirect and in some cases is controversial.

The points above show the high degree of complexity in the regulation of the haemopoietic system where different pathways may lead to the same response. The same mature cell type may be produced by the action of different cytokines, and deficiencies in production of a cytokine will not necessarily result in the cessation of a specific differentiation pathway. This has been demonstrated experimentally using mice where specific genes have been 'knocked out'; for example, in mice lacking the functional GM-CSF gene, the number of granulocytes and macrophages is practically normal. Nevertheless, this does not make for a redundant gene, since specific functional abnormalities of the mature cells were detected. However, there are no examples where cytokines are produced or act in isolation: there is a regulatory network of stimulatory and inhibitory cytokines that act together to give an overall biological response.

Responses to growth factors

It is obvious from the above that the responses to growth factors are varied and complex and that the growth factors act in a concerted fashion. Haemopoietic cell responses include survival, differentiation, proliferation and, in the mature cells, induction of specific functions.

Specific growth factor receptors are found in all haemopoietic cells up to and including stem and progenitor cells. It is also obvious from Tables 1.3 and 1.5 that haemopoietic cells must have receptors for more than just one cytokine. This too has been demonstrated, not only by labelled ligands but also by the biological responses of the cells. In addition to the survival response, the synergistic

actions are also obvious from many experiments. A number of examples of synergisms are illustrated in Table 1.3: progenitor cells respond to a combination of factors by expressing an increased proliferation capacity (as seen by progenitors producing bigger colonies) or by being recruited into proliferation (more progenitors produce more colonies). Thus, synergism in the latter instance is demonstrated as combinations of growth factors that can elicit a response from cells that are unresponsive to a factor acting alone. For example, stem cell factor (SCF) is, by itself, a poor stimulus for colony formation. However, in combination with G-CSF, it is a potent stimulus for colony growth. The joint action of different growth factors and their relative levels also have an influence on differentiation. This is seen when the relative levels of G-CSF and M-CSF acting together direct the differentiation of GM-CFC to produce varying proportions of neutrophilic granulocytes and macrophages within the colonies.

Growth factor receptors

Cytokines bind to specific receptors on the cell surface. Most of these receptors have been cloned and their structure analysed. They have been grouped into families (members sharing more than 50% homology) and superfamilies (for those with less than 50% homology, usually 15–25%). Evolutionary relationships and common or distinct mechanisms of action are being actively investigated at present.

Functionally, as discussed above, receptors are able to mediate different types of response. One of the mechanisms involved in allowing pleiotropic effects is that different but related cytokines share receptor components. The receptors for GM-CSF, IL-3 and IL-5 all share a common β subunit but each has a specific α subunit. Thus unique actions of these cytokines sharing a common β chain may be dictated by the cellular distribution of the α chain (defining the target cell), by the signalling domains of the α–β complexes or of the individual α component in the formation of the α-chain–ligand complex following ligand binding. It is also likely that the β chain may be the limiting factor in competing actions of GM-CSF, IL-3 or IL-5. Alternatively, synergism can be observed if there is an excess of the β chain. Other cytokines also sharing a common chain are IL-6, IL-11, LIF (and others), which share gp130 (a protein functioning as their signal transducer) (Table 1.5). Some cytokines also have soluble receptors, thus offering another mechanism for modulating cytokine responses.

The roles of stromal cells

In the bone marrow, haemopoiesis takes place in association with stromal cells. These have been shown to produce a variety of cytokines and chemokines either constitutively or in response to stimulation (Table 1.6). As discussed above, the harmonic and integrated action of multiple regulatory molecules results in tightly regulated normal or stress haemopoiesis. There are several roles that stromal cells may fulfil: (a) as producers and releasers of cytokines; (b) by retaining cytokines as cell-membrane bound; and (c) as producers of molecules that are constituents of the extracellular matrix. These molecules can, in turn, sequester and bind growth factors and present them to target cells in a biologically active form. From this it follows that interactions of stromal cells and haemopoietic cells, or cell–matrix interactions, are normal regulatory features (Fig. 1.2). Immunostaining has shown that cytokines are not evenly distributed and are localized preferentially to specific stromal populations. This supports the concept that there are discrete environments (niches) that promote preferential development of defined cell populations. This is also supported by the preferential localization of progenitor cells to certain areas of human bone marrow.

Table 1.6 Cell types producing cytokines or chemokines

Cell type	Cytokines[a]
Fibroblasts, reticular cells	GM-CSF, G-CSF, IL-3, -6, -8, M-CSF, SCF
Macrophages	IL-1, -6, -8, GM-CSF, G-CSF, IL-6, M-CSF, TNF, TGF-β, MIP-1α
T cells	IL-2, -3, -4, -5, -6, -8, -9, TNF, TGF-β, GM-CSF
Bone marrow stromal cells	SCF, IL-1, -6, -7, -11, M-CSF, G-CSF, GM-CSF, LIF, TGF-β
B cells	IL-1, -6
Neutrophils	IL-1
Natural killer cells	IL-1, -3
Basophils	IL-5
Endothelial cells	IL-3, -6, -8, GM-CSF, G-CSF, M-CSF, SCF
Kidney cells	EPO, TPO
Liver cells	TPO

[a] TNF, tumour necorsis factor; TFG, transforming growth factor; MIP, macrophage inflammatory protein; see Table 1.3 for other abbreviations.

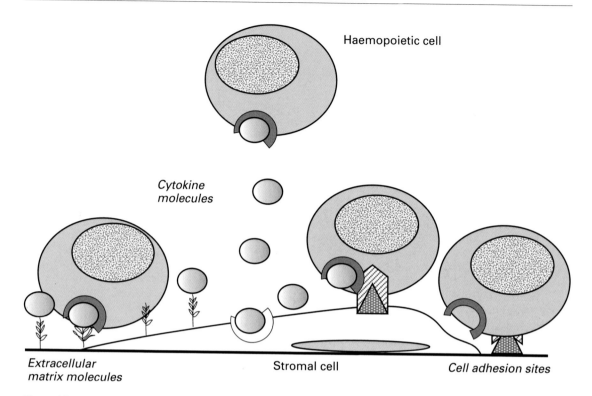

Haemopoietic cell

Cytokine molecules

Extracellular matrix molecules

Stromal cell

Cell adhesion sites

Figure 1.2

Model illustrating the interaction of haemopoietic cells and stomal cells with cytokines and extracellular matrix molecules.

NEW STEM CELLS

So far, we have discussed stem cells only in the context of haemopoietic cell development. At present, however, the concept that after the embryonic stage stem cells are committed to differentiation within their allocated tissue is being revised. It is now known that cells present in the bone marrow can develop into hepatocytes, brain or muscle cells. Furthermore, we have known for many years that stromal bone marrow cells are able to differentiate into bone, adipose, cartilage, endothelial and muscle tissue. Thus, the concept arose of the presence in the bone marrow not only of pluripotent haemopoietic stem cells but also of stromal cells with varied potential for differentiation. Proof of clonal development from a mesenchymal stem cell, however, is

not yet established, and it remains possible that different stromal cell populations give rise to the diverse cell types listed above. However, the concept is important, and proof of the potential clinical use of these cells is already available: osteogenesis imperfecta is improved following bone marrow transplantation. Conversely, it is also known that there are stem cells present in adult brain and muscle tissue that can develop into haemopoietic cells. However, the numbers of stem cells present in brain tissue that have haemopoietic potential are small and the numbers of bone marrow cells that are able to develop into brain cells (or into muscle) are also limited. The experimental data available so far certainly indicate that there is more developmental potential of some cells in adult tissues than had previously been assumed.

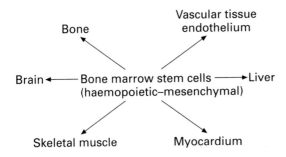

Figure 1.3

Potential targets for stem cell therapy, which may or may not involve genetic manipulation.

These new data have generated great enthusiasm about the potential of cell and genetic therapy for brain, muscle (including myocardial), hepatic and skeletal pathology (Fig. 1.3). While it is difficult to envisage the use of muscle or brain as cell sources for therapy, the availability of bone marrow cells (which may even be mobilized into the circulation) is obvious.

It is not yet clear, however, whether adult stem cells will be able to match the potential of embryonic stem cells. On the other hand, the ethical considerations (strongly held by part of the public) pertaining to the use of the latter do not apply to adult (i.e. non-embryonic, somatic) stem cells.

There remain, however, many questions to be answered before these new potential treatments materialize: can we manipulate differentiation (or de-differentiation followed by differentiation) across the defined embryonic origin of the target tissue? For example, can mesoderm-derived haemopoietic stem cells give rise to ectoderm-derived neuronal cells? Can we isolate, amplify and genetically manipulate these cells? Can we direct homing of stem cells to the target tissues? Assuming the latter is possible, can we prevent inappropriate differentiation of multipotential cells, either benign or malignant, in wrongly located tissue (for example, liver in muscle or muscle in brain)? Both adult stem cells and embryonic stem cells present these potential problems. In addition to these questions are the concerns associated with appropriate responses after genetic manipulation.

Nevertheless, we can envisage the revolution in treatment that these potential therapies may (will, as the optimists among us believe) bring in the medium-term future.

CONCLUSIONS

The advances in methodology that facilitated analysis of defined populations of stem and progenitor cells, and in turn allowed the detection of growth factors and their purification in recombinant form, have also allowed us to formulate sharp definitions of discrete steps concerning the regulation of blood cell production. In the last two decades, we learned much about cell proliferation. At present, progress is being made in our understanding of cell differentiation and the molecular steps involved in its regulation. We now have the ability to isolate and, to a certain extent, manipulate (either biologically or genetically) stem cells. This, together with our new glimpse into stem cell capacity for trans-tissue differentiation, defines the beginning of an exciting phase in which our knowledge of the haemopoietic system will be translated into new and exciting clinical applications, not only in haematology but also in a variety of other disciplines.

FURTHER READING

Collard R, Gearing A. (1994) *The Cytokine Facts Book*. London: Academic Press.

Metcalf D. (1988) *The Molecular Control of Blood Cells*. Cambridge, MA: Harvard University Press.

Phillips RL, Ernst RE, Brunk B et al. (2000) *Science* **288:** 1635–40.

Stem cells branch out (Editorial). (2000) *Science* **287:** 1417–46.

Testa NG, de Wynter EA, Weaver A. (1996) The study of haemopoietic cells in patients: concepts, approaches and cautionary tales. *Ann Oncol* **7** (Suppl 2): 5–8.

2 Normal coagulation

Owen P Smith

INTRODUCTION

Normal blood coagulation or haemostasis is a complex sequence of inter-related events by which the body prevents blood loss from the vascular tree. This is achieved by a multi-pathway interactive system with multiple negative- and positive-feedback loops, which ultimately ensure that blood is at all times fluid within the vasculature, but it also needs to be transformed into a clot when there is a breach in the integrity of the vascular tree. The protein and cellular components of this system have also been shown to be intimately involved in the inflammatory response, vasculogenesis, metastasis, cellular proliferation and tissue repair.

Tissue factor, a cell surface glycoprotein, is the principal biological initiator of blood coagulation. Exposure of circulating plasma VIIa to tissue factor triggers the coagulation cascade in vivo, which results in thrombin generation. Thrombin converts soluble fibrinogen to a fibrin network, activates platelets and stimulates coagulation by positive feedback activations of cofactors, factors V and VIII and the zymogens II, VII, IX, X, XII and XIII. Under physiological conditions, pro- and anticoagulant mechanisms are balanced in favour of anticoagulation; however, at sites of vascular damage resulting from inflammation, trauma etc., the anticoagulant system is downregulated and thus procoagulant forces prevail. This system maintains blood in its fluid phase while it allows rapid extravascular blood clotting to occur when needed. Over the past couple of decades, advances in our understanding of the details of the coagulation processes have begun to provide a variety of new approaches to the diagnosis, treatment and management of patients with haemorrhagic or thrombotic disease. Therefore, understanding the basic mechanisms of coagulation is likely to become increasingly important to those dealing with children with coagulation disorders.

PRIMARY HAEMOSTASIS

Under normal circumstances, the endothelium promotes blood fluidity by a number of interactions with platelets and the coagulation proteins. Following endothelial damage whether from trauma, inflammation etc., platelets rapidly adhere to the exposed 'damaged' subendothelium. This process is mediated primarily by von Willebrand factor protein (vWF), which binds to a specific protein on the platelet surface, glycoprotein Ib (GPIb). Following adhesion of platelets at the subendothelium, a series of physiological events occur that produce platelet activation. Activated platelets change shape from discs to irregular spiny processes, and the contents of the alpha granules and dense bodies (platelet organelles), such as calcium and the agonists adenosine diphosphate (ADP) and serotonin, are released (Table 2.1). The platelet agonist thromboxane A_2 synthesized from arachidonic acid is also released. During platelet activation, glycoprotein IIb, another integral platelet membrane receptor, undergoes conformational change that exposes recognition sites for soluble fibrinogen, fibronectin, vWF and vitronectin. The interaction between glycoprotein IIb, IIIa and fibrinogen is probably the most important in relation to the formation of an occlusive platelet plug in low-shear areas of the circulation, whereas the interaction of this receptor with vWF is key in areas of high shear. This

Table 2.1 Platelet granules and their content[a]

α granules	Dense granules	Lysosomes

Coagulation proteins
  Factor V
  Fibrinogen
  vWF
	Divalent cations
	  Ca^{2+}, Mg^{2+}
		Acid hydrolases

Growth factors
  PDGF
	Adenine nucleotides
	  ADP, ATP	

Platelet modulators
  Platelet factor 4
  β-thromboglobulin
	Platelet modulators
	  Bioactive amines
	  Serotonin	

Adhesive proteins
  Thrombospondin
  Fibronectin
  P-selectin		

[a] vWF, von Willebrand factor; PDGF, platelet-derived growth factor; ADP, adenosine diphosphate; ATP, adenosine triphosphate.

mechanism of primary haemostasis is often sufficient to stop bleeding. However, at other times, a more complex clot is required that involves platelet thrombus stabilization by fibrin, the process of secondary haemostasis.

SECONDARY HAEMOSTASIS

The conversion of soluble fibrinogen to insoluble fibrin is mediated by thrombin, which is generated following a series of linked proteolytic reactions in which zymogens are converted to trypsin-like enzymes (serine proteases) (Fig. 2.1). Each protease in turn then catalyses the subsequent zymogen/protease transition by cleavage of peptide bonds and in so doing amplifies the system, and in turn there is a rapid accumulation of fibrin. This highly efficient mechanism of fibrin formation is achieved through the formation of multimolecular complexes (zymogen, a cofactor and a converting enzyme).

The activation of the extrinsic pathway, also known as the tissue factor pathway, is by far the most important triggering mechanism to generate thrombin in vivo. This is achieved by a protein, tissue factor (TF), which is a cell surface glycoprotein that serves as a cellular receptor for factor VIIa (FVIIa). Normally TF is not exposed to blood, but if blood comes into contact with TF (vascular injury) then circulating factor VIIa together with TF triggers the coagulation cascade via activation of factor VII to factor VIIa, thereby generating more factor VIIa/tissue factor complexes and in turn amplifying the initial haemostatic response. The factor VIIa/tissue factor complex also activates factor X either directly or via activation of factor IX to factor IXa. Both factor IXa and Xa require their cofactors, factors VIIIa and Va respectively. The net result is that for factor Xa, Va converts prothrombin to thrombin, which in turn converts fibrinogen to fibrin, which in the normal situation is stabilized by factor XIII, via crosslinking fibrin molecules together. This final step completes the last stage of secondary haemostasis.

Tissue factor is expressed by many cells

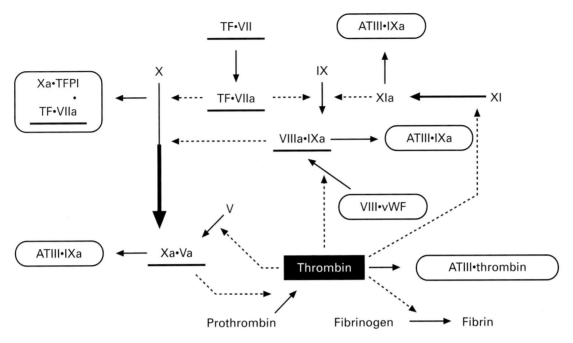

Figure 2.1

Coagulation is now seen as a network of interactions triggered by contact of blood with extravascular tissue factor (TF). The initial conversion of factor X to Xa by the tissue factor VIIa complex (TF•VIIa) leads to generation of small quantities of thrombin, which back-activate factor V and factor VIII. Rapid thrombin generation then proceeds with feedback to factor XI. Note that factor VIII bound to vWF is inactive until proteolysed by thrombin. (Reproduced with permission of Professor EG Tuddenham and Blackwell Science, from Tuddenham EG, Cox TM, Sinclair J eds. (1997) *Molecular Biology in Medicine*. Oxford: Blackwell Science.)

such as monocytes and endothelial cells but is not normally in contact with blood. Tissue factor expression can be induced in these cells by endotoxin, thrombin, tumour necrosis factor α (TNF-α), interleukin-1β (IL-1β) and other pro-inflammatory cytokines and growth factors. It is clear that most of these stimulatory agents are elevated in disease processes, especially inflammation and cancer, where thrombosis is a prominent feature.

The intrinsic pathway, also called the contact phase of coagulation, may have physiological importance, but the precise in vivo mechanism of initiation of this pathway is unclear and, to date, TF is considered the principal biological initiator of blood coagulation.

NATURAL ANTICOAGULATION CONTROL MECHANISMS

Several natural anticoagulant mechanisms have been discovered that exert damping effects upon procoagulation and in turn halt the generation of thrombin. Without these inhibitory mechanisms of coagulation, the physiological activation of clotting would result in inappropriate or enhanced thrombosis formation within intact blood vessels. The major inhibitors of blood coagulation include the tissue factor pathway inhibitor (TFPI) and antithrombin III (ATIII) (see Fig. 2.1), with elements of the protein C pathway (protein C, protein S and thrombomodulin). These highly complementary inhibitory processes serve to extinguish the generation of thrombin and quench thrombin once it is formed.

TFPI primarily inhibits factor Xa and factor

VIIa/tissue factor, while antithrombin decreases the rate of thrombin generation by inactivating factors Xa, IXa, XIa and VIIa but also, perhaps more importantly, inhibits the thrombin that is already produced. The protein C pathway cannot function in the absence of thrombin generation, and therefore once thrombin is generated it binds to thrombomodulin on the endothelial cell, which in turn activates protein C to activated protein C, which suppresses coagulation principally by the inactivation of factors Va and VIIIa (Fig. 2.2). These combinations of TFPI and antithrombin and TFPI and the protein C

pathway components contribute to a synergistic inhibitory mechanism of coagulation.

FIBRINOLYSIS

Fibrin deposition stimulates the release of tissue plasmin zymogen activator (t-PA) and the urokinase-type plasminogen activators (u-PA). These plasminogen activators convert inactive plasminogen to the active serine protease plasmin. The presence of fibrin accelerates t-PA generation of plasmin by a factor of 500, whereas urokinase-dependent plasmino-

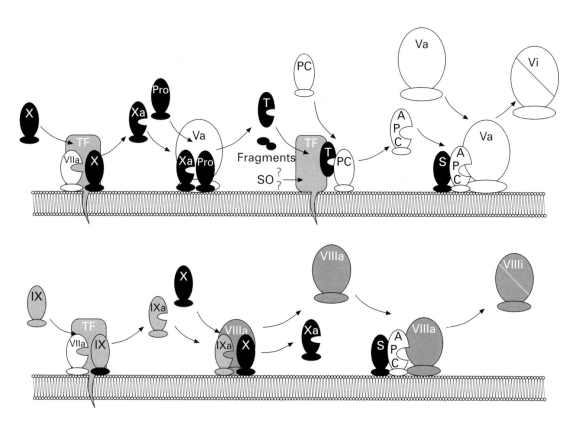

Figure 2.2

Interaction of the protein C pathway with the extrinsic coagulation system. This is a model in which the coagulation stimulus is tissue factor (TF). TF binds factor VIIa (VIIa) to activate either factor IX (IX) or factor X (X). Factor IXa or Xa then complexes with either factor X or prothrombin (Pro), respectively. Thrombin (T) interacts with thrombomodulin (TM) to activate protein C (PC), and the activated protein C (APC) then complexes with protein S (S) to inactivate factor Va and VIIIa. For simplicity, the activations of factors VII, V and VIII are not shown. (Reprinted with permission from Esmon CT. (1999) *Haematologica* **84:** 254–9.)

gen activation is only moderately affected. Once formed, plasmin rapidly digests fibrin and fibrinogen to yield fibrin and fibrinogen degradation products. These degradation products differ from the products produced following plasmin action on fibrin extensively cross-linked by factor XIII, in that D-dimers are produced from the latter.

Regulation of fibrinolysis also involves inhibitors such as plasminogen activator inhibitor 1 (PAI-1), which is the major physiological modulator of the fibrinolytic system. There is also evidence that PAI-2 and PAI-3 also play an important role. Activation of the fibrinolytic pathway may also be initiated by contact-phase interactions (intrinsic pathway) but the plasminogen/t-PA system is by far the most important.

ENDOTHELIUM

Endothelial cells also play a pivotal role, not only in propagating the coagulant process, but also in halting it through the natural anticoagulant mechanism as outlined above. Another interesting feature of endothelium is its inhibitory effects on platelet function. Endothelium produces prostacyclin (PGI$_2$) which is a cyclo-oxygenase product of arachidonic acid metabolism and has a potent inhibitory effect on platelet aggregation. Endothelium also produces a substance, previously known as endothelium-derived relaxing factor (EDRF), and now identified as nitric oxide. It inhibits both platelet adhesion and aggregation. Both nitric oxide and prostacyclin relax vascular smooth muscle, and in doing so these compounds have a dual role in keeping blood in the fluid phase, namely through platelet inhibition and vasorelaxant properties.

CLINICAL EVALUATION

The patterns of bleeding seen in children with defects in primary and secondary haemostasis are typically different. Those with a primary haemostatic defect usually present with small, superficial ecchymoses and mucosal bleeding ('wet purpura'), and characteristically ooze from minor cuts and have inappropriate bleeding at the time of surgical procedures. Those with defects in secondary haemostasis usually have a more florid presentation, with large-vessel bleeding with associated palpable subcutaneous ecchymoses, intramuscular haematomata and haemarthrosis.

It is essential that a careful bleeding history is taken from the child and/or parents, as this usually proves to be the strongest predictor of bleeding risk. Specific questions should include the time of the first bleeding episode, as this will help in differentiating inherited from acquired disorders. If there is a strong suspicion that there is an inherited component, a family tree should be constructed, as this is usually helpful in identifying the mode of inheritance. Other useful questions are: What is the frequency of bleeding? Are bleeds associated with trauma, and how much blood has been lost? Have blood transfusions needed to be given? Has the child had a haemostatic challenge, such as dental extraction, tonsillectomy, appendicectomy, or circumcision, and what was the outcome? Although less of a confounder in children, a drug history (to include herbs and homeopathic remedies) should always be taken.

The majority of children coming for evaluation have a normal physical examination. A minority will have cutaneous bruising, the pattern of which may prove to be the only clue that bleeding is of non-accidental injury in nature. The increased propensity to bleed may be part of a well-recognized syndrome such as Hermansky–Pudlak (oculocutaneous albinism), Chediak–Higashi (partial oculocutaneous albinism), Wiskott–Aldrich (eczema and recurrent infections) and TAR (thrombocytopenia with absent radii), where the bleeding is secondary to platelet dense granule storage pool disease and thrombocytopenia in the Wiskott–Aldrich and TAR patients.

As with bleeding disorders, the history is very important for evaluation of thrombotic disorders. Specific questioning relating to a family history of venous thromboembolic disease (VTE) may shed light on the fact that the child may have compound heterozygosity or homozygosity for one of the natural anticoagulant protein genes and thus is predisposed to VTE. This area is covered in Chapter 3.

LABORATORY COAGULATION TESTING

The sample

Laboratory testing of coagulation depends on the quality and freshness of the plasma specimen obtained. Whole blood, anticoagulated with sodium citrate in a 9:1 ratio, is a specimen of choice. Citrate is preferred, as EDTA can falsely increase the PT and APTT results. It must be remembered that the 9:1 ratio of blood:citrate is important, as altering this ratio will interfere with the test results. High haematocrit, traumatic venesection and a haemolysed sample may also alter this ratio, and if any of these are present then the coagulation laboratory should be informed.

The test

The usual screening tests for suspected coagulation disorder consist of the following:

1. **Prothrombin time (PT).** This tests the tissue factor pathway, namely deficiencies in factors VII, X, V, II and fibrinogen.
2. **Activated partial thromboplastin time (APTT).** This tests the contact factor pathway for further deficiencies in the factors prekallikrein, high-molecular-weight kininogen, and factors XII, XI, IX, X, VIII, V, II and fibrinogen.
3. **Thrombin time (TT).** This tests for deficiency or inhibition of fibrinogen. It should be remembered that a prolonged TT can occur in patients receiving therapeutic heparin, patients with increased fibrin degradation products and patients with disorders of hypofibrinogenaemia. The reptilase/R test, which is a variation on the thrombin time, is an alternative method to test for fibrinogen activity. In this test, reptilase reagent is added to plasma instead of thrombin to activate the proteolytic conversion of fibrinogen to fibrin. The reptilase time is not inhibited by heparin and demonstrates only minimal inhibition by fibrin degradation products (FDP). This test is useful in determining whether there is contamination with heparin.

4. **Quantitative fibrinogen assay.**
5. **Platelet count.**
6. **D-dimers.** This test is based on highly specific monoclonal antibodies directed against a unique neoantigen of covalently cross-linked D-fragments resulting from fibrinolysis. The D-dimer method has several advantages in detecting degradation fragments when compared with the standard FDP assay, perhaps the most important being its superior sensitivity and specificity profile.
7. **Substitution tests.** When a prolonged PT or APTT is observed, the question arises as to whether or not this prolongation is due to a deficiency or an inhibitor. The patient's plasma is incubated as a 50:50 mix with normal plasma. If there is a failure of full correction in a 50:50 mix with normal plasma then one should suspect an inhibitor of coagulation such as lupus anticoagulant. A direct screen with kaolin, clotting time and dilute Russell viper venom test (DRVVT) should then be performed to assess lupus anticoagulant status. If the patient's PT or APTT corrects in a 50:50 mix with normal plasma then the most likely diagnosis is a deficiency within the coagulation protein cascade. In order to delineate which factor is deficient there are two approaches: (a) screening for individual protein deficiencies with the relevant coagulation-deficient plasma, or (b) performing a number of assays with substitution tests as outlined below:
    Aged plasma. This lacks labile factors V and VIII but retains normal activity of all other coagulation factors. Therefore, if aged plasma does not correct the screening tests then deficiency in V and VIII is expected.
    Fresh absorbed plasma. This lacks the vitamin K-dependent factors (II, VII, IX and X) but retains normal activity of all the other coagulation factors. Therefore, if the addition of this plasma does not correct then one is dealing with a deficiency of these proteins.
    Aged serum. This lacks fibrinogen, factors II, V and VIII but retains normal activity over other coagulation factors. Therefore, if this plasma does not correct the clotting

---

Table 2.2 Laboratory tests of hypo- and hypercoagulable states

Global tests
PT, APTT, platelet count, D-dimer, fibrinogen

Specific hypocoagulation tests	**Specific hypercoagulation tests**
Intrinsic pathway protein assays	Activated protein C resistance ratio
Factors VIII, IX, XI, XII	Antithrombin III
	Protein C
Extrinsic pathway protein assays	Protein S (total and free)
FVII	Factor VIII
	Fibrinogen
Common pathway protein assay	Homocysteine
Factors V, X	Plasminogen activator inhibitor 1
Prothrombin	
Fibrinogen	*Genotypes*
Factor XIII	FV^{R506Q}, $FII^{G20210A}$, T1-MTHFR, PAI-1$^{4G/5G}$
von Willebrand assessment	
vWF:antigen	Lupus anticoagulant
vWF:ristocetin cofactor activity	
vWF multimer analysis	Anticardiolipin antibodies
	Anti-β_2-glycoprotein 1
Platelet aggregation	
Platelet nucleotide content and release	
Platelet immunophenotyping via Flow	
– Glanzmann's thrombasthenia (GPIIb-IIIa)	
– Bernard–Soulier syndrome (GPIb)	

---

times then one is dealing with a deficiency in one of the above.

A combination of clotting times using the above three plasmas usually suggests a deficiency in a specific coagulation factor. This suspected deficiency is then confirmed by a specific factor assay. Because of the advances in both automated coagulometers and plasma reagents over the past couple of decades, most coagulation laboratories now measure directly individual clotting factor activity within intrinsic, extrinsic and common pathways and avoid the indirect methodologies as outlined above.

Other tests that should be available when evaluating children with haemorrhagic (hypocoagulable) or thrombotic (hypercoagulable) disorders are shown in Table 2.2, and their clinical correlates will be discussed in more detail in Chapters 8 and 9 and in Chapter 10 respectively.

FURTHER READING

Christensen RD, ed. (2000) *Hematologic Problems of the Neonate*. Philadelphia: WB Saunders.

Coman RW, Hirsch J, Marder VJ, Salzman EW, eds. (1994) *Haemostasis and Thrombosis: Basic Principles in Clinical Practice*, 3rd edn. Philadelphia: JP Lippincott.

Esmon CT, Gu Jian-Ming, Xu Jun, Qu D, Stern-Kurosawa DJ, Kurosawa S. (1999) Regulation and function of the protein C anticoagulant pathway. *Haematologica* **84**: 363–8.

Hathaway WE, Goodney SH. (1993) *Disorders of Haemostasis and Thrombosis: A Clinical Guide*. New York: McGraw-Hill.

Loscalo J, Schafer A, eds. (1998) *Thrombosis and Haemorrhage*, 2nd edn. Baltimore: Williams and Wilkins.

3 Molecular biology and genetic manipulation

Mark Lawler

INTRODUCTION

Molecular biology plays a key role in our understanding of the mechanisms of human disease, and provides the technology to translate laboratory research into clinical practice. Haematology has benefited from this more than other clinical disciplines, due in no small part to the easy access to biopsy material. Molecular biological techniques have permitted the elucidation of the underlying molecular mechanisms in a variety of haematological disorders. Sickle cell anaemia and the thalassemias were among the first human genetic diseases for which mutations at single gene loci could be identified. The discovery of restriction enzymes and the development of DNA hybridization and Southern blotting techniques were key advances, providing the first molecular tools for human disease studies. Family studies to ascertain genetic linkage to particular loci were also aided greatly by the plethora of neutral variation that has been uncovered in the human genome in the last 10 years. The search for mutations in specific genes has also been advanced by the development of the polymerase chain reaction (PCR), by far the most significant development in this new discipline of molecular pathology. Mutation detection and polymorphic diversity studies have also allowed the identification of genetic determinants for the more common multifactorial diseases and the finding of the factor V Leiden mutation and its association with venous thromboembolism (VTE) has proved a watershed in our understanding of risk factors in thrombosis.

Changes at the gene level are also detectable in malignant diseases such as leukaemia, and it is perhaps here that the molecular revolution has had its most obvious influence. Defining the molecular lesion in a particular patient can aid in diagnosis, help stratify in terms of prognosis and allow assessment of the therapeutic benefit of conventional or experimental approaches. Molecular testing has come of age and is particularly relevant in the paediatric leukaemia context.

Molecular therapeutics are at a much earlier stage than molecular diagnostics, and initial gene therapy approaches have not been as successful as was initially hoped, for example in gene therapy for adenosine deaminase (ADA) deficiency. However, new advances in vector development, allied to better delivery of vector to the appropriate tissue, will undoubtedly improve gene therapy protocols, and antisense and antigene approaches may have particular relevance in paediatric malignancy, where inappropriately expressed oncogenes must be silenced to derive therapeutic benefit.

In this chapter, the impact of molecular biology and gene manipulation in paediatric haematology will be outlined. The search for disease genes has now become one that is highly active, both in the characterization of inherited disorders such as haemophilia and in providing clues to the genesis of multifactorial disease such as VTE. This new science of molecular pathology has also been important in the evolving classification of leukaemia, leading to the development of diagnostic tools for predicting 'good' and 'bad' responders to current therapeutic approaches.

Allied to these developments in understanding how defects in the genetic blueprint can influence disease pathology, this wealth of knowledge and technology may also provide therapeutic options in molecular medicine, and some of these 'gene therapy' approaches will undoubtedly become part of routine clinical practice in the new millennium.

MOLECULAR TECHNOLOGIES IN PAEDIATRIC HAEMATOLOGY

Restriction enzymes

As the human genome is very large ($3–6 \times 10^9$ base pairs (bp)), it is necessary to be able to reduce it to more convenient sizes for analysis of particular regions. This can be achieved through the use of restriction endonucleases (REs). These enzymes were isolated from various types of bacteria in the 1970s and were found to have sequence-specific targets in DNA. They usually recognize 4 or 6 bp palindromic sequence motifs, but REs exist that can cleave at 5, 7, 8 or 10 bp recognition sites. They are named according to the bacteria from which they were isolated: e.g. the enzyme *Eco*R1 (recognition site GAATTC) originates from the bacteria *Escherichia coli*. Over 1000 REs have been identified and characterized. Digestion with these enzymes cuts DNA into more manageable sizes and allows manipulation of the genetic material and electrophoresis through a gel matrix (agarose or acrylamide).

Nucleic acid hybridization and Southern blotting

Following digestion with the RE and gel electrophoresis, further manipulation may be necessary. Take for example, a situation where an individual may have a deleted α-globin gene leading to α-thalassaemia. How can this be detected? The procedure to identify such mutations uses a technique known as Southern blotting, which relies on the fact that an artificially created segment of DNA (termed a DNA probe) will bind to a single-stranded complementary sequence of DNA or RNA (a process called hybridization), just as if the complementary strand were its normal partner in a DNA double helix. Thus, if a panel of samples were being

tested for the presence of α-globin gene deletions (see Fig. 3.1), the samples would be prepared and digested with an RE that cuts outside the α-globin alleles. (Remember, in unaffected individuals, there are two α-globin gene copies on each allele inherited from the mother and father.) Electrophoresis would be performed to separate the samples based on their size, the DNA within the gel would be made single-stranded by incubation with alkali and the material would be blotted (transferred to a nylon membrane). This essentially creates a copy of the single-stranded material on the gel. The nylon membrane containing the single-stranded material is incubated with a solution containing the DNA probe. Hybridization occurs between regions of complementary nucleotide sequence, and if the probe is labelled with a radioactive nucleotide then the pattern of hybridization can be revealed after X-ray autoradiography (Fig. 3.1).

Polymerase chain reaction and mutation detection

While the technologies described above allowed greater understanding of the molecular basis of haematological disease, the requirement for 10–20 μg of DNA for a single analysis could be limiting. This is particularly relevant in the paediatric setting, where sufficient material for Southern blotting approaches may be difficult to obtain. The advent of PCR technology revolutionized molecular pathology in this area, both by providing large amounts of material for analysis of genetic or acquired genetic defects and in delivering a new source of hitherto unaccessible material: retrospective material including paraffin-embedded sections and stored haematological slides. Ten to twenty years of stored haematological material suddenly became accessible to molecular analysis!

PCR relies on the same hybridization technology indicated above for REs but in addition exploits the ability of the DNA polymerase to copy large amounts of DNA from a defined nucleic acid template. Two artificial pieces of DNA of approximately 20 nucleotides length each (termed primers) are chosen for their ability to hybridize to and

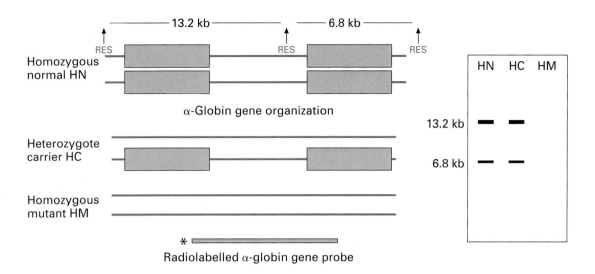

Figure 3.1

Southern blot analysis to detect α-globin gene deletions. The α-globin gene organization is shown on the left of the figure with a map of the region indicating three restriction enzyme sites (RES) that bracket the two copies of the gene at each allele and yield fragments of 13.2 kb and 6.8 kb respectively. On the right of the figure is a representation of a Southern blot analysis indicating the patterns observed in cases of a homozygous normal (HN) individual, a heterozygous (HC) individual and a homozygous mutant (HM) individual. * indicates the radio label.

'bracket' a target sequence. They each bind to different complementary strands and provide a starting point for the DNA polymerase to initiate copying of the DNA template (Fig. 3.2). Multiple rounds of DNA strand separation, primer annealing and primer extension lead to an exponential accumulation of the target sequence. While PCR can only be performed directly on DNA, it is also possible to analyse RNA, provided it is first converted into DNA by reverse transcriptase (RT), which in its natural form performs this function in the retrovirus life cycle. Analysis of RNA is particularly useful in the detection of leukaemia-specific RNA fusions generated by translocation events in which reverse transcription is followed by PCR (RT-PCR), allowing molecular detection of the acquired genetic lesion.

While PCR can be formatted to allow detection of known mutations in genes implicated in haematological disease, usually in a dot/slot blot format, it can also be used to determine the presence of new mutations in a DNA sequence. This can be particularly useful in analysing genes for dominant mutations where direct sequencing techniques allow analysis of both alleles simultaneously. In addition, screening techniques such as single-strand conformational polymorphism analysis (SSCP) or denaturing gradient gel electrophoresis (DGGE), both of which rely on PCR, allow candidate mutation regions within genes to be identified prior to DNA sequencing.

These new molecular technologies can aid in diagnosis, permit prognostic classification of risk groups or determine response to therapy in paediatric patients who have a molecular component to their disease. The molecular basis of these disorders will be described briefly and the role of molecular

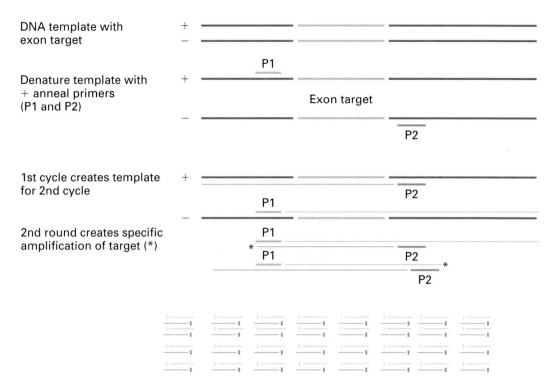

Figure 3.2

Principles of PCR amplification. An exon target for PCR analysis is indicated and the primers P1 and P2 are designed to bind to complementary sequences on each strand of the target DNA. Cycles of denaturation of the template, primer annealing and primer extension by the DNA polymerase lead to an exponential accumulation of the DNA target. Use of a thermostable DNA polymerase such as *Thermus aquaticus* (*Taq*) polymerase and thermal cycling apparatus has made this procedure semi-automated, and subsequent developments such as nucleic acid extraction apparatus and real-time PCR aim to automate the process.

biology and gene manipulation illustrated by relevant examples.

MOLECULAR MECHANISMS IN SINGLE-GENE DISORDERS

Indirect gene tracking

The search for the disease genes that contribute to Mendelian single-gene disorders may appear straightforward in the light of current molecular technologies and the Human Genome Project (the race to deter-

mine our entire genetic blueprint by 2005, or 2003 at the rate of progress of the new technologies – a first draft has already been achieved), but it has been a long and arduous one, requiring painstaking research in the pre-molecular pathology days. In some instances, a biochemical clue as to the nature of the gene defect, for example an easily measurable enzyme defect, provides a useful starting point for characterizing the mutant gene. However, most situations are not so fortuitous and an indirect method is required to provide a clue to the location of the mutant gene. There are three basic requirements for this 'indirect gene tracking' approach: (i) good diagnosis with defined criteria to ensure that all the individuals under study have the same genetic condition, (ii) collection of family pedigrees and ascertainment of mode of inheritance (autosomal dominant, autosomal recessive, X-linked, mitochondrial) of the disease and access to a blood sample to study the condition, and (iii) informative genetic markers. Genetic markers are variations in human DNA (preferably ones whose chromosomal locations are known) that can allow precise determination of the segregation of the disease trait through a family pedigree. Only 1% of the human genome codes for RNA that is translated into protein. While the regions encoding genes (exons) are conserved between individuals in a population, the intervening regions are not held under the same evolutionary constraints. Thus these regions, both within genes (the introns) and between genes (intergenic), can have widely different nucleotide sequences allowing differences, or polymorphisms, between individuals in a pedigree to be identified.

Types of genetic marker

Protein polymorphisms

These include the highly polymorphic classical HLA antigens, blood groups, and a variety of enzyme or structural protein polymorphisms. However, they are inevitably rare since all proteins are derived from the 1% of the human genome that is under selective pressure to conserve coding DNA sequence and biological function. DNA polymorphisms are much more numerous, and now that the technology is available to study them (Southern blotting and the PCR), they have replaced protein polymorphisms for genetic studies.

DNA markers

Most DNA markers define neutral polymorphisms in the large non-coding DNA component of the human genome. They include restriction fragment length polymorphisms (RFLPs), minisatellite or variable number tandem repeat sequences (VNTRs) and

microsatellite or short tandem repeat (STR) polymorphisms (Fig. 3.3).

RFLPs were the first DNA polymorphisms to be characterized. As the name suggests, they involve variations in RE sites. The variation can involve either the creation of a new RE site or the loss of an RE site by a DNA base change. The polymorphism is revealed after Southern blotting with a DNA probe or can be detected using a PCR-based assay.

Genetic markers are given a score based on the degree of polymorphism that they uncover in a population (the polymorphism information content or PIC value). A PIC value of 0 implies that no polymorphism is revealed by the marker (i.e. it is monomorphic) while a PIC value of 1 indicates that the marker is polymorphic between all individuals tested. In a simple allele RFLP system, the maximum possible PIC value is 0.5. The search for more informative markers gave rise to two types of genetic marker that are fundamentally different from RFLPs.

VNTRs or **minisatellites** (the first-generation DNA fingerprinting tools) are DNA repeat sequences whose core ranges from 9 to 70 bp and that are arranged head-to-tail in tandem array. The number of repeats varies between individuals from 10 to 150 copies. Although polymorphic, their non-random distribution limits their use in mapping the full length of a chromosome. They can be detected using Southern blotting or PCR.

Microsatellites or **short tandem repeats** (STRs) are di-, tri- or tetra-repeat nucleotide sequences (e.g. of the nucleotide sequences CA, CAG or TTTA) with a variable unit from 10 to 60 copies. STRs can only be detected by PCR amplification and analysis on high-resolution gel matrices, owing to the small variation in size between alleles. STRs are abundantly scattered throughout the genome and are therefore currently the most widely used hypervariable systems for gene tracking. A complete high-resolution linkage map of the genome based on STRs is now available, allowing saturation mapping for particular genetic traits.

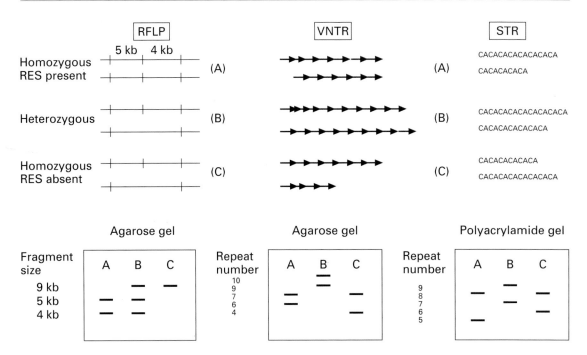

Figure 3.3

Types of DNA polymorphisms. Genomic organization and gel electrophoresis patterns are shown for each of the common types of DNA polymorphic marker: restriction fragment length polymorphisms (RFLPs), variable number tandem repeats (minisatellites: VNTRs) and short tandem repeats (microsatellites: STRs). Fragment size refers to the fragments generated by restriction enzyme digestion and repeat number refers to the number of tandem repeats (either VNTRs or STRs) in the different examples shown. RES, restriction enzyme site.

Genetic linkage

Given that panels of genetic markers are now available, it is possible to perform a 'genome-wide scan' to determine which chromosomal sublocation might harbour a gene that when mutated leads to the development of the Mendelian disorder. Markers are used in genetic linkage analysis to trace the possible association between the genetic marker and the disease in a pedigree. While a detailed description of genetic linkage is beyond the scope of this chapter, the basis of the approach is that if, for example, a particular polymorphic allele always segregates with individuals within the pedigree that have haemochromatosis, then the polymorphic marker probably lies close to the chromosomal location of the mutant gene. Genetic markers are not implicated in the development of the disease, they simply point to a possible chromosomal location for the mutant gene.

Finding the disease gene

Genetic linkage analysis indicates the region of the genome where the mutant gene resides. However, this region may be as large as 10^6 bp and contain a variety of genes. A candidate gene approach involves a search for mutations in genes already identified in this region, which through knowledge of their biological function might implicate them in the disorder. More complex approaches, again beyond the scope of this chapter, but involving techniques such as chromosome walking, chromosome jumping and gene trapping, may be employed to identify potential genes in this region if no candidate gene is available for analysis.

Identification of the disease-causing gene and the specific mutation(s) that give rise to the condition not only provides us with increasing knowledge of the condition, but also allows the development of a molecular test that can help in diagnosis or assessment of carrier status (in recessive disorders) or allow prenatal testing. Depending on the condition, this can be a straightforward or a difficult process. In sickle cell anaemia, a single nucleotide base change (A→T) leading to the substitution of a valine for a glutamine in the β-globin gene (and creating a diagnostic Dde-1 RE site) is responsible for all cases of sickle cell anaemia. Contrast this with β-thalassemia, where a variety of different mutations in the same β-globin gene can give rise to different forms of β-thalassemia with different severities. The molecular complexity can be further increased by situations where mutations in more than one gene can account for an identical or similar phenotype (e.g. retinitis pigmentosa).

Molecular medicine into practice: haemophilia A and flipping the tip of X

Haemophilia A is the most common and severe bleeding disorder in humans. The cloning of factor VIII (F8), the protein whose deficiency causes the disease, in 1984, was a triumph for the biotechnology industry and led to the detection of mutations that cause the disease. However, its large size (26 exons, 189 kb) meant that detection of mutations was a slow and tedious process, and large deletions or single base changes only accounted for 5–10% of known mutations. Use of the PCR scanning methods described earlier led to an increase in the number of mutations detected; however, even with the use of DGGE, only half of the mutations in severely affected patients could be detected by this highly sensitive technique.

This surprising observation led to a more detailed study of the F8 gene structure in severely affected individuals, and it was found that within the largest intron (between exon 22 and 23), which is 32 kb long, there is a second copy of the F8 gene called factor VIIIA (*F8A*). *F8A* differs from its normal counterpart in only one respect: it lacks any introns. Further study indicated that two other copies of this *F8A* gene lie approximately 500 kb upstream of the *F8* gene. In addition, a smaller gene termed *F8B* has an exon within intron 22 that is fused to exons 23–26 to give a short transcript. This gave rise to the concept of the *flip tip mutation* as a new mutational mechanism in haemophilia (Fig. 3.4).

Molecular confirmation of this hypothesis has allowed characterization of this unusual mutation strategy as the cause of 45% cases of severe haemophilia A. Direct characterization allows study of patients who have a de novo mutation without any family history of haemophilia A. It also provides a direct Southern blot test, and, given the high incidence of this mutation in severe forms of haemophilia A, this test should probably be the first screening method in patients who have factor VIII levels of less than 1%. Recently, a complex PCR-based assay has been developed to detect this inv (22) (IVS 22) mutation.

MOLECULAR MECHANISMS IN COMPLEX DISORDERS

In many common human diseases, both genetic and environmental influences may be important in the development of the disease phenotype. Some of these diseases are polygenic, with minor contributions of several gene loci to the disease. Use of association studies and sib pair analysis in population studies and the collection of family trios for transmission disequilibrium testing (TDT) have provided the statistical basis to analyse the contribution of genetic polymorphisms to common multifactorial diseases. One area where disease risk has been associated with increased incidence of mutations/polymorphic variants in DNA is in thrombosis. Studies over the last 4–5 years have identified certain genetic variants associated with increased risk to VTE, especially in association with other environmental risk factors, including smoking and the oral contraceptive pill.

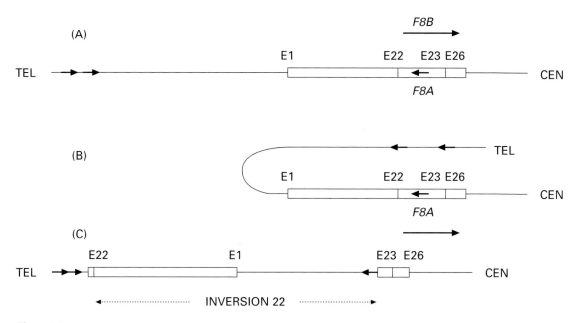

Figure 3.4

The IVS 22 mutation in haemophilia A. The structure of the haemophilia gene region is shown, with the normal *F8* gene and the positions of the *F8A* and *F8B* genes indicated (A). One of the upstream *F8A* genes combines by homologous recombination with the intron 22 *F8A* gene that is on the same chromosome (B). A crossover (genetic exchange of material) between these two regions results in inversion of the intervening sequences. Thus the factor VIII gene is divided into two parts, with an intact promoter and exons 1–22 greatly separated from and in the opposite orientation to exons 23–26 of the gene (C). TEL, telomere; CEN, centromere; E, exon.

Factor V Leiden

Factor V (FV) is a crucial component of the clotting cascade, and when it is cleaved to its active form FVa, it is involved in the pathway that leads to the generation of thrombin. In 1994, a mutation in the *FV* gene was identified independently by three research groups. The mutation leads to a 10-fold decrease in the rate of FVa degradation by activated protein C, thereby leading to excessive thrombin generation. This single point mutation has been termed factor V Leiden (FVL). This particular mutation accounts for 95% of the hereditary forms of activated protein C resistance (APCR). The mutation is a G-to-A transition at position 1691 in exon 10, which leads to a replacement of R at position 506 by Q (glutamine). FVa:Q-506 is not cleaved at position 506 by APC, resulting in a general hypercoagulation state. FVL is highly prevalent in Caucasian populations: the mean allele frequency throughout Europe has been estimated to be 2–7%, although in Scandinavian populations it may be as high as 12%. Heterozygotes have a 5- to 10-fold and homozygotes an 80-fold increased risk of developing VTE. In groups of thrombosis patients, deficiencies of antithrombin III, protein C or protein S were together found in 5% of the patients, indicating APCR (found in 40% of thrombotic patients) to be at least ten times more common than any of the other known genetic defects. Apart from VTE, FVL has been associated with pulmonary embolism, arterial thromboembolism in children and moderation of haemophilia A.

The APC-resistance phenotype was originally demonstrated as a resistance to the anticoagulant activity of APC in an activated partial thromboplastin time (APTT)-based assay. The assay results are not reliable, however, when tested patients are receiving anticoagulants or have long baseline APTTs due to antiphospholipid antibodies. DNA-based assays, such as PCR amplification followed by RFLP analysis are more reliable, but also more expensive and can only be carried out by laboratories with the appropriate equipment. There have been discussions concerning the establishment of FV genotype screening programmes, since VTE is a significant cause of morbidity and mortality in hospitalized patients. Carriers of the mutation could avoid being exposed to known risk factors and take prophylactics, such as anticoagulant therapy (e.g. with warfarin) against thrombosis in risk situations, such as oral contraception, surgery, shock, pregnancy and trauma.

The prothrombin variant (20210 G-to-A)

In 1996, a second genetic risk factor for VTE was identified. Examination of the prothrombin (FII) gene in a group of patients with a history of thrombophilia was performed by PCR, and subsequent direct sequencing revealed a G-to-A transition at position 20210 (3' untranslated region) in 18% of these cases. This correlates with a 2.8-fold increased risk of developing VTE for heterozygotes for the FII variant. Consequently, the FII variant (G20210A) is a risk factor for VTE second only to factor V Leiden. FII is the circulating precursor of the serine protease thrombin, a key enzyme in the processes of haemostasis and thrombosis, which exhibits procoagulant, anticoagulant and antifibrinolytic activities. G20210A is associated with elevated FII levels; thus carriers of this allele have significantly higher FII levels than non-carriers, suggesting that G20210A acts through the elevated FII levels. Studies in families presenting with VTE indicated that the presence of more than one mutation (FVL, G20210A) with or without the presence of environmental factors may increase the risk of thrombotic disease, and many thrombosis clinics now perform genetic testing for these two variants.

MOLECULAR BASIS OF ACQUIRED GENETIC DISEASE

Paediatric leukaemia

Molecular pathology has greatly increased our knowledge of the involvement of genetic lesions in the pathogenesis of leukaemia. Leukaemia is an acquired genetic disorder as somatic mutations can be detected in the bone marrow or peripheral blood. The majority of these changes involve translocation events leading to activation of an oncogene or anti-apoptotic gene. Molecular analysis indicates that leukaemia can be a differentiation-blockade disorder – in acute promyelocytic leukaemia (APL), the t(15;17) translocation involving the retinoic acid receptor is implicated. Leukaemia can also involve the expression of a specific anti-apoptotic gene, for example, *BCR–ABL* in chronic myeloid leukaemia (CML) and Philadelphia-positive acute lymphoblastic leukaemia (ALL).

In acute leukaemia, many of the genes that are involved in translocation events are transcription factors, and a small number of these genes may have different translocation partners (translocational promiscuity), leading to the concept of master genes – genes whose products regulate many different processes in normal haemopoiesis and which when mutated can thus give rise to different forms of leukaemia depending on their promiscuous partner. Several different translocation events have been shown to target the 21q22 region and disrupt the *AML-1* gene. *AML-1* encodes a DNA-binding protein that is part of a core binding factor protein (CBF) complex implicated in the transcriptional regulation of a variety of genes involved in haemopoiesis, including GM-CSF, myeloperoxidase, among others. In the normal situation, *AML-1* interacts with a transactivator (TA) and core binding factor β (CBFβ) (Fig. 3.5). In the t(3;21) and t(8;21) translocations, the TA portion is replaced by the *EAP, MDS-1* or *EVI-1* genes (chromosome 3) or the *ETO* gene (chromosome 8) respectively. Replacement of the TA domain means that although AML-1–ETO or AML-1–EVI-1 can bind to target genes, they cannot activate them. In addition, inv(16) generates a core binding

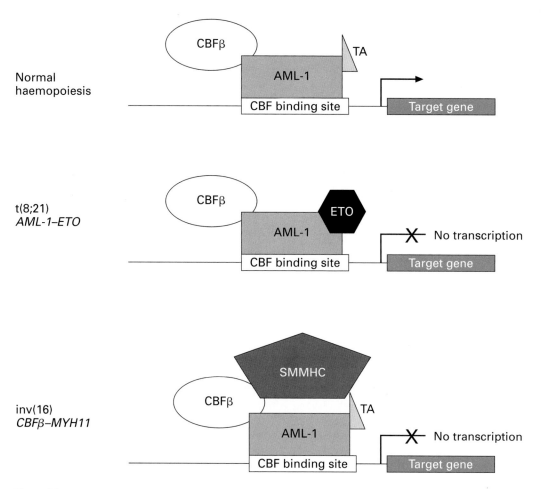

Figure 3.5

AML-1 and leukaemogenesis. The three panels show how gene expression occurs at core binding factor (CBF)-responsive promoters in the normal, t(8;21) and inv(16) situations. In both t(8;21) and inv(16), AML-1 can bind to the CBF binding site but transactivation of the target gene cannot occur. TA, transactivator; SMMHC, smooth muscle myosin heavy chain; *MYH11*, SMMHC gene.

factor β/smooth muscle myosin heavy chain (CBFβ–SMMHC) fusion that similarly cannot activate target genes (Fig. 3.5). Other mechanisms may also perturb *AML-1*, as the t(12;21) generating a TEL–AML-1 fusion protein involves a virtually intact AML-1 protein, complete with its transactivating domain. Other genes also function as 'master genes',

the most prominent being the mixed-lineage leukaemia (*MLL*) gene, which shares homology to the *Drosophila* gene *trithorax*, which when mutated by translocation can lead to a variety of acute leukaemias (11q23 abnormalities, t(9;11)). In the paediatric setting, t(4;11), involving an *MLL–AF4* gene fusion, is particularly common in infants under one year of age and conveys an extremely bad prognosis.

The value of molecular biology in leukaemia

Determination of the molecular defect in particular forms of leukaemia is highly relevant in patient management. Advances have meant that we can speak in terms of 'good' and 'bad' molecular prognostic factors and treatment of patients can be stratified according to molecular indicators. Examples of good molecular prognosis markers include the t(15;17) in APL, as this indicates that all-*trans*-retinoic acid (ATRA) should be used to induce remission, while the presence of the Philadel-phia chromosome in ALL (Ph-positive ALL) is a bad molecular prognostic indicator. The common molecular aberrations in childhood ALL together with their prognostic significance are shown in Table 3.1. Molecular assays not only aid diagnosis and prognosis but can also be particularly useful in assessing the ability of chemotherapy or allogeneic stem cell transplantation (SCT) to achieve remission in patients receiving treatment for leukaemia. The molecular approaches have defined a concept of *minimal residual disease* (MRD), where detection of 'leukaemia-specific' DNA or RNA or 'leukaemia-associated' antigens is achievable at degrees of sensitivity where morphological or karyotypic analysis is normal (Fig. 3.6). A variety of methods are available to

Table 3.1 The common structural alterations in childhood ALL	
Chromosomal rearrangement	**Comment**
t(9;22)(q32;q11)	Occurs in 5% of childhood ALL; high leukocyte count; *BCR–ABL* fusion
t(4;11)(q21;23)	Frequent in infants; involves the *MLL–AF4* fusion; dismal prognosis
del(9)(p21)	About 10% of childhood ALL; T-ALL involves p16 cyclin-dependent kinase inhibitor; poor prognosis
Chromosome 14 abnormalities	All involve the T-cell receptor (TCR): t(1;14)(p34;q11): *TAL-1* t(8;14)(q24;q11): *MYC* t(10;14)(q24;q11): *HOX-11* t(11;14)(p13;p11): *RTBN-2*
t(12;21)(p12–13;q22)	20–30% of B-lineage ALLs; *TEL–AML-1*; excellent prognosis
t(1;19)(q22;p13)	B-lineage ALL; high leukocyte count; *E2A–PBX1* gene fusion; unfavourable prognosis, but improving with intensive chemotherapy
dic(9;12)(p11–12;p12)	B-precursor ALL; 5-year disease-free survival rate 80–90%
Chromosome 8 abnormalities	B-cell ALL with FAB-L3 t(8;14)(q24;q32-3) *MYC–IgH* t(2;8)(q12;24) *Igλ–MYC* t(8;22)(q24;q11) *MYC–Igκ*

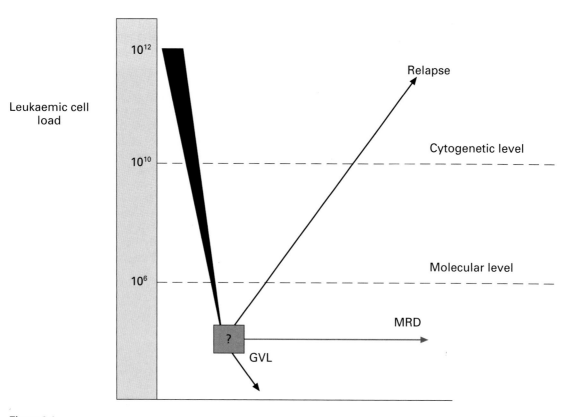

Figure 3.6

Minimal residual disease (MRD). When a patient presents with leukaemia, there are approximately 10^{12} leukaemia cells on board. While chemotherapy and/or total body irradiation and bone marrow transplantation may reduce this by 4- to 6-fold depending on the agents used, there is still the question of a significant number of malignant cells persisting. Conventional technologies could only detect 1% leukaemia cells as the minor cell population, and patients were said to be in remission even though 10^9–10^{10} leukaemia cells could still be present, below the limit of detection of these techniques. Molecular techniques have lowered this detection threshold significantly, allowing detection of the minor cell population at 10^{-6} or 10^{-7}. This has given rise to the concept of minimal residual disease and allows us to distinguish between classical haematological remission and molecular remission. In allogeneic stem cell transplantation, the presence of a graft-versus-leukaemia effect (GVL) may eradicate the residual leukaemia cells or allow immunological control of disease. If residual leukaemia cells can escape this donor immune control, then relapse may occur.

detect MRD and are summarized below, with particular reference to the paediatric population.

Cytogenetic analysis is used when a non-random chromosomal abnormality is present, and has a sensitivity of 10^{-2} in the detection of the leukaemia cell. Cytogenetic analysis requires dividing cells to generate metaphase spreads, and may be difficult in the paediatric setting, particularly in the immediate post-treatment phase when obtaining sufficient metaphases may prove technically difficult. Combining cytogenetics and fluorescence in situ hybridization (FISH) technology, particularly when applied to interphase nuclei, avoids the need for dividing cells and increases the sensitivity of detection of leukaemic cells by at least one log-fold.

Immunophenotyping techniques are based on the occurrence of aberrant or unusual patterns of antigen expression on leukaemia cells. Multiparameter flow cytometry allows the use of 2–4 different labels, permitting detection of both surface antigen and intracellular markers, and sensitivities can range from 10^{-3} to 10^{-5}.

Polymerase chain reaction analysis can be used to detect the disease-specific chromosomal rearrangements, but can also detect 'clone-specific' rearrangements such as the re-arranged immunoglobulin heavy chain (IgH) or T-cell receptor (TCR) genes; this is particularly relevant for MRD detection in acute leukaemia as many cases without chromosomal aberrations have rearranged IgH or TCR genes. Sensitivities range from 10^{-3} to 10^{-6}, depending on the type of leukaemia.

MRD detection by immunophenotyping

In precursor B-cell ALL, CD10 and terminal deoxynucleotidyl transferase (TdT) expression are the two main phenotypic markers used. Overall, leukaemia-associated phenotypes can be detected in 70–90% of childhood precursor B-ALLs. Over 90% of T-ALLs can be detected using TdT and other T-cell markers (e.g. CD2, CD3, CD5 and CD7), usually by double immunofluorescence staining. Other immuno-phenotypic targets include leukaemia-specific antigens resulting from chromosomal trans-location events (e.g. TAL-1 protein). In AML, the incidence of leukaemia-associated pheno-types ranges from 30% to 85% and involves detection of combinations of myeloid antigens that are undetected or at very low back-grounds in normal cells. These include CD34 in association with CD14, CD20, CD22 and CD56. In addition, overexpression of myeloid-related markers contributes to approximately 20% of AML phenotypes.

MRD detection by PCR

IgH/TCR fingerprinting

This is one of the more common technologies used to detect MRD, particularly in childhood ALL, as it does not require the presence of a leukaemia-specific marker. The variable (V), diversity (D) and junctional (J) regions of both the *IgH* and *TCR* genes undergo rearrange-ment to generate the diverse primary antigen-specific repertoire of the immune system. In normal lymphoid cells, there is a huge diver-sity of possible rearrangements, whereas in lymphoid malignancies, a clonal population of cells derived from the precursor leukaemic clone will carry the same *IgH* or *TCR* rearrangement. Thus a PCR-based detection system can be used in each patient to develop a clone-specific MRD detection system. Con-sensus PCR primers for V-family and J-family segments of the *IgH* or *TCR* locus are designed to amplify a target of 400–500 bp around the junction from the patient at diagnosis. DNA sequencing of the PCR product allows the design of junction-specific oligonucleotide probes that can be used for MRD analysis in serial samples from the patient during and post therapy (Fig. 3.7). The sensitivity of the technique is high (10^{-4} to 10^{-6}), depending on the type of malignancy analysed, but clonal evolution can give rise to false-negative results and it is usually necessary to perform both an *IgH* and *TCR* assay where possible.

PCR of chromosomal aberrations

The majority of cases as indicated above involve chromosomal translocation events. If translocation breakpoints occur within a 2–3 kb region, then DNA is used as the tem-plate; however, for more diverse translocation breakpoints, for example t(4;11)(q21;q23) involving *MLL* and *AF4* in precursor B-ALL, RT-PCR is performed from the mRNA target. RT-PCR can be applied to 40–45% of child-hood precursor B-cell ALLs but is only rele-vant in 15–25% of T-ALLs. In AML, detection of the t(15;17) translocation in APL is relevant at diagnosis, as it indicates that treatment with retinoic acid is appropriate, and also in the MRD scenario in assessing response to retinoids. In most diseases, the presence or absence of a leukaemia-specific target is not sufficient to indicate relapse or disease-free survival, and quantitative techniques using either competitive PCR or 'real-time' PCR are required.

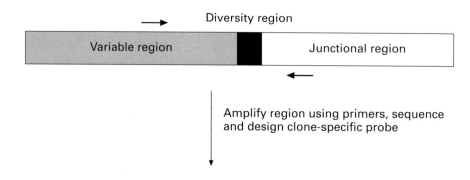

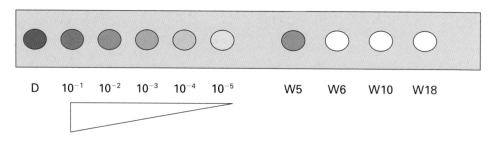

Figure 3.7

MRD assessment by PCR of *IgH* gene rearrangements. Consensus primers allow amplification of a 'clone-specific' fragment from a diagnostic marrow sample (D), which is sequenced to allow design of a clone-specific probe. PCR amplification of post-treatment samples and comparison with limiting dilutions of the diagnostic amplified fragment allows semi-quantitative analysis of MRD. In the example shown, the sensitivity of detection of the minor cell population is 10^{-5}, and while the initial week 5 (W5) sample shows MRD positivity at a level of 10^{-2}, subsequent aspirates (weeks 6, 10 and 12) are PCR-negative, suggesting that the patient is in long-term molecular remission.

Significance of MRD in acute leukaemia

Most large MRD studies to date in children have focused on childhood ALL, both during and after treatment. Low levels or absence of MRD after completion of induction therapy appear to predict good outcome in both immunophenotyping and PCR clonality studies. However, it is important to note that quantitation of levels of MRD can be relevant in particular types of leukaemia, and a steady decrease of MRD levels during treatment is associated with a good prognosis, whereas persistent high levels or increases in MRD positivity generally lead to clinical relapse.

Several prospective studies have indicated that sequential sampling, preferably using a quantitative approach, allows stratification of patient risk of relapse. However, it is important to note that while MRD studies show trends in relation to relapse or good outcome, MRD negativity at the end of chemotherapy does not unequivocally equate with leukaemia-free survival. MRD analysis is also useful in assessing the success of allogeneic SCT for this disease; however, it is important to use at least two different primer assays to avoid the problem of clonal evolution, which can occur in 20–30% of childhood ALLs. In addition, the use of chimaerism studies (where PCR-based assays can be used to follow the fate of donor and recipient cells post SCT) are useful in the management of paediatric patients in the post-transplant setting and can help predict relapse, graft rejection or disease-free survival.

Detection of leukaemia-specific markers using RT-PCR, for example the *PML–RARα* rearrangement in APL, particularly by serial analysis post ATRA therapy, can allow the true relevance of MRD in this clinical setting to be addressed. Other leukaemia-specific translocations, for example, *AML-1–ETO* in t(8;21) and *CBF–MYH11* in inv(16), are also amenable to PCR-based MRD analysis. In addition, PCR-based tests can be used to assess the degree of contaminating leukaemia cells in peripheral blood stem cell autografts.

NEW DEVELOPMENTS

Molecular therapeutics: gene therapy and antisense therapy

Molecular diagnostics have a key role to play in paediatric haematology. But what of molecular therapeutics? Somatic gene therapy has been the goal of many scientists and clinicians for the last 10 years. What is the progress to date? Somatic gene therapy involves the amelioration of a disease by introduction of genetic material with therapeutic potential into a somatic tissue. It is only in the last 5–10 years that gene transfer could be contemplated in the clinic. Gene therapy has benefited from (i) the gene transfer and expression techniques of molecular genetics, (ii) the natural ability of retroviruses to infect foreign replicating cells and stably integrate their genetic material into the host genome, and (iii) the fact that SCT provides a straightforward delivery of in vitro manipulated material into the blood stream. Thus a retrovirus (the most commonly used gene vector to date) can be engineered to contain an appropriate segment of DNA, and ex vivo transduction of haemopoietic cells allows subsequent introduction of foreign material into the host by the SCT route.

One of the first criteria for a suitable gene therapy model is for the corrected cells to have a growth advantage in the patient. Obvious candidates would be mutations in DNA metabolism, as corrected cells would show more efficient cell division. Evidence from allogeneic SCT of adenosine deaminase (ADA)-deficient patients indicated that T cells from the donor easily outgrow ADA-deficient cells – therefore ADA was chosen as the initial model system for gene therapy. The finding that individuals can have as little as 5% or as much as 50 times the standard levels of ADA are also important factors for a preliminary gene therapy protocol, as the level of expression need not be under stringent control.

Gene therapy, the ADA story

On 14 September 1990, the first child was treated for this disease by gene therapy. Blood was taken from the patient, a 4-year-old girl with no immune function. Red cells were given back by leukapheresis and mononuclear cells isolated by Ficoll centrifugation. These cells were grown in tissue culture, stimulated with interleukin-2 and infected with a third-generation retrovirus containing the ADA gene and a *neo* marker gene. The girl received 8 infusions of the transduced cells in an 11-month period and was also on weekly injections of polyethylene glycol (PEG)–ADA. PCR showed gene-corrected T cells (20–25%) in the mononuclear cell population. Her clinical condition had improved, so subsequently she received maintenance gene therapy infusions at 6-month intervals. Gene-corrected cells maintained their function for over 2.5 years. A second patient (a 9-year-old girl) received 11 infusions of gene-corrected autologous T cells from January 1991. Results in both patients were highly encouraging.

However, these studies were complicated by the fact that these patients were receiving PEG–ADA also. Removal of PEG–ADA indicated that sufficient long-term expression of ADA in gene-corrected T cells could not significantly alter the phenotype, an extreme disappointment for the proponents of gene therapy. Current work is concentrating on getting the ADA gene into primitive cells, either by manipulation of the microenvironment through the use of molecules such as fibronectin or by using other sources of stem cells such as cord blood. A variety of clinical trials are underway using some of these newer approaches.

Other candidates for haematology gene therapy protocols

Other metabolic disorders are also good candidates for gene-therapy-based approaches, as 5–25% of normal enzyme activity will normally suffice for protection from clinical disease in disorders such as haemophilia B. Several metabolic disorders are caused by absence of specific lysosomal enzymes that degrade specific compounds. The inability to degrade these compounds can lead to organ dysfunction, both visceral and in the central nervous system. Gaucher's disease, a deficiency of β-glucocerebrosidase, is treatable with enzyme-replacement therapy and SCT, thus showing the potential for a gene-therapy-directed approach. Clinical trials involving the introduction of retroviral vectors containing the β-glucocerebrosidase cDNA into bone marrow or stem cells are ongoing. Animal studies in Sly's syndrome (mucopolysaccharidosis VII), where β-glucurondidase deficiency results in accumulation of sulphated glycosaminoglycans, has indicated that autologous fibroblasts transfected with appropriate vectors and transplanted in mice can correct the lysosomal storage problems and serve as a model for the human situation. Recent studies in the haemophilic dog model also suggest that gene therapy approaches may be useful in the treatment of this disorder in humans.

Gene marking studies

Gene marking studies, which were initially used to demonstrate the safety of the technology, have also been shown to be useful in the assessment of cancer therapy. In September 1991, two children with AML were given autologous marrow that had been marked with the neomycin-resistance gene (*neo*) . The objective was to see if the re-emerging leukaemia originated from the infused autologous marrow or if relapse in the patient was due to residual leukaemia in the patient's own marrow. The marker gene is lost when

transduced cells die – thus the detection of marked malignant cells after transplantation indicated that the reinfused marrow contributed to relapse. This has important ramifications for a purging protocol, at least for autologous bone marrow transplantation in AML patients, and subsequent trials have begun for other leukaemias and neuroblastoma, where the effects of purging can be analysed in a randomized clinical trial using two different retroviral vectors.

Antisense studies

The methods described so far have involved the use of vector systems to deliver genes/gene products to the tissue(s) of interest and are particularly useful in restoring old functions or providing new functions to cells. However, in some situations, we may wish to block expression of a disease-specific gene, particularly in the treatment of malignancy, where cancer-specific fusion genes contribute to the disease phenotype. This can be achieved by the use of antisense oligodeoxynucleotides (ODNs). The principle of antisense technology involves blocking normal translation of mRNA. An oligonucleotide sequence is designed that will be coding for the same sequence as the mRNA but in the opposite direction. The antisense ODN binds to RNA, forming an RNA–DNA hybrid. This RNA–DNA hybrid blocks translation through activation of the RNase H pathway. RNase H recognizes RNA–DNA hybrids and degrades them rapidly within the cell. Antisense strategies have been employed successfully in vitro and in animal models, while phase I clinical trials in both CML and non-Hodgkin's lymphoma have been performed. Recent studies have also indicated that ribozymes, molecules that can cleave RNA directly, can be used as antisense agents.

SUMMARY AND CONCLUSIONS

Molecular pathology and molecular medicine have key roles to play in paediatric haematology. The technology that has developed over the last number of years has given greater access to primary material and allowed large-scale prospective and retrospective studies to be performed. In addition, it has provided us with the tools for molecular testing of inherited haematological diseases. The recent discovery of mutations in genes that result in an increased risk of DVT is extremely important, as both the disease and the genetic change(s) are common and so will impact greatly on world health. Acquired genetic changes play a key role in the development of leukaemia, and our evolving picture of the molecular landscape of haematological malignancy is providing key information that aids in the clinical management and stratification of these patients.

Advances in gene therapy at the preclinical and experimental therapy level are impressive but there are still major problems to be addressed. The treatments described thus far have in general concentrated on ex vivo gene therapy using viral vectors. The main problem with expanding gene therapy to treat large numbers of patients is the complexity of the current protocols. Ex vivo protocols require the extraction and manipulation of patient-specific cells and their re-introduction into the patient. This is probably only feasible in highly specialized institutes. Gene therapy is perhaps a natural progression from blood transfusion and stem cell transplantation; indeed the blood transfusion centres of today may be the gene therapy centres of the future. Some transfusion centres already collect stem cells for treatment of leukaemia, so their metamorphosis to centres for gene therapy vectors is not too far-fetched. The recent advances in antisense technology also look promising.

It is necessary of course to temper our excitement not only with a degree of realism but also with a high regard for the safety aspects of this new therapy. Gene therapy is at a very early stage, so we have no idea of what long-term side-effects may ensue. If we think about it, the long-term aim of any protocol would be a type of 'genes in a bottle' approach where the gene of interest could be injected just like a pharmaceutical drug. Thus, it could be injected intravenously much as insulin is delivered in diabetics. Perhaps the 'gene-drug' is on the horizon. Whatever the case, molecular biology has a key role to play in paediatric haematology in the new millennium.

FURTHER READING

Antonarakis SE. (1998) Molecular genetics of coagulation factor VIII gene and haemophilia A. *Haemophilia* **4** (Suppl 2): 1–11.

Brenner MK. (1998) Applications of gene transfer in hematologic malignancy. *Recent Results Cancer Res* **144**: 60–9.

Martinez-Climent JA, Garcia-Conde J. (1999) Chromosomal rearrangements in childhood acute myeloid leukemia and myelodysplastic syndromes. *J Pediatr Hematol Oncol* **21**: 91–102.

Morgan GJ. (1998) Modern molecular diagnostics and the management of haematological malignancies. *Clin Lab Haematol* **20**: 135–41.

van Dongen JJM, Szczepański T, Langerak AW, Pongers-Willemse MJ. (1999) Detection of minimal residual disease in lymphoid malignancies. In: Degos L, Linch DA, Löwenberg B, eds. *Textbook of Malignant Haematology*. London: Martin Dunitz: 685–724.

GLOSSARY OF GENETIC AND MOLECULAR TERMS

Allele The particular form of the gene that is inherited from one parent.

Dominant The presence of one allele of a pair is sufficient to provide the phenotype of the individual. Cf. *recessive*.

DNA Deoxyribonucleic acid, a double-stranded molecule containing a deoxysugar phosphate backbone and consisting of nucleotide base pairs that specify the genetic alphabet. In DNA, the four bases are adenine (A) and guanine (G) (the purine bases) and cytosine (C) and thymine (T) (the pyrimidine bases).

Dot blotting A process by which DNA or RNA is immobilized on a nylon membrane and hybridized with a probe to determine the presence or absence of a particular nucleic acid sequence.

Denaturing gradient gel electrophoresis (DGGE) A gene-scanning technique to detect potential areas of mutation. A segment of DNA is amplified by PCR and electrophoresed through a gel matrix where there is a gradient established that allows DNA segments of different sequence to be distinguished.

Direct sequencing A PCR-based approach that allows definition of the nucleic acid sequence of both alleles in the one assay. It is based on the classical sequencing approach of Frederick Sanger, which uses dideoxynucleotides (ddNTPs) in the protocol.

Exon The coding region of the gene. Genes may be composed of many exons.

Gene The molecular blueprint of cells; it is composed of a coding region (exons and introns) and a control region (promoter region and upstream activating elements or enhancers).

Genotype The genetic composition of an individual.

Heterozygote The alleles of a gene inherited from male and female parents are different.

Homozygote Both alleles of a gene inherited from male and female parents are identical for the trait of a particular gene.

Intron The intervening sequence between exons, which does not code for protein and must be spliced out prior to translation. One or a few introns may be present in one and the same gene.

Locus The physical position of the gene.

Phenotype The physical expression of the genotype.

Recessive The presence of both alleles is required to provide the phenotype of the individual. Cf. *dominant*.

RNA Ribonucleic acid, a single-stranded molecule containing a sugar phosphate backbone, and in which uracil (U) replaces thymine (T) of DNA. The intermediate product of the gene before it is expressed in a protein is messenger RNA (mRNA).

Splicing The process of removing introns from the premessenger RNA prior to translation.

Single-stranded conformational polymorphism (SSCP) analysis A simple mutation scanning technique, which relies on amplified DNA fragments of different sequence exhibiting different mobilities through a gel matrix.

Transcription The process by which the coding region of the gene is converted from DNA to messenger RNA.

Transcription factors DNA-binding proteins that recognize motifs or DNA signatures in the promoter region of target genes and act to control transcription.

Translation The process by which messenger RNA directs the synthesis of protein at the ribosome with the aid of transfer RNAs and amino acids.

Translocation Generally refers to the movement of genetic material from one chromosome to another.

4 Management of infections

Ian M Hann

INTRODUCTION

Progress with the cure of cancer and blood disease in children depends upon concomitant improvements in supportive care, and in particular the control of infection. Some progress has been made with preventative measures, and the building of air-filtered facilities and prevention of pneumocystis infection with co-trimoxazole have been the most important advances in prophylaxis of fungal infection. Progress with antibacterial prophylaxis has been bedevilled by a failure to properly assess the available antibiotics and the serious risk of subsequent development of resistant organisms. At present, as a consequence, no firm recommendations can be made. In the area of systemic fungal infection, amphotericin B and its lipid forms remains the gold standard, but the newer drugs such as voriconazole, posaconazole and caspofungin are worthy of further investigation. The various lipid formulations of amphotericin are now available, the best tested of which is the liposomal preparation, AmBisome, which has been shown to reduce the incidence of breakthrough systemic fungal infection, and at the same time produces less nephrotoxicity, less hypokalaemia and less serious infusion-related reactions. It can also be used at much higher dosages than conventional amphotericin, as can other lipid preparations, in patients with unresponsive infection. Herpes simplex infection can be prevented by acyclovir prophylaxis in high-risk patients and zoster immunoglobulin prevents serious zoster infection in patients who have been in contact with the virus. Ganciclovir and high-dose immunoglobulin have had an impact on cytomegalovirus infection and are of value in patients who have evid-

ence of infection on specific testing. A great deal of work has gone into identifying groups of neutropenic patients who are at low risk of infection and who could receive a single antibiotic such as ceftazidime, ceftriaxone or meropenem, and possibly be discharged from hospital early or even be treated at home. Children with a temperature below 39°C, short prior and predicted neutropenia and no evidence of shock fall into this category, but are only about a fifth of the whole cohort. Large trials of the approach are now justified. The best evidence at present is that the remainder of the patients, which includes most patients with acute myeloid leukaemia (AML), bone marrow transplant (BMT) recipients, high-risk acute lymphoblastic leukaemia (ALL) patients and non-Hodgkin's lymphoma (NHL) and neuroblastoma patients, should be treated with an aminoglycoside and piptazobactam or ceftazidime. If a patient fails to respond to this regimen, then either appropriate antibiotics should be given, if a causative organism is grown, or the aminoglycoside should be dropped and a form of amphotericin B started at 4–7 days from the beginning of fever, if the patient remains neutropenic.

When the reader goes through the chapters of this book, he or she should be struck by one thing above all others. Huge steps forward have been made in the cure of previously dreaded diseases. Probably the best example is AML, from which 90% of patients died 20 years ago. Now more than half will survive, at the cost of multiple infections and severe gut and organ toxicity. Almost invariably, the advances have been achieved by the use of very intensive chemotherapy protocols. Such achievements would not have occurred without the improved management of infections, in much the same way as most surgical advances follow upon improvements in anaesthetic techniques. However, now is not the time to sit back on our laurels. To do so would be negligent, because we still lose patients from fatal infection and, for instance, in the area of BMT much of the additional antileukaemic benefit of the graft is lost because of the approximately one-in-ten chance of overwhelming infection. We also face the burgeoning problem of systemic fungal and viral infection and the modern scourge of multiresistant organisms. Thus, we must be vigilant and not adopt regimens of treatment that increase the risk to subsequent generations of patients. Recent examples of worrying trends include the emergence of bacterial resistance following the widespread use of ciprofloxacin prophylaxis, such that 45% of isolates from patients in the large European series (International Antimicrobial Group of the European Organization for Research into the Treatment of Cancer, IATG-EORTC) had become resistant to ciprofloxacin within a decade. Also, the presence in our hospitals of vancomycin-resistant enterococci (VRE) should warn us strongly against the profligate use of the glycopeptide antibiotics vancomycin and teicoplanin. Most of all, we should resist the urge to use multiple concoctions of what we naively think are safe antimicrobial agents, in a panic-stricken attempt to treat an unresponsive infection. Nowhere is ignorance more prevalent and nowhere is insight more lacking than in the treatment of these patients. The answer is to do what we did before 'evidence-based medicine' was invented and rely on knowledge from large randomized clinical trials wherever possible. On a more optimistic note, between 1978 and 1994 the overall mortality from infection in neutropenic patients within the IATG-EORTC studies fell from 21% to 7%, and over the last 35 years the mortality from Gram-negative bacteraemia has fallen from 90% to below 10%.

PROPHYLAXIS

Prevention of bacterial infection

Progress in this area has been depressingly slow and fraught with difficulties. The biggest problem has been the inability of study groups to carry out large randomized trials with appropriate controls and adequate follow-up. Despite this, antibiotic prophylaxis is in widespread use and has almost certainly contributed to the increase in culture-negative infections and a gradual shift from Gram-negative towards Gram-positive infections such that the latter account for more than two-thirds of bacteraemias in most series. The latter effect has undoubtedly been enhanced by the use of indwelling right atrial catheters. Although this type of access has revolutionized intravenous therapy as well as fluid and nutritional support, it has also increased the incidence of Gram-positive organisms in particular, and especially coagulase-negative staphylococci, which have a propensity to stick to plastic. It is also possible that the use of H_2-blockers and other antacids has increased colonization of the gastric and oesophageal flora by oral streptococci.

Ever since anticancer therapy became more effective and infections became a problem, the prevention of infection has been considered a very attractive option, with its potential to decrease infection rates and improve the patient's quality of life. Various physical methods have been proposed and have led to great attention from the media, because 'life-bubbles' and the like are very attractive to everyone except those who have to try to survive in the emotional and sensory deprivation that they produce. Add to that the administration of gruesome antibiotic prophylactic regimens and one has an inhumane regimen that is in any case ineffective and thankfully has been abandoned. Semmelweiss would have approved of the only important measure – which is handwashing and strict aseptic technique, especially when handling intravenous catheters. High-efficiency air filters have been shown to reduce the risk of *Aspergillus* and possibly other airborne infections, and should probably be incorporated in all facilities wherein high-intensity therapeutic protocols are administered.

Chemoprophylaxis of bacterial and fungal infections was introduced when it became clear that more than 80% of the infective bacterial pathogens originated from the patient's own endogenous flora – a fact that should always be borne in mind when considering ineffective measures such as masking and gowning of visitors and banning of pets at home. Various gut decontamination methods have been examined and are remarkable either for their impalatability or the difficulties in monitoring the colonizing flora, which in any case showed development of resistance. Thus, this was another impractical and largely intolerable development that failed the test of time. Co-trimoxazole was initially used for this purpose and is palatable, although it can very rarely produce severe skin reactions and commonly suppresses the blood count. It does prevent *Pneumocystis carinii* pneumonia when it can be tolerated – and when it can't, there is some evidence that monthly pentamidine inhalations or oral dapsone may be a useful alternative. There has been a rather tedious debate as to the nosological classification of this organism, and the current belief is that it is a fungus.

The other vogue is to liberally dispense a fluoroquinolone drug for prophylaxis of bacterial infection, and ciprofloxacin is the most commonly used of these agents. The trials performed have shown a consistent reduction in the incidence of Gram-negative bacteraemia and no effect, or even an increase, in Gram-positive bacteraemias. After the initial euphoria, a degree of healthy scepticism has fallen over this approach. It must also be remembered that these agents are not currently licensed for this use in children because of possible toxicity on growing bones. It has also been realized that the reduced incidence of Gram-negative bacteraemia has not been translated into a decreased incidence of febrile episodes, nor by a reduction in the use of antibiotics. It has, however, been accompanied by an increased incidence of staphylococcal and streptococcal infections and there has been no clear reduction in overall mortality. The impression is

that the result of ciprofloxacin prophylaxis has not been an absolute reduction in the incidence of Gram-negative bacteraemias, but rather a change in the relative proportions of Gram-positive and Gram-negative bacteraemias and of unexplained (i.e. 'masked') fevers. Whether or not this is a beneficial effect is very uncertain, and it certainly makes the clinical management tricky. What is more, there is no doubt that the use of this type of prophylaxis has led to the development of resistance amongst bacteraemia organisms. In the IATG-EORTC series between 1983 and 1990, all 92 strains of *Escherichia coli* were sensitive to quinolones, and between 1991 and 1993, 27% were resistant, all from patients receiving quinolone prophylaxis, whereas only one resistant organism occurred in 29 patients with *E. coli* bacteraemia who had not received quinolone prophylaxis. The message is twofold: only use this prophylaxis in highly selected children known to be at real risk from Gram-negative infection; and whenever prophylaxis is instituted, this should be done with a healthy degree of scepticism and intensive long-term monitoring. Also, consideration should be given to the combined use with antibiotics such as colistin that may deal with the Gram-positive organisms.

Prevention of fungal infection

At the present time, it is known that air filtration reduces the risk of *Aspergillus* infection and oral fluconazole reduces the incidence of oropharangeal candidiasis, at a dose of 3 mg/kg/day. However, this type of prophylaxis should only be used in higher-risk patients, who are essentially BMT and AML patients. Several reports have shown an increasing rate of colonization and infection due to the fluconazole-resistant species *Candida krusei* and *C. glabrata* and also the development of azole resistance within *Candida* strains. Fluconazole is ineffective against filamentous fungi such as *Aspergillus*, which are the biggest worry in patients receiving steroids and undergoing allogeneic BMT. A new oral itraconazole preparation with improved bioavailability is being investigated, but it is too soon to decide whether or not it is effective and other methods such as intranasal amphotericin B have proven to be ineffective in recent randomized studies. The next area for investigation would be the prophylactic use of low-dose amphotericin B or AmBisome, or one of the newer agents such as voriconazole or posaconazole and the echinocandins such as caspofungin. It is crucially important that these studies should be carried out in trials admitting large numbers of high-risk patients, and ideally these would be carefully controlled.

At present, all that we can do in addition is to try to avoid the use of steroids as much as is possible (e.g. abandoning conventional amphotericin B when steroids are needed to control reactions), to advise patients to avoid high risk of contact with spores (e.g. in dung heaps) and to ensure that hospital diets, including spices, herbal teas and condiments, are clear of spores along with the hospital air that patients breathe.

Prevention of viral infection

Acyclovir prophylaxis prevents the emergence of herpes simplex peri-oral infections in high-risk patients and in particular in BMT recipients. There is some evidence that disruption of the mucosal barriers by this virus leads to the ingress of bacterial and fungal organisms, and the hope in future is that this type of prophylaxis plus positive use of mucosal growth factors may reduce symptoms and the risk of systemic infection. Other than that, it can only be said that the risk of cytomegalovirus (CMV) infection is probably reduced by transfusion of blood products that are leukodepleted and from screened CMV-negative blood donors. The risk of infection with this organism in children is low, but various manoeuvres in allogeneic BMT recipients may be of value and appear to have been associated with a reduced incidence and severity of infection. These regimens include the use of prophylactic ganciclovir and high-titre CMV immunoglobulin, and their pre-emptive use when there is evidence of infection on regular antigen testing of blood and/or broncho-alveolar lavage fluid.

Use of haemopoietic growth factors

Here we have a group of compounds that are currently of limited value and yet whose use is widespread and profligate. The use of granulocyte–macrophage colony stimulating factor (GM-CSF) is restricted because of increased toxicity compared with granulocyte colony stimulating factor (G-CSF). However, it may have additional benefit in the therapy of established systemic fungal infection because of enhanced monocyte numbers or functions, and randomized studies are allegedly under way. G-CSF is of some value in very high-risk patients undergoing allogenic BMT because it shortens the period of severe neutropenia by up to a week and may allow earlier recovery from infection. Its most common use is in the unresponsive febrile neutropenic patient, the area in which information is most limited. Until we have firmer results, its use should be restricted to allogeneic BMT patients, clinical trials of safety and efficacy (both against infection and in enhancing the anticancer effect of cytotoxic agents) and patients who are deteriorating and unresponsive to broad-spectrum antimicrobial agents. In the past, these patients were those who would have been given so-called white cell transfusions. In the future, we look forward in the hope that combinations of granulocyte cytokines plus thrombopoietin plus mucosal protective agents (e.g. glutamine) will be valuable.

MANAGEMENT OF THE FEBRILE AND NEUTROPENIC PATIENT

Diagnosis

The mainstay of specific diagnosis in a febrile patient is repeated blood cultures. Physical examination and chest x-ray do add some useful information on occasions, and, for instance, if there is evidence of an interstitial pneumonic process then the usual approach nowadays would be to treat the patient as if they had a *Pneumocystis*, *Mycoplasma* or *Legionella*, or, an atypical organism, with high-dose co-trimoxazole and erythromycin or clarithromycin. Then, if there is no response within 48 hours, a broncho-alveolar lavage will often give more information and allow a 'homing-in' of therapy. If there is no response to co-trimoxazole in a proven *Pneumocystis* infection, then the addition of pentamidine and steroids may well help. In totally unresponsive pneumonia, surfactant therapy has sometimes proved life-saving. One of the major advances has been the ready availability of ultrasound and computed tomography (CT) scans to pick up hepatosplenic candidiasis and lung CT, which can identify early lesions of invasive aspergillosis.

Various surrogate markers of infection have had their champions over the years. The CRP (C-reactive protein) is, in the view of the present author, little more than a fancy ESR and adds nothing to patient management. Various fungal antigen tests for *Candida* and *Aspergillus* are in a developmental stage and show some promise which requires validation in prospective studies. In the end, except in the rare case where a culture is positive from a definitely infected site, one has to rely on blood cultures or simply on the progress of fever.

Planned progressive therapy

Every unit that manages children with cancer and blood diseases should try to construct a team approach to the problem, with experts in infectious diseases, microbiology and respiratory disorders involved wherever possible in the decision-making process. The policy towards antimicrobial use depends on the local flora and fauna, and in particular on whether or not resistant organisms are a local problem. A suggested scheme is included in Figs 4.1 and 4.2, and Tables 4.1 and 4.2. This information is an adaptation of a scheme devised by the author's friend and colleague, Dr Harry Gaya and is reproduced with his kind permission. Clearly these recommendations are controversial but based on the best available current evidence. The choice between monotherapy and combination therapy is not an easy one because of limited evidence, but the IATG-EORTC series allowed an analysis of infectious episodes in 759 children. The best predictor for a poor outcome and the existence of bacteraemia was a temperature of 39°C or over, presence of shock, and long previous or predicted course of severe neutropenia. The majority of these patients were undergoing transplant procedures or intensive chemotherapy for AML, ALL, neuroblastoma or high-stage

---

Table 4.2 Single daily aminoglycoside dose adjustments

Gentamicin

$$\text{New dose}^a = \frac{\text{Old dose} \times 2.5}{\text{Conc. (8 h) mg/l}}$$

Amikacin

$$\text{New dose}^a = \frac{\text{Old dose} \times 10}{\text{Conc. (8 h) mg/l}}$$

[a] Day 2, then twice weekly.

Table 4.1 Antibiotic dosage levels for empirical regimens

Antibiotic	Dose (mg/kg body weight)	Schedule
Piperacillin + tazobactam[a]	80 + 10	q8h
Meropenem[b]	20	q8h
Gentamicin[c]	5	o.d
Amikacin[c]	20	o.d.

[a] If body weight > 50 kg, give adult dose: 4 g + 0.5 g q8h.
[b] If body weight > 50 kg, give adult dose: 1 g q8h.
[c] Follow instructions for dose adjustment.

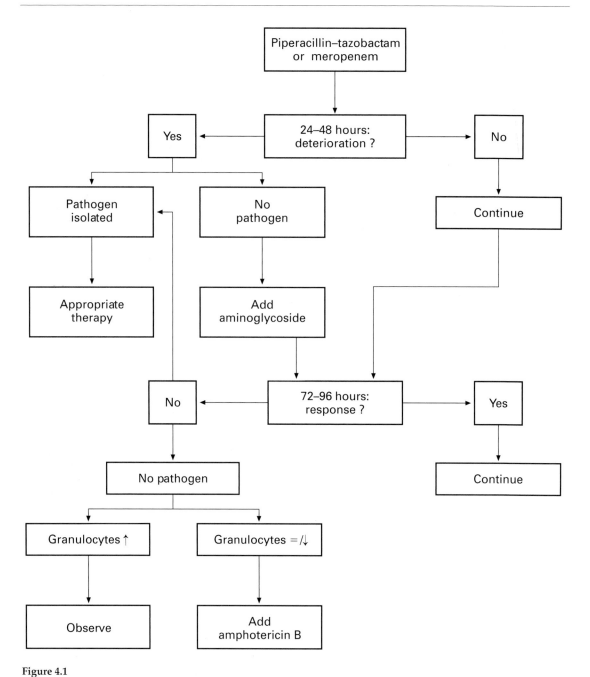

Figure 4.1

Scheme for monotherapy.

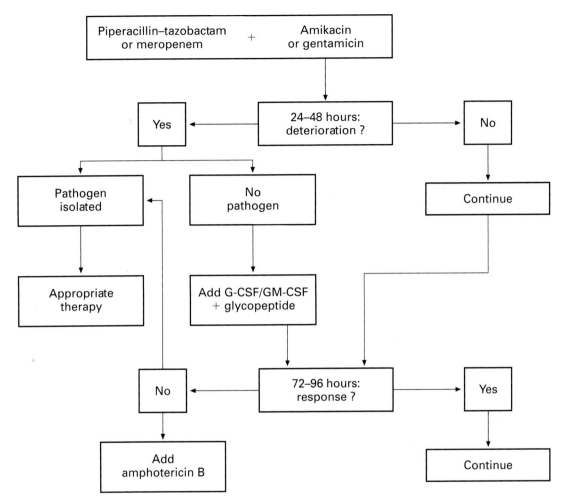

Figure 4.2

Scheme for combination therapy.

NHL. Thus, patients with neutrophil counts $> 0.1 \times 10^9/l$ that are unlikely to fall and those who are expected to have a short duration of neutropenia, and those who do not have the adverse features shown above, would come into the group in whom the monotherapy guidelines in Fig. 4.1 could be followed.

Whilst considering risk factors, it is useful to realize that children are different from adults and that their management may be affected by this knowledge. Children less frequently have a defined site of infection than adults, and where they do have a defined site

there are more upper respiratory but fewer lung infections. The incidence of shock is similar to adults, occurring in only 2% of cases, and the incidence of bacteraemia is also similar at about 22% overall. Clinically documented infection is less common in children (19% versus 28% for adults) and fever of unknown origin commoner (49% versus 38%). More importantly, children develop more streptococcal and fewer staphylococcal bacteraemias than adults, but the relative incidence of Gram-negative bacteraemia (29% of the total bacteraemias) is similar. Children have a lower mortality (1%) from infection than adults (4%) and the time to defervescence tends to be shorter.

The question arises as to whether patients can be discharged earlier than in the past, to complete courses of antibiotics at home or even to have the whole course on an outpatient basis. Various regimens have been devised, and very small series that tend to include mainly good-risk patients have been reported. All that can be said at present is that monotherapy and even combination therapy can be given at home, but large prospective trials are required. One in 50 patients still develops shock and a high proportion of higher-risk patients do not have early resolution of fever. It is possible to consider early discontinuation of intravenous antibiotics in a patient in the good-risk group whose fever responds promptly, whose blood cultures remain negative and whose general condition is very good. Courses as short as two days have been given and patients even discharged with zero neutrophil counts. However, the approach must remain cautious in patients whose neutrophil counts are likely to remain very low for more than a few days.

The use of glycopeptides (teicoplanin and vancomycin)

A great deal has been written on this subject and a great deal more heat than light has been generated as a consequence. The IATG-EORTC proved the most important points in a large randomized trial: that it is not necessary to use these agents in an empirical fashion and that therapy with these agents must not be widely adopted without awareness of the very serious consequences of the greater problems with multiresistant organisms that already exist. At present, there is no convincing evidence from large randomized trials that teicoplanin or vancomycin have advantages over each other, apart from the major advantage of single daily dosing with teicoplanin, which can thus facilitate its use at home. On this point, a once-daily regimen of teicoplanin and ceftriaxone, with or without a single daily dose of aminoglycoside, covers most organisms extremely well, apart from perhaps *Pseudomonas* strains, and

is easy to administer.

Various hospitals have adopted various policies to deal with what they call 'line infections'. As there is rarely any proof that this was or remained the site of infection, it is an unhelpful term. There is a correlation between marked reddening of the right atrial catheter entry site or tunnel and the existence of Gram-positive organisms, especially coagulase-negative staphylococci. Thus it may be justified to add in a glycopeptide to the initial empirical regimen when this exists and there has not been defervescence within 48 hours. However, it is probably more sensible to use glycopeptide therapy only when Gram-positive organisms are found that are not sensitive to other agents, or in patients who are clinically deteriorating. These microbes very rarely cause serious infections and usually grow in blood cultures within a few days, and thus it is not usually necessary to use these antibiotics in an empirical fashion. At the present time, there is conflicting evidence that leaving glycopeptides in the intravenous catheter or using them as flushes is effective.

Once-daily aminoglycosides (see Table 4.2)

There is a wealth of evidence that efficacy may be enhanced and toxicity reduced by single daily dosage of aminoglycosides, and many countries have adopted this approach. Some would advise caution in using this dosing in children before more information is available, but it has already become standard treatment in major centres in a number of countries and facilitates home therapy. No doubt we will hear a great deal more about this over the next few years.

Use of therapeutic antifungal agents (see Table 4.3)

The biggest problem with the management of fungal infection is the difficulty with diagnosis. Patients with unresponsive serious infections should be regarded as having fungal infection unless proved otherwise, until mycologists come up with some better tests. Molecular biological (polymerase chain reaction, PCR) techniques for *Aspergillus* antigen are giving encouraging results. Any patient with cellulitis or necrotic lesions of the face, and particularly those in whom infection of the upper airways becomes evident, is most likely to have an infection with *Aspergillus* or *Mucor* species – not anaerobic infections, which are very rare in this group of patients. Thus, the widespread use of metronidazole is unjustified and it should only be used in the rare instances where anaerobes are found and are not sensitive to agents such as piptazobactam. Patients with cavitating lung lesions probably have an *Aspergillus* infection, which is associated with typical changes in the lung detectable on CT scan. Patients with isolated splenomegaly often turn out to have a viral infection such as CMV or Epstein–Barr virus (EBV), but those with persistent hepatosplenomegaly probably have *Candida* infection if their primary disease is not the cause. Again, CT or ultrasound of the liver and spleen showing changes of a Gruyère cheese type appearance can be typical. In all instances, it is extremely difficult to prove a diagnosis without tissue biopsy, and the dangers of such may preclude that approach. As a consequence, much antifungal therapy is empirical (see Figs 4.1, 4.2 and Table 4.3).

A number of new antifungal agents are under investigation, such as voriconazole. There are three lipid-associated amphotericin compounds, and the liposomal preparation AmBisome has been extensively studied in randomized trials of pyrexia of unknown origin in adults and children. It is safer, causing less nephrotoxicity, hypokalaemia and infusion related-reactions and there are fewer breakthrough systemic fungal infections. The other major advantage is that the dose can easily be escalated to at least 5 mg/kg/day, and trials of its use in prophylaxis and therapy of systemic fungal infection is under way. All three lipid-associated compounds are worthy of further head-to-head studies in patients with proven infection.

Table 4.3 Possible criteria for use of liposomal amphotericin B (AmBisome)[a]

- *If the patient is receiving cyclosporin A or tacrolimus*
  Dose for empirical therapy: 1 mg/kg/day or 3 mg/kg/day (see Walsh and Prentice papers)
  Dose for systemic fungal infection clinically or microbiologically documented):
  3 mg/kg/day
- *If the patient has existing nephrotoxicity*
  Serum creatinine > 1.5 times upper limit of normal for age
- *If the patient has existing hepatotoxicity*
  Liver function tests > 3 times upper limit of normal for age
- *If the patient is on three or more nephrotoxic agents*
  Aminoglycoside, vancomycin, furosemide, cisplatin, carboplatin, melphalan etc.

To convert a patient from amphotericin deoxycholate to liposomal amphotericin (AmBisome), the patient should have one of
- Severe infusion-related reactions (fevers, chills, rigors) persisting for > 72 hours
- One episode of hypotension (persisting despite slowing infusion rate to 6 hours)
- One episode of hypoxia
- Hypokalaemia of ≤ 2.5 mmol/l persisting despite supplemental potassium up to 3 mmol/kg/day and use of amiloride or spironolactone
- Serum creatinine ≥ 2 × upper limit of normal for age
- Clinical evidence of infection progression

[a] The same criteria could apply to other lipid preparations but there is limited current evidence available for children.

CONCLUSIONS AND OUTLOOK

Infection management has been a great success story of the last 25 years, but the challenges are greater than ever. Newer and ever more intensive cytotoxic regimens have faced us with a Pandora's box of problems. Barely a month goes by without reports of infections with organisms never previously known to produce problems in humans. It is essential to remain vigilant, work with the new drug developments and construct randomized clinical trials that will allow rational and economically justified therapy decisions to be made.

FURTHER READING

Hann I, Viscoli C, Paesmans M, Gaya H, Glauser M (1997). A comparison of outcome from febrile neutropenic episodes in children compared with adults; results from four EORTC studies. *Br J Haematol* **99**: 580–8.

Hargrave DR, Hann IM, Richards SM et al (2001). Progressive reduction in treatment-related deaths in Medical Research Council childhood lymphoblastic leukaemia trials from 1980–1997 (UKALL VIII, X and XI). *Br J Haematol*, **112**: 293–9.

Lowis SP, Oakhill A (1997). Management of acute complications of therapy in paediatric oncology. In: Pinkerton CR, Plowman PN, eds. *Paediatric Oncology*. London: Chapman & Hall: 677–702.

Patrick CC (1992). *Infections in Immunocompromised Infants and Children*. Edinburgh: Churchill Livingstone.

Prentice HG, Hann IM, Herbrecht R et al (1997). A randomized comparison of liposomal versus conventional amphotericin B for the treatment of pyrexia of unknown origin in neutropenic patients. *Br J Haematol* **98**: 711–8.

Riley LC, Hann I, Wheatley K et al. (1999) Treatment-related deaths during induction and first remission of AML in children treated on MRC AML10. *Br J Haematol* **106**: 436–44.

Viscoli C, Castagnola E. (1998) Planned progressive antimicrobial therapy in neutropenic patients. *Br J Haematol* **102**: 879–88.

Walsh TJ, Finberg RW, Arndt C et al (1999). Liposomal amphotericin B for empirical therapy in patients with persistent fever and neutropenia. National Institute of Allergy and Infectious Diseases Mycoses Study Group. *N Engl J Med* **340**: 764–71.

5 Blood transfusion in children and neonates

Helen Enright

INTRODUCTION

Although mystical properties had been attributed to blood for many centuries, the first documented successful transfusion was carried out in 1667 when blood was transfused from a lamb to a child with anaemia by Denis, philosopher and physician to King Louis XIV of France. Denis followed this by a successful transfusion to a 34-year-old patient, who unfortunately died following a subsequent transfusion some months later – and the first haemolytic transfusion reaction was thus documented. Subsequent attempts at transfusion was carried out by Blondell in the early 1800s using human donor blood. However, it was the discovery of ABO blood groups by Landsteiner in 1900 and the identification of the Rhesus antigen system in 1939 that allowed a scientific approach to transfusion. The development of anticoagulant solutions, plastic storage bags, preservative solutions and facilities to maintain blood at 4°C allowed the evolution of transfusion science from the 1950s onwards. During the 1970s and 1980s, component therapy became standard transfusion practice, and the knowledge that human immunodeficiency virus (HIV) and hepatitis viruses could be transmitted by blood transfusion profoundly altered the course of transfusion history. This resulted in an increasing awareness of safety issues, avoidance of unnecessary blood transfusion, and emphasis on prevention and documentation of the adverse effects of transfusion. Today, the collection and processing of blood components is a highly complex process similar to manufacturing processes in the pharmaceutical industry, with an emphasis on ensuring appropriate transfusion with component therapy and a safe blood supply.

This chapter will discuss the laboratory procedures involved in pre-transfusion testing, the components available for transfusion to children, the indications for their use and the adverse effects of transfusion. In addition, specific clinical situations and special issues related to neonatal transfusion are discussed.

TRANSFUSION MANAGEMENT AND PRACTICE

The recognition that blood products can transmit viral infections, particularly HIV infection, has changed dramatically the approach to modern transfusion. Consequences include the implementation of measures to increase the safety of blood transfusion, increased testing of blood products for evidence of transmissible infection, a shift to component therapy, and increased use of recombinant coagulation factors and transfusion substitutes. Key components of transfusion management now include transfusion audit, haemovigilance, and centralized reporting of transfusion reactions and adverse events. Transfusion audit involves the development, implementation and assessment of transfusion policies and guidelines at local, national and international levels, and the assessment of the appropriateness of blood transfusion. Most hospitals now have a multidisciplinary transfusion committee to consider local transfusion needs, practice and policies. Education, cooperation and open communication between the laboratory and clinical staff and patient education are of utmost importance.

Blood groups

The red cell phenotype of an individual is determined by antigens of two types present on the red cell membrane: those where the antigen specificity is determined by carbohydrate moieties attached to membrane proteins or lipids (e.g. the ABO, Lewis and P systems) and those where the epitope is a membrane protein (e.g. the Rhesus, Duffy, Kell, Kidd and MNSs systems). Of the many families of antigens described, only some are of clinical importance. This is related to (a) their degree of antigenicity, (b) the frequency of the antigen in the population, and (c) the activity of the antibody at 37°C. The ABO group is of particular importance, as the antibodies occur naturally in patients lacking the corresponding antigen (Table 5.1), are IgM and activate complement, thus readily causing haemalysis. The importance of the Rhesus system is related to the immunogenicity of the Rhesus antigens, the fact that 85% of the (Caucasian) population are Rhesus (D)-positive, and the activity of antibodies at 37°C. Other clinically important antigens in transfusion medicine are Cc and Ee of the Rhesus system, and the Kell (Kk), Duffy (Fy^a, Fy^b), Kidd (Jk^a, Jk^b), Lutheran (Lu^a, Lu^b), MNSs, P and Lewis (Le^a, Le^b) systems.

Testing of donated blood

Following careful selection of donors, donated blood is subjected to extensive testing, usually at the regional blood transfusion centre (Table 5.2). These tests are performed to determine the ABO and Rhesus group of the donated blood, to detect any antibody present in donor serum, and to exclude infective or potentially infective components. Routine tests are performed for hepatitis B, hepatitis C, HIV (-1 and -2), human T-cell leukaemia/lymphoma virus (HTLV-I and -II) and syphilis, with optional additional testing for cytomegalovirus (CMV).

Prescribing blood products and identification of the patient

Most transfusion fatalities are due to transcription (i.e. clerical) errors and/or failure to properly identify the patient when obtaining blood or at the time of transfusion. It is therefore critical that appropriate procedures to ensure safe transfusion practice are adhered to. The transfusion should be appropriately *prescribed*, including documentation of the *reason for transfusion*. There should be a record of patient or parent *informed consent*, including an explanation to the patient and/or parent of the reason for transfusion and the

Table 5.1 ABO antigens and antibodies					
ABO type	Frequency[a]	Antigens on red cells	Antibodies in plasma	Preferred donor	Acceptable donor[b]
A	0.45	A	Anti-B	A	O
B	0.09	B	Anti-A	B	O
O	0.43	H	Anti-A Anti-B	O	None
AB	0.04	A + B	None	AB	A > B > O
[a] Caucasian populations. [b] Red cell transfusions only.					

Table 5.2 Laboratory testing prior to transfusion

Tests performed on donated blood[a]

ABO and Rhesus group	HIV-1 and -2 antibody
Red cell antibody screen	HIV antigen
Red cell phenotyping (optional)	HTLV-I and -II antibody
Hepatitis B surface antigen (HBsAg)	*Treponema* antigen
Hepatitis B core antibody (anti-HBc)	CMV (optional)
Hepatitis C antibody (anti-HCV)	

Pre-transfusion testing[b]

Recipient blood	**Donor blood**
ABO and Rhesus group	ABO and Rhesus group
Antibody screen	
Antibody identification if antibody screen is positive	

Donor and recipient blood
Crossmatch (donor red cells + recipient serum)

[a] Usually performed at the regional donor centre. [b] usually performed at the hospital blood bank where the transfusion is planned.
CMV, cytomegalovirus; HIV, human immunodeficiency virus; HTLV, human T-cell leukaemia/lymphoma virus.

---

potential side-effects involved. The patient must be identified at the bedside at the time of sample taking and also at the time of transfusion. The sample drawn must be clearly labelled with, at a minimum, the patient's full name, date of birth, hospital number, date and the signature of the person performing the phlebotomy. This information must be handwritten – addressograph labelling of samples is not acceptable. The details on the sample must comply with those on the request form. It has become critically important to ensure the traceability of transfused blood products for 'look-back' programmes, so all transfusions must be properly documented in the patient's medical record.

Routine blood bank procedures

When a request for crossmatched blood is received by the blood bank, the following laboratory testing is performed: ABO and Rhesus testing of the recipient and donor red cells, screening of the recipient and donor serum for anti-red-cell antibodies, and crossmatching of donor red cells with recipient serum. The antibody screen involves testing the recipient serum against test cells from at least two individuals, the combined antigen profile allowing detection of all clinically important antibodies. If the antibody screen is negative and the crossmatch shows compatibility, the red cells are released for transfusion. If the antibody screen is positive, the antibody requires identification and cells must be selected that lack the corresponding antigen. A 'type and screen' should be ordered if it is not very likely that the patient will need transfusion. In this case, the blood bank will perform the ABO and Rhesus testing and screen the serum for antibodies: if the antibody screen is negative, no further testing is done, but blood can be made available within a short period of time if required. Most hospital blood banks will agree a maximum blood order schedule (MBOS) with their clinical users to guide ordering and appropriate transfusion and to help predict transfusion needs and therefore manage the blood bank inventory. In an absolute emergency, type-specific or group O Rhesus-negative units may be used while awaiting the results of the crossmatch.

BLOOD TRANSFUSION COMPONENT THERAPY: PREPARATIONS AND CLINICAL INDICATIONS

Component therapy is the preferred approach in transfusion medicine, and the use of whole blood is rarely indicated. Following collection, whole blood is centrifuged and separated to yield red cells, platelets and plasma, which is frozen to provide fresh-frozen plasma and cryoprecipitate, or pooled and fractionated to prepare specific factor concentrates, albumin and immunoglobulin preparations (Table 5.3). These latter preparations are treated to inactivate viruses by dry heat, pasteurization or solvent–detergent methods.

Cellular blood components

Red blood cells

Red blood cell units are derived from a single donation of blood that is centrifuged, the plasma removed and the red cells suspended to a haematocrit of approximately 0.75 in an additive anticoagulant and nutrient solution (e.g. SAG-M: saline, adenine, glucose and mannitol). Units are stored at 1–6°C for 35–42 days, depending on the additive solution. The volume of one unit of red cells is approximately 260–280 ml. Units contain little residual plasma (approximately 20 ml) and may also be depleted of leukocytes. Special paediatric packs are available in most centres

The decision to transfuse a child should always take into account the age and clinical condition of the patient, the diagnosis and cause of the anaemia, complicating factors, anticipated further blood loss, and the nature and timing of any planned surgical procedures. Packed red cells are used for the correction of symptomatic anaemia and in situations of acute blood loss. Transfusion may be necessary in acute blood loss that amounts to 10–20% or more of the blood

Table 5.3 Blood and blood components used in clinical blood transfusion
Red cells
Packed red cells
Frozen/deglycerolized red cells
Platelets
Single random-donor platelet concentrates
Pooled random-donor platelet concentrates
Apheresis (single-donor) platelets
HLA-matched apheresis platelets
Modifications to red cell and platelet preparations
Gamma-irradiation
Leukocyte depletion
CMV-tested (seronegative)
Plasma and plasma-derived products
Fresh frozen plasma
Cryoprecipitate
Cryoprecipitate-poor plasma
Prothrombin complex concentrate
Factor VIII
Factor IX
Factor XIII
Fibrinogen
Antithrombin III
Protein C
Albumin
Intravenous immunoglobulin
Disease-specific immunoglobulin
$Rh_0(D)$ immunoglobulin
Recombinant products
Recombinant factor VIII
Recombinant factor IX
Recombinant factor VIIa

volume or that is sufficient to induce hypovolaemia as manifested by tachycardia, tachypnea and/or hypotension. In infants, other symptoms that may influence the decision to transfuse include respiratory distress, cardiomegaly, increasing liver size, poor feeding or apnoea.

In chronic anaemia, transfusion of red cells is indicated for symptomatic patients regardless of the aetiology of anaemia and for asymptomatic patients with haemoglobin of 7–8 g/dl or less if no other medical therapy (such as iron or folate) is likely to correct the anaemic state. Transfusion may also be warranted in asymptomatic patients with haemoglobin less than 8 g/dl prior to emergency surgery, when time precludes evaluation of the anaemia or specific replacement therapy, or for surgical procedures where significant blood loss is expected. In a non-bleeding child, a dose of 4 ml/kg should result in a 1 g/dl increase in the haemoglobin level. The red cells should be transfused through the largest-gauge needle possible, as haemolysis may occur when using small-gauge needles.

Frozen deglycerolized red cells

Red cells may be stored frozen for prolonged periods in cytoprotectant solutions containing glycerol. Deglycerolized red cells (washed to remove glycerol) are rarely indicated except in patients with rare blood types or with multiple red cell antibodies, for storage of autologous cells for patients with antibodies to high-frequency antigens, and occasionally for patients with IgA deficiency and antibodies to IgA who have experienced severe transfusion reactions.

Transfusion of patients with sickle cell anaemia and haemoglobinopathy

Asymptomatic patients with uncomplicated sickle cell anaemia generally do not require transfusion. It may be desirable to transfuse patients to decrease the concentration of haemoglobin S (HbS) and increase haemoglobin A in specific clinical situations. These include symptomatic anaemia, impending cerebrovascular thrombosis, splenic sequestration crises, priapism, acute chest syndrome and preparation for surgery involving general anaesthesia. In these acute situations, exchange transfusion may be required to decrease the HbS level to 30%. For general anaesthesia, reduction of the HbS level to 60% may be sufficient. Repeated transfusion results in red cell immunization, and antigen-negative blood may be difficult to procure.

In thalassaemic patients, the problems of chronic iron overload should be balanced against the potential benefits of transfusion. 'Hypertransfusion' regimens may be instituted to decrease endogenous erythropoiesis (and the complications of medullary expansion and extramedullary haemopoiesis).

Platelet preparations

Available platelet preparations include platelets suspended in plasma prepared by the centrifugation of a unit of blood (random-donor platelet concentrates, which are usually pooled for transfusion), and single random-donor units collected by apheresis. HLA-matched apheresis platelets (usually matched at two HLA antigens) are also available. Patients are transfused at a dose of one unit of random donor platelet concentrate per 10 kg of body weight. One unit of random-donor platelets contains approximately 5×10^{10} platelets in 60 ml of plasma. The volume of one apheresis unit is approximately 350–400 ml, containing approximately 2.4×10^{11} platelets (if used for small patients, the dose, i.e. the volume infused, should be adjusted accordingly). Platelets are stored at 22°C on a mechanical agitator and have a shelf-life of 5 days. Platelet units should be ABO-compatible as the platelets are suspended in plasma, with a risk of haemolysis if there is a high-titre anti-A or anti-B antibody present. Rhesus-negative female children should receive Rhesus-negative platelets.

There is no absolute platelet count level or 'trigger' for transfusion, and the decision to transfuse is a clinical one taken following assessment of the bleeding risk in conjunction with the patient's platelet count. Prophylactic transfusion is generally undertaken for patients without bleeding where the platelet count is less than $10 \times 10^9/l$. Therapeutic transfusion of platelets is indicated when the platelet count is less than $30 \times 10^9/l$ with active bleeding, or less than $50 \times 10^9/l$ if the patient is a neonate, if there are compounding factors (including coagulopathy, fever or severe infection) or if the patient has recently received drugs known to cause platelet dysfunction.

Platelet transfusion is also indicated if the platelet count is less than $50 \times 10^9/l$, if the patient is undergoing major surgery, or if the platelet count is less than $100 \times 10^9/l$ following cardiopulmonary bypass with excessive bleeding or prior to neurological or ophthalmic surgery. Occasionally, platelet transfusion may be used for patients with platelet dysfunction (but a normal count) with active bleeding. However, in this situation, the use of antifibrinolytic agents or desmopressin (DDAVP) should be considered.

The response to platelet transfusion may be assessed by documenting an increment in the patient's platelet count 1 hour after transfusion. The corrected count increment (CCI) is defined as:

$$\frac{(\text{post-transfusion} - \text{platelet count pre-transfusion count}) \times \text{body surface area}}{\text{platelets transfused}}$$

The expected CCI at 1 hour post transfusion is approximately 15 000. Patients with a CCI at 1 hour following transfusion of <5000–7500 are considered refractory to transfusion. Refractoriness develops in up to 80% of multiply transfused patients. Factors contributing to failure to respond appropriately to platelet transfusion include infection, splenomegaly, coagulopathy (e.g. disseminated intravascular coagulation, DIC) and alloimmunization. In alloimmunized patients, platelet transfusions from a HLA-matched donor may be helpful, and leukocyte depletion of platelets has been shown to reduce the incidence of alloimmunization.

Granulocyte concentrates

Since the advent of recombinant growth factors (such as granulocyte and granulocyte–macrophage colony stimulating factors, G-CSF and GM-CSF) for clinical use, granulocyte concentrates are now rarely indicated. Granulocyte concentrates may, however, very occasionally be considered in patients with life-threatening infections with neutropenia or granulocyte dysfunction. The absolute neutrophil count should be less than $0.5 \times 10^9/l$ (or less than $3 \times 10^9/l$ in neonates) and there should be evidence of progressive infection with failure to respond to broad-spectrum antibiotics, culture-specific therapy, and cytokines.

Modification of cellular blood components

Leukocyte-depleted blood components

Blood products depleted of leukocytes may be produced by differential centrifugation or by bedside or in-laboratory filtration. Pre-storage leukodepletion is increasingly performed routinely in blood centres to reduce accumulation of cytokines in stored products (which contribute to febrile transfusion reactions) and to decrease the incidence of alloimmunization. These products do not require additional bedside leukodepletion. Filtration leukodepletion removes over 99.9% of leukocytes: red cell units contain less than 5×10^6 leukocytes and retain over 80% of the original red cell content. Platelet loss of 20–25% of the original content of platelet concentrates also occurs.

Leukodepleted red cells and platelets are indicated for patients with documented recurrent febrile non-haemolytic transfusion reactions. There is increasing use of such components for the prevention of platelet alloimmunization in patients where multiple transfusions are anticipated and to decrease CMV transmission by transfusion. Leukocyte-depleted products do not prevent transfusion-associated graft-versus-host disease (GVHD) or transfusion-associated lung injury. Leukocyte-depleted products are recommended for intra-uterine exchange transfusion and for haemolytic disease of the newborn, and are generally advisable where lifelong transfusion is required (e.g. in sickle cell anaemia and thalassaemia).

Cytomegalovirus (CMV)-seronegative cellular blood products

Blood products that have tested negative for CMV are indicated for transfusion to immunosuppressed patients at risk of CMV disease. These include neonates of CMV-seronegative mothers (although many centres provide all neonates less than four months of age and all pregnant women with CMV-seronegative blood products), patients with severe combined immunodeficiency and other primary congenital immunodeficiency states, CMV-seronegative patients who are to receive solid organ transplants, and CMV-seronegative bone marrow transplant recipients (and potential recipients). In addition, CMV-seronegative products should be used for all patients with haematological malignancy until their CMV serostatus is known, CMV-seronegative HIV-positive patients, and intra-uterine transfusions. In areas where the supply of CMV-tested products is limited, leukocyte depletion by filtration may be an acceptable alternative approach to decreasing the transmission of CMV disease.

Gamma-irradiated components

The presence of immunocompetent lymphocytes in transfused blood products may cause transfusion-associated GVHD in immunosuppressed patients. Transfusion-associated GVHD is characterized by skin rash, elevated liver enzymes, and (unlike transplant-associated GVHD) bone marrow aplasia. The mortality rate approaches 90–100%. Gamma irradiation of blood products to prevent lymphocyte proliferation effectively prevents this complication, and is therefore indicated for patients with bone marrow and peripheral blood stem cell transplants, those with severe combined immunodeficiency or other congenital immunodeficiency syndromes, and after therapy-induced immunosuppression, aggressive chemotherapy (especially with fludarabine or for Hodgkin's disease), immunotherapy or extensive radiation therapy. Other indications include homologous components for bone marrow transplant donors, neonatal intensive care patients until their immune status is clarified, low-birth-weight infants, exchange transfusion in the neonate, and for directed donations from family members.

Plasma and plasma-derived products and components

Fresh frozen plasma

A unit of fresh frozen plasma contains the plasma derived from one blood donation.

Units are stored at $-30°C$, and thawed at $37°C$ when required. It takes approximately 15–20 minutes to thaw units of fresh frozen plasma. Each random-donor unit contains approximately 220–250 ml of plasma, and apheresis packs (500–600 ml) are now available. Fresh frozen plasma contains the coagulation factors normally contained in plasma. The use of fresh frozen plasma should be limited to correction of documented coagulopathy due to deficiency of coagulation factors in a patient who is bleeding or is scheduled for invasive medical or surgical procedures, reversal of warfarin therapy complicated by bleeding, plasma exchange treatment of thrombotic thrombocytopenic purpura (TTP) and haemolytic uremic syndrome (HUS), massive blood transfusion complicated by coagulopathy and bleeding, and treatment of congenital factor deficiencies where a concentrate is not available (e.g. factor V). The response to an initial dose of 10–12 ml/kg should be assessed by repeating the coagulation screen. Fresh frozen plasma is not recommended for volume expansion in hypovolemia or as a source of nutritional support. Adverse effects associated with the use of fresh frozen plasma include volume overload, urticarial and anaphylactic reactions, and occasionally haemolysis due to the presence in plasma of anti-A and anti-B antibodies. Units used should therefore be ABO-compatible. Infection transmission is also a risk, and may be reduced by the use of viral-inactivated plasma (VIP).

Cryoprecipitate

Cryoprecipitate, prepared from thawing of fresh frozen plasma, contains factor VIII (80–100 units of factor VIII:C per unit), and fibrinogen (150–300 mg/unit). Cryoprecipitate may be considered for therapy or prophylaxis of bleeding complications in patients with von Willebrand's disease documented by a positive history and supporting laboratory studies. The usual dose in moderate to severe von Willebrand's disease is 1 unit/10 kg body weight (each unit contains 10–20 ml), and infusions are given 8-hourly. Cryoprecipitate transfusions should be ABO-compatible. However, virus-inactivated factor VIII concentrates enriched in von Willebrand's factor (such as Haemate P) are generally preferred, and cryoprecipitate should not be used in patients with haemophilia A or B, who should receive specific clotting factor concentrates. Other indications for cryoprecipitate include documented hypofibrinogenemia (<1 g/l) in an actively bleeding patient and treatment of bleeding or prophylaxis prior to surgical procedures in hepatic or renal failure patients with prolonged bleeding times. The alternative use of desmopressin should be considered.

Purified factor VIII concentrate

The major indication for human factor VIII concentrate is for a patient with a confirmed history of haemophilia A (i.e. a documented hereditary deficiency in factor VIII) who is bleeding or scheduled for an invasive medical or surgical procedure, or as planned prophylaxis for such a patient. Patients with mild or even moderate deficiency may respond to desmopressin. Recombinant factor VIII is now available and is preferred by many centres. The dose required can be determined from the calculated plasma volume and the desired factor VIII increment. As an approximate guide, a dose of 1 unit/kg will increase the levels of factor VIII in the recipient by 2%. Infusions may be intermittent (every 8–12 hours) or continuous during a bleeding episode. The response to therapy should be assessed by measuring factor VIII levels, and patients should be monitored for the development of antibodies inhibitory to factor VIII, which occur in up to 15% of patients. Patients who develop inhibitors may require treatment with very large doses of factor VIII concentrate, recombinant factor VIIa, or prothrombin complex concentrates. Efforts to decrease the level of inhibitor antibody include plasma exchange and various immunosuppressive regimens.

Purified factor IX concentrate

Factor IX concentrate is indicated for patients with hereditary deficiency of factor IX (haemophilia B) who are bleeding or who are scheduled for invasive medical or surgical procedures. A dose of 1 unit/kg will increase the factor IX level in the recipient by approximately 1%. Doses are usually repeated at 12-hourly intervals. Recombinant factor IX is now available and is widely used. The incidence of inhibitor development is lower than in factor VIII deficiency.

Prothrombin complex concentrates

Prothrombin complex concentrates contain factors II, IX and X and may be used in patients with multiple clotting factor deficiencies. However, owing to potential thrombotic complications, fresh frozen plasma is generally preferred. The use of prothrombin complex concentrates in haemophiliac patients with factor VIII inhibitors has largely been superseded by the use of activated recombinant factor VIIa, as has the use of factor VIII inhibitor bypassing activity (FEIBA) preparations.

Fibrinogen

Fibrinogen preparations may be used for the selective replacement of fibrinogen in congenital or acquired hypofibrinogenaemia complicated by bleeding, although, owing to the risk of transmission of hepatitis associated with earlier preparations, cryoprecipitate is often preferred as a source of fibrinogen. A dose sufficient to increase the fibrinogen level to 100 mg/dl (approximately 100 mg/kg body weight) is recommended in bleeding patients.

Recombinant VIIa

Patients with haemophilia A with high-titre factor VIII inhibitors who are bleeding or scheduled for invasive medical or surgical procedures are now generally treated with recombinant factor VIIa.

Factor XIII

Patients with congenital factor XIII deficiency and active bleeding may be treated with factor XIII concentrate or, alternatively, with fresh frozen plasma. The recommended initial dose of factor XIII to control bleeding complications in deficient patients is 10–20 units/kg body weight.

Antithrombin III (ATIII) concentrate

Antithrombin III (ATIII) concentrate may be indicated for patients with congenital ATIII deficiency with thrombosis or at high risk for thrombosis (e.g. when undergoing surgical procedures). Occasionally, concentrate may be used for patients with acquired ATIII deficiency with thrombotic disorders (e.g. patients with acute lymphoblastic leukaemia receiving asparaginase therapy or patients with the nephrotic syndrome).

Protein C

Protein C concentrate is derived from plasma pooled from donors. Protein C therapy has replaced plasma infusions in congenital homozygous protein C deficiency. Its use has also been described in severe coagulopathy with associated purpura fulminans complicating meningococcal septicaemia where the protein C level is 0.20 IU/ml or less.

Human albumin

Human albumin prepared from pooled plasma donations has been used as volume replacement in severe hypovolaemic shock and in severe hypoalbuminaemic states (such as liver failure) with oedema. The use of albumin in hypovolaemic shock is, however, extremely controversial. Preparations are depleted of red cell antibodies, so may be used regardless of donor and recipient ABO or Rhesus group. Albumin is used in preference to fresh frozen plasma as a replacement fluid for plasma exchange procedures (except in TTP/HUS, where plasma should be used). Adverse effects include circulatory overload, allergic reactions and the risk, albeit very low, of transmission of viral infection.

Intravenous immunoglobulin

Preparations of pooled human immunoglobulin may be indicated as replacement therapy in hypogammaglobulinaemia (congenital or acquired), for therapy of autoimmune thrombocytopenia (ITP), neonatal alloimmune thrombocytopenia, neonatal thrombocytopenia secondary to maternal ITP, and autoimmune haemolytic anaemia, and for prophylaxis and therapy of CMV infection in bone marrow and solid organ transplant recipients. Preparations available are derived from large numbers of donors and are usually heat-treated for viral inactivation. The half-life of transfused immunoglobulin is 21–25 days. The most commonly used doses for ITP treatment are 1 g/kg/day for 2 days or 0.5 g/kg/day for 5 days. In replacement therapy for hypogammaglobulinaemia, an appropriate regimen is 0.2 g/kg every 4 weeks. Intravenous immunoglobulin may also be indicated in parvovirus-induced bone marrow aplasia in patients with chronic haemolytic states (due to the high titre of parvovirus neutralizing antibody). Side-effects include febrile reactions, transient rashes and headache. Transmission of viral infections, including hepatitis B and C, has been documented.

Other immunoglobulin preparations prepared from pooled human plasma include CMV immunoglobulin, hepatitis B immunoglobulin, varicella zoster immunoglobulin, tetanus immunoglobulin, rubella immunoglobulin and rabies immunoglobulin, all of which are used in some clinical situations for the passive immunization of patients exposed to the respective illnesses. $Rh_0(D)$ immunoglobulin is an important agent for the prevention of haemolytic disease of the newborn (HDN) due to feto-maternal Rhesus incompatibility.

PROCEDURES IN BLOOD TRANSFUSION

Exchange transfusion

The two major indications for exchange transfusion in clinical practice are for sickle cell anaemia patients where simple transfusion is unlikely to decrease the haemoglobin S concentration to the desired level, and for haemolytic disease of the newborn. Special considerations in neonatal exchange transfusion are considered elsewhere in this chapter. In older children, exchange may be carried out manually as in the 'push-pull' technique used in neonates or by cell separators. Central venous access with a suitable catheter may be required.

Plasma exchange

Plasma exchange may be considered for patients with TTP or HUS, immune thrombocytopenia, haemophilia A complicated by factor VIII inhibitors, or rapidly progressive glomerulonephritis, and for selected patients with severe coagulopathy. Plasma should be replaced using albumin, except in TTP/HUS, where plasma replacement is essential.

Leukapheresis

In patients presenting with acute leukaemia with markedly elevated white cell counts causing central nervous system (CNS) or cardiovascular compromise, emergency leukapheresis may be instituted to temporarily remove white cells from the circulation while commencing more definitive chemotherapy. Very rarely, platelet apheresis may be indicated for patients with severe thrombocytosis.

NEONATAL BLOOD TRANSFUSION: SPECIAL CONSIDERATIONS

The haemoglobin and haematocrit generally decline in the first 3 months after birth. This decline is exaggerated and anaemia is extremely common in low-birth-weight and premature infants. This is contributed to by blood sampling for laboratory testing and by intercurrent illness, especially in the neonatal intensive care setting.

During the first few weeks of life, symptomatic babies with a haemoglobin of 8–10 g/dl or haematocrit of 23–25% may require red cell transfusion. Symptoms of anaemia may include tachypnoea, tachycardia and poor feeding, but these should be correlated with the laboratory findings when deciding if transfusion is required. Acute or chronic blood loss may also require red cell transfusion. An initial dose of 15 ml/kg at a rate of 2–5 ml/kg/h is usual. All infants should be monitored for fluid overload, and diuretics should be used as appropriate. A rate of 2 ml/kg/h should be used if the patient is at risk of congestive cardiac failure. Blood warming is indicated for exchange transfusions and for transfusions given at a rapid rate (>10 ml/kg/h). Erythropoietin may be considered in an effort to decrease transfusion requirements in premature neonates, although this is controversial.

Special blood packs derived from red cell concentrates are available for neonatal use. Alternatively, aliquots from the same unit separated into a number of bags or dispensed into a syringe immediately prior to transfusion may be used to decrease donor exposure. Units should be group O Rhesus-negative and from a donor with low anti-A and anti-B antibody titres. Generally, fresh blood (within 7 days of collection) is recommended for transfusion to neonates, as with increased storage, red cell units show increased potassium, lactate, plasma haemoglobin and decreased pH, 2,3-DPG and ATP levels. The immaturity of the neonatal immune system is associated with an increased risk of transfusion-associated GVHD and of CMV infection. Therefore, all cellular blood products (platelets and red cells) should be from CMV-seronegative donors and have been gamma-irradiated.

Compatibility and blood group testing in the neonate

Due to the immaturity of the neonatal immune system, the anti-red-cell antibodies present are those of the mother, and infants generally do not form allo-antibodies in the first few months of life. Care must be taken during typing, as neonatal red cells may show only weak expression of the ABO antigens. It is conventional to use group O Rhesus-negative donor cells with a low anti-A and anti-B titre, and, traditionally, maternal serum is used for the crossmatch until the age of 6 months. The maternal serum should be screened for antibodies. If the maternal antibody screen and the infant's direct antiglobulin test are negative, group O Rhesus-negative units can be given without further testing.

Neonatal thrombocytopenia

Thrombocytopenia develops in up to 20% of special care unit babies and is often multifactorial in origin (Table 5.4). Immunological causes include maternal autoimmune thrombocytopenia and neonatal alloimmune thrombocytopenia.

The treatment of neonatal thrombocytopenia involves recognition and correction of the underlying cause. In general, prophylactic transfusion should be given at platelet counts of less than $30 \times 10^9/l$ in term babies, but in low-birth-weight or preterm infants, prophylactic transfusion may be appropriate at counts of less than $50 \times 10^9/l$ to protect against the risk of intraventricular haemorrhage. The appropriate dose is one random–donor unit (containing 5×10^{10} platelets in 50 ml volume) per 10 kg body weight (or, as an approximation, 10 ml/kg). The platelets should be fresh, and it may be necessary to reduce the unit for transfusion to a minimum volume of approximately 15 ml.

Neonatal alloimune thrombocytopenia (NAIT)

Neonatal alloimmune thrombocytopenia (NAIT) is due to maternal sensitization to platelet-specific antigens, either by transfusion or (more commonly) by transplacental haemorrhage of fetal platelets. The antiplatelet IgG that is formed crosses the placenta, causing thrombocytopenia in the fetus and neonate. The commonest antibody implicated is an anti-HPa-1a antibody (formerly known as PLA-1) formed in HPA-1a antigen-negative mothers with HPA-1a-positive infants. Ninety-eight percent of the adult population are HPA-1a antigen-positive and their infants are therefore not at risk. The incidence is 1 in 5000–10 000 births and the mortality is approximately 10%, primarily from CNS haemorrhage.

The differential diagnosis includes other causes of neonatal thrombocytopenia, including maternal ITP with transplacental passage of maternal antiplatelet antibody (Table 5.4). In NAIT, the mother has a normal platelet count and usually no history of ITP. The infant has a normal coagulation screen. The maternal serum contains anti-HPA-1a antibodies and maternal platelets are HPA-1a antigen-negative. Post partum, rapid serological diagnosis should be followed by treatment with antigen-negative platelets (e.g. washed maternal platelets re-suspended in compatible plasma). Alternatively, intravenous immunoglobulin may increase the platelet count, and exchange transfusion has also been used. In subsequent pregnancies, affected infants may be identified ante partum by PCR-amplified RFLP analysis (see Chapter 3) of material from chorionic villous biopsy, or alternatively fetal blood may be collected for platelet antigen typing and platelet count. If there is severe third-trimester thrombocytopenia, intrauterine transfusion or maternal therapy with intravenous immunoglobulin may be attempted. In the presence of known very low platelet counts in the fetus ($<50 \times 10^9/l$), some authorities recommend elective delivery by Caesarean section, although this remains controversial.

Table 5.4 Differential diagnosis of neonatal thrombocytopenia

Immune-mediated	Non-immune
Neonatal alloimmune thrombocytopenia (NAIT)	Sepsis
Secondary to maternal autoimmune thrombocytopenia	Congenital viral infection
	Disseminated intravascular coagulation
	Massive transfusion
	Congenital amegakaryocytic thrombocytopenia

Neonatal thrombocytopenia secondary to maternal autoimmune thrombocytopenia

This is commonly a concern in pregnancies where the mother has a history of ITP or has thrombocytopenia due to ITP during pregnancy. The outcome following birth is good and serious thrombocytopenia or intracranial haemorrhage are rare. Affected infants may be thrombocytopenic at birth, but the platelet count may not reach its nadir until a few days after birth, and platelet counts at 1, 3 and 5 days at least are indicated.

Maternal intravenous immunoglobulin and/or steroid therapy have not been proven to have any effect on the neonate's platelet count but may be helpful in raising the mother's platelet count prior to delivery. Vaginal delivery is advised if the maternal platelet count is greater than $50 \times 10^9/l$. If the neonate has or develops a count less than $50 \times 10^9/l$, the infant should be treated with intravenous immunoglobulin. In the presence of bleeding complications, although it may not produce an appropriate increment, platelet transfusion may provide some haemostatic benefit.

Coagulation factor replacement

The newborn has decreased contact activation and vitamin K-dependent factors (40–60%) compared with adult values. Factor VIII and von Willebrand's factor are usually in the normal adult range. There may be a moderate deficiency at birth of antithrombin III and protein C. Vitamin K is given routinely to neonates in many countries at a dose of 0.5–1 mg intramuscularly or 2 mg orally, and this practice should be strongly encouraged. In bleeding infants, fresh frozen plasma may be used while awaiting the response to vitamin K.

Neonatal thrombosis

Neonatal thrombosis due to congenital or acquired protein C deficiency, although rare, may be associated with multivessel thrombosis with multi-organ infarction, and may be treated with protein C concentrate infusion.

Similarly, antithrombin III concentrate is available for therapy of congenital antithrombin III deficiency complicated by thrombosis.

Haemolytic disease of the newborn (HDN)

Haemolytic disease of the newborn (HDN) is due to maternal allo-antibodies directed against fetal red cell antigens (commonly Rhesus antigens) causing haemolytic anaemia in the fetus or neonate. The formation of allo-antibodies is stimulated by transplacental leakage of fetal red blood cells or prior blood transfusion. Sensitization of a Rhesus-negative mother by a Rhesus-positive infant results in passage of antibody across the placenta. In milder forms, HDN may be detected by a positive direct antiglobulin test in the infant and allo-antibodies in the maternal serum. In severe cases, there may be intra-uterine death or anaemia and haemolysis at birth. Amniotic fluid analysis and fetal umbilical blood sampling may predict the severity of HDN in the infant and guide therapeutic decisions regarding intervention, including intrauterine transfusion. The incidence of Rhesus (D)-associated HDN has been very much reduced by the use of $Rh_0(D)$ immunoglobulin.

Exchange transfusion in the neonate

Indications for exchange transfusion in the neonate include hyperbilirubinaemia (including that due to HDN), sepsis, disseminated intravascular coagulation (DIC), removal of toxins, hyperammonaemia, polycythaemia, respiratory distress syndrome (to increase oxygen delivery by decreasing the level of haemoglobin F), anaemia, and NAIT. The objective in patients with HDN is correction of the anaemia and hyperbilirubinaemia and replacement of Rhesus-positive with Rhesus-negative red cells. Indications to proceed with exchange transfusion include a cord blood indirect bilirubin level of more than 4 mg/dl, an indirect bilirubin level of more than 20 mg/dl within 72 hours of birth, or a rapidly rising bilirubin. The procedure is generally carried out using the umbilical vein and, if it is feasible to canulate the artery, can be performed in a continuous manner, the artery being used for withdrawal and the vein for transfusion. Alternatively, using a three-way stop-cock and a 'push-pull' technique, the vein alone can be used. Generally, aliquots of 10–20 ml are withdrawn and replaced; care should be taken to ensure that the aliquot removed does not exceed 5–10% of the infant's total blood volume. One blood volume exchange may be expected to replace 65% of the original intravascular component (two blood volume exchanges will replace 85%).

Partial exchange transfusion may be used in situations where it is desirable to correct anaemia but necessary to avoid fluid overload. It is often also the course of action when correction of neonatal polycythaemia is necessary.

Problems encountered during exchange transfusion may include hypo- or hypervolaemia (including congestive cardiac failure), catheter site complications (including sepsis), hypothermia, initial hyperglycaemia with rebound hypoglycaemia, acidosis, hyperkalaemia, and acute transfusion reactions. Hypocalcaemia secondary to citrate toxicity is of particular importance in the neonate who has a decreased ability to metabolize calcium. Calcium levels should therefore be monitored and treatment given as appropriate with calcium gluconate. Blood should be warmed before use if the exchange is being carried out at a rate that is greater than 0.5 ml/kg/min.

ADVERSE EFFECTS OF TRANSFUSION

Acute transfusion reactions

Immediate adverse events to transfusion include acute haemolytic transfusion reactions, febrile transfusion reactions, urticarial reactions and, rarely, septic shock due to contamination of the blood component with endotoxin-producing organisms.

The most important causes of acute haemolytic transfusion reactions are transfusion of incorrect blood and transfusion of blood to a recipient with an undetected antibody. Less common are haemolytic reactions due to the presence of anti-red-cell antibodies in the donor plasma, bacterial contamination, excessive blood warming, or the addition of drugs or intravenous solutions to the transfusion. The most important cause of transfusion of incorrect blood is clerical or transcription error, and the commonest cause of fatal transfusion reactions is administration of ABO-incompatible red cells. The *Serious Hazards of Transfusion (SHOT)* report indicated that the incidence of transfusion of incorrect blood in the United Kingdom was approximately 1 in 30 000 transfusions. By chance, two-thirds of these will not be ABO-compatible and 1 in 10 ABO-incompatible transfusions will be fatal. Anti-A and anti-B antibodies are IgM antibodies that readily activate complement, and therefore haemolysis may be immediate and severe. Clinical features of acute haemolytic transfusion reactions include chills, fever, hypotension, dyspnoea, back pain and haemoglobinuria. Complications include coagulopathy and oliguria with acute renal failure. A suspected haemolytic transfusion reaction should be managed as an emergency, with discontinuation of the transfusion, appropriate hydration, attention to oxygenation and maintenance of an adequate urinary output. The transfusion pack and giving set should be returned to the laboratory for serological testing and investigation of the reaction.

More common are mild febrile transfusion reactions, complicating 0.5–1% of red cell transfusions. These reactions are likely related to cytokines (e.g. tumour necrosis factor α, TNF-α) and leukocytes contained in stored blood products, and are characterized by chills, fever, headache and nausea, but no evidence of haemolysis. Leukocyte depletion of blood products may decrease the incidence of febrile transfusion reactions, and pre-storage leukodepletion has been shown to be effective. In addition, pre-medication with antipyretic agents and/or hydrocortisone may be used for patients with recurrent febrile transfusion reactions. Other acute reactions include urticarial and hypotensive reactions, including anaphylaxis.

Other acute complications of transfusion include fluid overload and acute pulmonary oedema, air embolism, citrate toxicity, and acid–base and electrolyte disturbances.

Special problems associated with massive transfusion include thrombocytopenia, coagulopathy, hypothermia, acidosis, hypocalcaemia and acute respiratory distress syndrome (probably due to microaggregates in stored blood).

Transfusion-related acute lung injury (TRALI)

Transfusion-related acute lung injury (TRALI) is a rare but serious complication of transfusion, characterized by dyspnoea, fever and the development of diffuse lung infiltrates, generally within 4 hours of transfusion. It is believed to be mediated by antileukocyte antibodies in the donor plasma (most of which are anti-HLA antibodies) interacting with recipient leukocytes, with resultant complement activation, release of cytokines and pulmonary endothelial injury.

Delayed haemolytic transfusion reactions (DHTR)

Delayed haemolytic transfusion reactions (DHTR) typically occur 7–10 days following transfusion and are usually due to a low-titre anti-red-cell antibody undetected by pre-transfusion testing. Transfusion is followed by an anamnestic antibody response with resultant haemolysis. The antibodies involved are commonly Rhesus (anti-E, anti-c), anti-Fy^a, anti-Jk^a or anti-K. Classically, there is delayed hyperbilirubinaemia with a falling haemoglobin, but clinical signs may be subtle, particularly in the postoperative phase. Appropriate investigations include a direct antiglobulin test and documentation of haemolysis, including indirect bilirubin and haptoglobin measurements. Often, a delayed haemolytic transfusion reaction is identified only following repeat blood testing for subsequent transfusion when an antibody is detected (the so-called 'delayed serological transfusion reaction').

Alloimmunization

Alloimmunization to red cell antigens with the formation of multiple red cell antibodies commonly occurs in multiply transfused patients, causing delay in identifying compatible blood for transfusion. Often the antibodies formed have Rhesus specificity. As the Kell antigen is particularly antigenic, patients for whom multiple transfusions are anticipated should receive Kell antigen-negative blood.

Reactions to platelets

Febrile non-haemolytic transfusion reactions are more common after platelet transfusion than after red cell transfusion, complicating between 5% and 30% of all platelet transfusions. They are believed to be primarily mediated by cytokines present in the donor plasma, which increase on storage of the product. Leukocyte depletion of platelet preparations reduces the incidence of febrile transfusion reactions, and pre-storage leukodepletion may be advantageous. Allergic reactions may also complicate transfusion of platelets. Hypotensive reactions secondary to activation of bradykinins by leukocyte-depletion filters have been described recently.

Transfusion-associated graft-versus-host disease (GVHD)

Graft-versus-host disease (GVHD) is a rare but frequently fatal complication of transfusion in patients who are immunosuppressed. For this reason, patients receiving myeloablative or immunosuppressive therapy or those with congenital immunodeficiency should receive gamma-irradiated blood products to prevent engraftment of contaminating lymphocytes and associated GVHD. The probability of developing GVHD is increased in premature and low-birth-weight infants, and blood products destined for such recipients should also be routinely gamma-irradiated.

Transfusion transmitted infection

Transmission of bacterial infection by transfusion is uncommon, but viral infection is the subject of much concern and has changed the face of transfusion practice in the last two decades. Viral infections that may be transmitted by transfusion include hepatitis A, B, C and G, HIV, HTLV (-I and -II), CMV,

Epstein–Barr virus (EBV) and parvovirus B19. Hepatitis A is rarely transmitted by transfusion, and the risks of hepatitis B and C have been decreased by mandatory testing of all donor blood. The current risk of contracting HIV infection from a blood transfusion is less than 1 in a million, that of contracting hepatitis C is 1 in 500 000 and hepatitis B is 1 in 100 000. Donor selection processes now include an extensive medical history to identify risk factors for infectivity with hepatitis and HIV. That transfusion-associated infection still (albeit rarely) occurs, despite extensive screening of donors and testing of donated blood, is due to false-negative test results, transcription errors in the testing laboratory, and the existence of a 'window period' shortly after infection where the donor is infective but has yet to form antibodies. Recently, parvovirus B19 infection has been shown to be transmissible by transfusion. CMV infection is particularly important in CMV-seronegative patients who are immunosuppressed (especially those who are undergoing bone marrow or peripheral blood stem cell transplantation), neonates in whom the immune system is not yet fully developed and recipients of solid organ transplants. HTLV-I causes adult T-cell leukaemia and can be transmitted by transfusion. HTLV-II infection, which could theoretically be transmitted by transfusion, causes HTLV-associated myelopathy, but no transfusion-associated case has been identified to date. There is no proven risk of transmission by blood transfusion of new variant Creutzfeldt–Jacob disease.

Bacterial infections of concern include contamination of blood products with staphylococci or *Pseudomonas* species. *Yersinia* can survive in refrigerated anticoagulated blood, and the production of endotoxin may cause severe illness in the recipient. Other infections that may be transmitted by transfusion include syphilis, trypanosomiasis (Chagas' disease), babesiosis and malaria.

Iron overload

The prevention of transfusion-related iron overload should be considered in children receiving multiple red cell transfusions, especially in those with thalassaemia or other haemoglobinopathies where it is anticipated that transfusion requirements will be lifelong and there is defective utilization of iron. Transfusional iron overload should also be considered in patients with bone marrow failure syndromes such as aplastic anaemia, Fanconi anaemia or myelodysplastic syndrome. Chelation therapy should be considered before the advent of iron overload and associated organ (heart, liver and pancreas) damage.

Iron chelation therapy is generally carried out using the parenteral iron chelator desferrioxamine, usually administered by subcutaneous pump for 18 hours daily. Side-effects include neuropathy, cataract formation and sensory hearing loss. It is anticipated that new orally active iron chelation agents such as L1 (hydroxypiridone) will become available in the near future.

ALTERNATIVE APPROACHES TO TRANSFUSION

In the late 1980s, the advent of growth factors, including granulocyte colony stimulating factor (G-CSF) and erythropoietin, dramatically altered transfusion practice, essentially eliminating the use of granulocyte transfusions and decreasing red cell requirements in some patients with chronic anaemia. In addition, the development of recombinant coagulation factor products has greatly influenced the management of patients with inherited bleeding disorders such as haemophilia. Erythropoietin therapy should be considered as an alternative to red cell transfusion in patients with chronic anaemia, especially in patients with chronic renal failure. In selected patients, appropriate therapy with erythropoietin can reduce or even abolish the need for regular blood transfusion and the dangers associated with lifelong transfusion. Most studies in adults report a significant improvement in energy levels, well-being and quality of life for treated patients, but few studies in children have been reported. Recombinant G-CSF and granulocyte–macrophage colony stimulating factor (GM-CSF) preparations are now widely used in neutropenic patients following high-dose chemotherapy or bone marrow or peripheral blood stem cell transplantation. Thrombopoietin and megakaryocyte growth and development factor are developmental agents not yet in routine clinical use. Although they may shorten the duration of thrombocytopenia in some patients following high-dose chemotherapy, current agents under study are unlikely to eliminate the need for platelet transfusions.

Possible future developments include the provision of haemoglobin and platelet substitutes, ex vivo expansion of haemopoietic progenitor cells, and gene therapy, perhaps eventually obviating the requirement for transfusion of donor blood products.

FURTHER READING

McClelland DBL. (1999) *Handbook of Transfusion Medicine.* London: HMSO Publications Centre.

Serious Hazards of Transfusion (SHOT) Annual Report 1996–1997. Manchester: SHOT Office, Manchester Blood Centre.

Voek D, Cann R, Finney RD et al. (1994) Guidelines for administration of blood products: transfusion of infants and neonates. British Committee for Standards in Haematology Blood Transfusion Task Force. *Transfusion Med* **4:** 63–9.

6 Anaemia

Irene Roberts and George Vassiliou

INTRODUCTION

Anaemia is normally defined as a haemoglobin (Hb) concentration below the lower limit of the 'normal range' for a population of age- and sex-matched individuals. This limit is conventionally set at two standard deviations below the population mean. Normal values of Hb (and mean cell volume, MCV) for age are shown in Table 6.1. From birth to 3 months of age, the mean Hb concentrations decrease progressively to reach a nadir at 3 months of about 11.5 g/dl. There follows a modest rise to about 12.0 g/dl by the age of 6 months, after which the Hb remains stable up to the age of 6 years. From 6 to 12 years, the mean Hb rises to 13.5 g/dl.

Anaemia is the commonest haematological abnormality presenting to paediatricians and haematologists. The most important causes are hereditary and nutritional, although immune haemolysis must always be considered, especially in the newborn, and in individual patients the cause is often multifactorial. Advances in molecular biology have greatly increased our understanding of the pathophysiology of most types of anaemia, from haemoglobinopathies to membrane abnormalities and bone marrow failure syndromes. This great expansion in knowledge, however, has not as yet led to significant progress in therapy.

In the management of many severe anaemias, the consequences of the disease are exchanged for the problems and complications of long-term blood transfusions. Specific treatment is only available for a minority of anaemias, and even then it is only curative in the nutritional ones. The worst forms of anaemia can be cured by allogeneic bone

Age	Hb (g/dl)		MCV (fl)	
	Mean	±2 SD	Mean	±2 SD
Birth	16.5	13.5–19.5	108	98–118
1 week	17.5	13.5–20.5	107	88–127
1 month	14	10.0–18.0	104	85–123
2 months	11.5	9.0–14.0	96	77–115
3–6 months	11.5	9.5–13.5	91	74–108
6–24 months	12.0	10.5–13.5	78	70–86
2–6 years	12.5	11.5–13.5	81	75–87
6–12 years	13.5	11.5–15.5	86	77–95
12–18 years: F	14.0	12.0–16.0	90	78–103
M	14.5	13.0–16.0	88	78–98

Table 6.1 Normal range for haemoglobin (Hb) and mean cell volume (MCV) by age[a]

[a] Modified from *Blood Reviews* (1998) **12**: 106–14.

marrow transplantation (BMT), but this procedure has a significant mortality and complication rate, making it a realistic option only in the most debilitating of cases.

As mentioned above, anaemia is often multifactorial, and elucidating its causes is akin to detective work. A logical way of approaching this is to recognize that anaemia must arise as a result either of reduced red cell production, of increased red cell destruction, of blood loss, or of a combination of these factors. This scheme is followed for all the anaemias discussed in this chapter and is summarized in Table 6.2 (for neonatal anaemias) and Table 6.3 (for anaemias in older infants and children).

Anaemia in the neonatal period has distinct physiological features and a distinct patho-genesis. Interpretation of results has to be made on a background of ontogeny-related changes in the red cell membrane, red cell enzymes and Hb production, which vary according to the gestational age as well as the postnatal age of the baby. In addition, haematological abnormalities in the baby are often attributable to pregnancy-related or pre-existing disorders in the mother; diseases such as haemolytic disease of the newborn, for example, are unique to the neonate. For all of these reasons, features specific to neonatal anaemia are considered separately at the beginning of each section in this chapter.

The greatest change to the spectrum of causes of neonatal anaemia over the last 50 years has been the increasing numbers of surviving pre-term infants. Most neonatal inten-

---

Table 6.2 Causes of neonatal anaemia

A. Impaired red cell production
- Congenital infection, e.g. cytomegalovirus (CMV), rubella
- Diamond–Blackfan anaemia: 25% may be anaemic at birth
- Pearson's syndrome
- Congenital dyserythropoietic anaemia
- Transient erythroblastopenia of childhood (rare in neonates)
- Congenital leukaemia

B. Increased red cell destruction (haemolysis)
- Alloimmune; haemolytic disease of the newborn (Rh, ABO, Kell, other)
- Autoimmune, e.g. maternal autoimmune haemolysis, drug-induced
- Infection, e.g. bacterial, syphilis, malaria, CMV, toxoplasma, herpes simplex
- Red cell membrane disorders, e.g. hereditary spherocytosis
- Infantile pyknocytosis
- Red cell enzyme deficiencies, e.g. pyruvate kinase deficiency
- Some haemoglobinopathies, e.g. α-thalassaemia major, HbH disease
- Macro/microangiopathy, e.g. cavernous haemangioma, disseminated intravascular coagulation (DIC)
- Galactosaemia

C. Blood loss
- Occult haemorrhage before birth, e.g. twin-to-twin, feto-maternal
- Internal haemorrhage, e.g. intracranial, cephalhaematoma
- Iatrogenic: due to frequent blood sampling

D. Anaemia of prematurity
- Impaired red cell production plus reduced red cell lifespan

---

Table 6.3 Causes of anaemia in infants and children

A. Impaired red cell production
- Nutritional deficiencies
  - Iron
  - Folate/vitamin B_{12}
- Bone marrow failure syndromes
  - Aplastic anaemias: acquired
    - inherited/congenital, e.g. Fanconi anaemia
  - Pure red cell aplasias: acquired, e.g. transient erythroblastopenia of childhood (TEC)
    - inherited/congenital, e.g. Diamond–Blackfan anaemia
  - Dyshaemopoietic anaemias: acquired
    - inherited/congenital, e.g. Pearson's syndrome, congenital dyserythropoietic anaemias (CDA)
- Bone marrow infiltration, e.g. leukaemia, metastatic tumours, osteopetrosis

B. Increased red cell destruction (haemolysis)
- Red cell membrane disorders, e.g. hereditary spherocytosis
- Red cell enzyme deficiencies, e.g. pyruvate kinase deficiency
- Haemoglobinopathies, e.g. β-thalassaemia major, HbH disease
- Immune
- Miscellaneous, e.g. infections, paroxysmal nocturnal haemoglobinuria (PNH)

C. Blood loss
- Gastrointestinal, e.g. Meckel's, oesophagitis, gastritis, inflammatory bowel disease
- Infections, e.g. hookworm, *Helicobacter*, schistosomiasis
- Menstruation

---

sive care units now care for newborns of gestational ages as low as 23 weeks. All such infants need prolonged inpatient treatment, anaemia is universal and severe, and multiple blood transfusions are always required. At the same time, the numbers of cases of haemolytic disease of the newborn have fallen dramatically since the introduction of prophylactic anti-D in 1969. Blood transfusion remains the only treatment for nearly all cases of neonatal anaemia, since erythropoietin has been shown to be of limited practical value in this setting and its use is confined to prevention or amelioration of the late anaemia of prematurity. There have, however, been many changes to transfusion practice in neonates over the last 10 years as efforts have focused on safer transfusion, particularly via strategies to reduce the numbers of donors to which each baby is exposed.

Worldwide, the prevalence and causes of anaemia in older infants and children have changed little over the last 50 years. However, in many countries, changes in the size of different ethnic groups have led to increases in inherited causes of anaemia in parts of the world where they were previously rare. In the UK, for example, estimates of the numbers of children with sickle cell anaemia have more than doubled over the last 10 years. In addition, life expectancy for sickle cell anaemia, and also for thalassaemias, has dramatically improved: childhood mortality from sickle cell disease has fallen from 15% 30 years ago to 3% since the introduction of prophylactic penicillin V; similarly, with the introduction of iron chelation therapy, the median life expectancy for β-thalassaemia major has increased from 20 years to over 40 years over the same time period. In addition, molecular characterization of the severe inherited disorders has made prenatal diagnosis possible for the majority of severe anaemias; in some countries, accurate available prenatal diagnosis has completely transformed the prevalence of the disease; for example, β-thalassaemia major, once common in Sicily and Cyprus, has almost been eliminated as a cause of childhood anaemia in these countries.

AETIOLOGY, INHERITANCE AND EPIDEMIOLOGY

Neonatal anaemia

The principal causes of anaemia in the term and preterm baby are shown in Table 6.2. In the vast majority of cases, anaemia is due to acquired disorders, for example blood loss, or to anaemia of prematurity; nevertheless, several inherited abnormalities do present in the newborn period.

Inherited disorders

Inherited disorders that can cause anaemia presenting in the neonatal period include:

- Diamond–Blackfan anaemia (DBA)
- Pearson's syndrome
- Congenital dyserythropoietic anaemia (CDA)
- Some red cell membrane disorders: mainly hereditary spherocytosis and hereditary pyropoikilocytosis
- Some red cell enzyme deficiencies: pyruvate kinase deficiency and rare severe forms of glucose-6-phosphate dehydrogenase (G6PD) deficiency
- Some haemoglobinopathies: HbH disease and α-thalassaemia major (*not* β-thalassaemia major).

Haemoglobinopathies that cause neonatal anaemia are (i) α-thalassaemia major (Hb Bart's hydrops fetalis) and (ii) HbH disease, which are due respectively to deletion of four

and three of the normal complement of four α-globin genes, and (iii) rare mutations of the γ-globin gene (e.g. Hb Poole) that cause the production of an unstable haemoglobin with resultant haemolytic anaemia. The aetiology and inheritance of the other disorders is discussed below.

Acquired disorders

Acquired disorders unique to the neonatal period that cause neonatal anaemia include the following.

Alloimmune haemolytic anaemia ('haemolytic disease of the newborn')

This is caused by transplacental passage of maternal allo-antibodies. The most common allo-antibodies causing severe haemolytic disease of the newborn are anti-D, anti-c and anti-Kell, which produce haemolysis in fetuses that carry the D, c and Kell antigens, respectively. These allo-antibodies are acquired either as a result of blood transfusion prior to or during pregnancy or as a result of allo-immunization during pregnancy. Allo-immunization due to anti-D affects around 1200 pregnancies per year and causes at least 50 deaths every year in the UK. The most common allo-antibodies associated with mild anaemia due to haemolytic disease of the newborn are anti-A and, less often, anti-B. Most group O women have naturally occurring IgM anti-A and anti-B antibodies that do not cross the placenta; haemolytic disease of the newborn only occurs in the 1% of women of blood group O who by chance have naturally occurring high-titre IgG anti-A/B antibodies that are able to cross the placenta. The vast majority of cases of haemolysis occur in group O women who are carrying a group A baby. While mild cases of haemolytic disease of the newborn due to anti-A occur in 1 in 150 births, severe cases are uncommon (1 in 3000 births).

Autoimmune haemolytic anaemia

This is uncommon and occurs where the mother has auto-immune haemolytic anaemia. Maternal auto-antibodies cross the placenta (analogous to neonatal thrombocy-topenia secondary to maternal idiopathic thrombocytopenic purpura, ITP).

Infantile pyknocytosis

This transient acquired disorder is a not uncommon cause of moderate anaemia in the first few weeks of life, usually in term infants. The cause is unknown but some cases appear to be due to selenium deficiency.

Neonatal anaemia due to blood loss

Anaemia due to blood loss is the commonest cause of neonatal anaemia in preterm infants. In most cases, this is iatrogenic and due to frequent blood sampling. In term infants, blood loss is also a not uncommon cause of anaemia and is often occult. This is the commonest cause of otherwise unexplained neonatal anaemia. Blood loss may occur: before or around delivery due to feto-maternal haemorrhage or to twin–twin transfusion; it may occur as a result of bleeding from a ruptured cord or abnormal placenta; or there may be bleeding into the baby itself (e.g. intracranial, intra-abdominal), particularly if delivery is traumatic.

Anaemia of prematurity

This anaemia is universal in preterm infants and is of multifactorial aetiology. The two most important factors in the pathogenesis are thought to be reduced red cell lifespan and inappropriately low erythropoietin production.

Anaemia in infants and children

The principal causes of anaemia in infants and children are shown in Table 6.3.

Anaemia due to impaired red cell production

Nutritional deficiencies

Nutritional deficiencies are the commonest anaemias in childhood, with iron deficiency being the most frequent. Megaloblastic anae-mia due to folate deficiency is seen most often in association with malabsorption, and vitamin B_{12} deficiency is rare in children.

Iron deficiency Absorbable iron (ferrous) is mostly derived from animal food. The unavailability of animal food and prevalence of hookworm infection make iron deficiency the commonest cause of anaemia worldwide, affecting half a billion people. In the UK, poor dietary intake is the most common cause of iron deficiency. Other causes of iron deficiency in childhood are summarized in Table 6.4. Toddlers and adolescents are the age groups most commonly affected; iron deficiency in infants <4 months of age is rare in term babies as iron stores at birth are around 80 mg/kg.

Megaloblastic anaemia: folate/vitamin B_{12} deficiency Megaloblastic anaemia results from impaired synthesis of nucleic acids usually secondary to abnormalities in the folate–vitamin B_{12} metabolic pathway. The resulting anaemia is macrocytic and associated with characteristic megaloblastic changes in bone marrow and peripheral blood cells. Inadequate dietary intake or absorption of folate (folic acid) or vitamin B_{12} (cobalamin) underlie most cases of anaemia at all ages. Increased requirement is also commonly seen in preterm babies and in children with chronic haemolytic anaemia (e.g. sickle cell anaemia). Causes of folate and vitamin B_{12} deficiency are summarized in Table 6.5.

Bone marrow failure syndromes

Anaemia due to bone marrow failure is detailed in Chapter 7, and only dyshae-mopoietic anaemias will be covered here.

Dyshaemopoietic anaemias are characterized by low blood counts in the presence of *hyper*cellular bone marrows, in contrast to aplastic anaemias, in which the low blood counts are the result of a *hypo*cellular bone marrow. In dyshaemopoietic syndromes, the cells within the hypercellular bone marrow are unable to proliferate and differentiate normally, which leads to increased cell death at all stages of haemopoietic cell differentiation

Table 6.4 Causes of iron deficiency by age group		
Group	**Inadequate iron absorption**	**Blood loss**
Infants (<12 months)	Increased demand: • rapid growth • prematurity Diet: • weaning diet • vegetarians	Uncommon
Toddlers/preschool children (1–4 years)	Increased demand: • rapid growth Diet: • excess cow's milk • tea drinking • low iron diets (rice/maize based) Malabsorption: • coeliac disease • Crohn's disease	Inflammatory bowel disease: • ulcerative colitis • Crohn's disease Infection: • hookworm • *Helicobacter*
Prepubertal school children (5–10 years)	Diet: • excess cow's milk • quirky diets Malabsorption: • coeliac disease • Crohn's disease	Meckel's Diverticulum Reflux oesophagitis: e.g. cerebral palsy Gastritis ± peptic ulcer Tropical infections: • schistosomiasis • hookworm
Adolescents	Increased demand: • growth (peak: girls 12 years; boys 14 years) Diet: • anorexia nervosa/slimming • vegetarian Malabsorption: • as for younger children	Menstruation: • plus causes listed for younger children

Table 6.5 Causes of megaloblastic anaemia		
Causes	**Folate**	**Vitamin B$_{12}$**
Inadequate intake	Malnutrition Special diets Goat's milk Breast feeding from folate- deficient mothers	Vegans Maternal deficiency
Malabsorption	Coeliac disease Tropical sprue Jejunal resection HIV infection Intestinal lymphoma	Lack of instrinsic factor (IF): • pernicious anaemia • gastrectomy • atrophic gastritis • IF mutations Small-bowel disease: • terminal ileal resection • stagnant loop • chronic tropical sprue • Crohn's disease[a] • Coeliac disease[a]
Increased requirement	Chronic haemolysis Prematurity Pregnancy Malaria Dialysis Rare: homocystinuria and Lesch–Nyhan syndrome	—

Drugs which inhibit or
compete for absorption
	Anticonvulsants
	   e.g. promidone
	Sulphonamides
	   e.g. sulphasalazine
	Co-trimoxazole
	Methotrexate
		Slow K[a]
		Metformin[a]
		Cholestyramine[a]
		Neomycin[a]

Rare disorders	Tetrahydrofolate reductase deficiency	Transcobalamin II deficiency

[a] May cause cobalamin deficiency but rarely megaloblastic anaemia.

and low blood counts as a result. Where the dyshaemopoiesis is confined to the erythroid series, there are two main disorders: congenital dyserythropoietic anaemias (CDA) and sideroblastic anaemias. Where the dyshaemopoiesis affects all the main blood cell lineages, the two main disorders are Pearson's syndrome and myelodysplasia.

Congenital dyserythropoietic anaemias (CDA)
This is a group of uncommon inherited disorders of erythropoiesis characterized by chronic anaemia, ineffective erythropoiesis and distinctive morphological appearances of the erythroid series in the bone marrow. At least six different types of CDA have been distinguished. Types I to IV are well charac-

terized. Genes for types I and III have been localized to chromosome 15q and for type II, the commonest CDA, to chromosome 20q; however, none of the genes responsible for CDA have yet been identified or cloned. Types I, II and IV are autosomal recessive; type III is autosomal dominant and the other types are heterogeneous.

Sideroblastic anaemias This is a group of mostly refractory anaemias characterized by the presence of excess iron and 'ring' sideroblasts in the bone marrow. (Ring sideroblasts are abnormal erythroblasts in which there is failure to incorporate iron into haem, hence the anaemia.) Sideroblastic anaemia is rare in children. It can be acquired but more often is inherited in children, usually in an X-linked pattern. Most X-linked cases are due to mutations of the *ALAS-2* gene (*a*minolaevulinic *a*cid *s*ynthase). The most important causes of acquired sideroblastic anaemia are lead poisoning and pyridoxine deficiency.

Pearson's syndrome This is covered in detail in Chapter 7.

Myelodysplasia In childhood, myelodysplasia may be inherited or acquired. Both forms are rare, with an estimated incidence of 0.5–4 per million children per year. In both acquired and familial cases, the haemopoietic stem cell is abnormal, and anaemia, thrombocytopenia and neutropenia result from abnormal differentiation. The genetic basis is heterogeneous; cytogenetic abnormalities of chromosomes 5, 7 and 8 are quite frequent, but the responsible genes on these chromosomes have neither been identified nor cloned.

Bone marrow infiltration

Infiltration of the bone marrow with malignant cells or connective tissue may cause anaemia, but rarely in isolation – there is nearly always accompanying thrombo-cytopenia and/or neutropenia. The commonest clinical situation in childhood is anaemia secondary to acute leukaemia. Other tumours that metastasize to the marrow are rhabdomyosarcoma, neuroblastoma and Ewing's sarcoma. The two important hereditary disorders are osteopetrosis and myelofibrosis.

Osteopetrosis (Albers–Schonberg disease) This rare disease may be autosomal recessive or autosomal dominant. The autosomal dominant form has no haematological manifestations. The autosomal recessive disease is caused by failure of bone resorption by abnormal osteoclasts, leading to a progressive reduction in the space for normal marrow haemopoiesis.

Myelofibrosis This disease is very rare in children. The marrow is replaced by abnormal fibrous tissue, leading to pancytopenia and a leukoerythroblastic blood film. Some cases are familial, others acquired. The genetic basis for myelofibrosis has not been identified.

Anaemia due to increased red cell destruction (haemolysis)

Most of the haemolytic disorders that cause clinical problems in childhood are inherited. These disorders can be classified in a number of ways. The simplest way of approaching the causes of increased red cell destruction is to consider firstly abnormalities intrinsic to the red cell that cause it to be prematurely destroyed (i.e. red cell membrane disorders, red cell enzymopathies and abnormal haemoglobins) and secondly extrinsic mediators of red cell destruction (i.e. immune mechanisms and physical fragmentation).

Red cell membrane disorders

The main membrane disorders that produce haemolysis severe enough to cause anaemia in the neonatal period are hereditary spherocytosis and hereditary pyropoikilocytosis.

Hereditary spherocytosis This is the commonest cause of haemolytic anaemia in Northern Europe, affecting 1 in 5000 people. It is usually autosomal dominant and is caused by specific mutations in the spectrin, ankyrin or Band 3 genes, which encode red cell membrane proteins essential for maintaining normal red cell integrity. While hereditary spherocytosis may present in the neonatal period, the milder forms do not present until later in childhood or even adulthood.

Hereditary pyropoikilocytosis (HPP) This un-common disease almost always presents in the neonatal period. HPP can be considered an autosomal recessive condition since it is nearly always due to inheritance of mutations in genes that encode red cell membrane pro-teins from *both* the mother and the father. Usually, the mother and father are completely well but have a minor abnormality on their blood film that hints at the diagnosis. The genes involved are spectrin, ankyrin and/or Band 4.1.

Hereditary elliptocytosis Straightforward her-editary elliptocytosis is autosomal dominant, and though elliptocytes are clearly visible on the blood film from birth onwards, anaemia is uncommon. Hereditary elliptocytosis is common, being similar in frequency to hered-itary spherocytosis. Most cases of hereditary elliptocytosis are due to specific mutations in the spectrin or ankyrin genes.

Red cell enzymopathies

The two commonest red cell enzymopathies that may cause anaemia are glucose-6-phos-phate dehydrogenase (G6PD) deficiency and pyruvate kinase (PK) deficiency.

G6PD deficiency It is important to note that although neonatal jaundice due to G6PD defi-ciency is common, severe neonatal anaemia is rare and largely confined to rare specific mutations of the *G6PD* gene (e.g. G6PD Nara) rather than the common type of G6PD defi-ciency (G6PD A−). The *G6PD* gene is on the X-chromosome and therefore G6PD defi-ciency is an X-linked condition. There are more than 300 different mutations of the *G6PD* gene with varying degrees of clinical severity. G6PD deficiency in childhood is typ-ically associated with two types of anaemia: the first type, chronic non-spherocytic haemolytic anaemia, is less common and is due to class 1 mutations of the *G6PD* gene; the much more common second type, acute haemolytic episodes on a background of a completely normal blood count, is precipit-ated by certain drugs/toxins (e.g. anti-malarials, fava beans) or by infection. G6PD deficiency is found all over the world but varies in prevalence from 20% in Central

Africa to 10% in parts of the Mediterranean and <0.5% in Northern Europe.

PK deficiency This is a much less common disease; however, it is the most common red cell enzymopathy that causes anaemia. The *PK* gene is on chromosome 1q. PK deficiency is autosomal recessive and more than 80 dif-ferent mutations of the *PK* gene have been described. The incidence of PK deficiency is around 1 in 1000 and, unlike G6PD defi-ciency, varies little worldwide.

Haemoglobinopathies

The three main types of haemoglobinopathy are α-thalassaemias, β-thalassaemias and sickling disorders. In general, abnormalities of the α-globin gene (α-thalassaemias) present in the fetal/neonatal period while abnormali-ties of the β-globin gene (β-thalassaemias and sickle cell disorders) present later in infancy or childhood.

α-thalassaemias The α-thalassaemias are most common in south east Asia, Africa, India and the Mediterranean. α-thalassaemia results from deletion of one or more of the four α-globin genes on chromosome 16. Dele-tion of one or two genes causes the α-thalas-saemia trait, which causes very mild or no anaemia; deletion of three α-globin genes causes HbH disease; and deletion of all four α-globin genes causes α-thalassaemia major (Hb Bart's hydrops fetalis). Where all four α-globin genes are deleted, it is not possible to synthesise any HbA (α2β2) or HbF (α2γ2), and therefore α-thalassaemia major is incom-patible with life except in rare circumstances where intra-uterine transfusion is started in the second trimester. The most severe forms of α-thalassaemia are usually seen in indi-viduals from the Far East, where the fre-quency of carriers with two-gene deletions is >5% and can be as high as 80%, and also in the Mediterranean, where the carrier fre-quency is 1–15%; several cases of α-thalas-saemia major are seen in the UK every year.

β-thalassaemias The β-thalassaemias are most common in the Indian subcontinent, Mediter-ranean, Middle East and to a lesser extent in Africa. β-thalassaemia major occurs when both of the two β-globin genes are abnormal; that is, the child inherits an abnormal β-globin gene from each parent. Usually, it is caused by point mutations rather than deletions in the β-globin gene on chromosome 11. Over 150 different mutations have been described. The effect of having two β-globin gene mutations is that the child is unable to make any HbA (α2β2); however, as they are able to make HbF (α2γ2), children with β-thalassaemia major remain well in utero and usually until 6–12 months of age, when the rate of HbF production drastically reduces just as it does in healthy children. In the UK, there are more than 300 children with β-thalassaemia major and around 30–40 new cases are diagnosed every year, mostly in families who originate from the Indian subcontinent.

Sickle cell syndromes The sickle cell syndromes are most commonly seen in children of African and Caribbean origin, although they are also seen in the Middle East, India and the Mediterranean. Sickle cell syndromes

are characterized by the inheritance of HbS, which is produced as a result of a point mutation in the β-globin gene (valine is replaced by glutamic acid at position 6). For this to cause disease, the HbS from the carrier parent has to be co-inherited with an abnormal β-globin gene from the other parent. The 3 most common types of sickle cell disease are summarized in Table 6.6; all are associated with chronic haemolytic anaemia. Where both abnormal β-globin genes produce HbS, the child has homozygous sickle cell disease, usually known as sickle cell anaemia. Where the child inherits HbS from one parent and HbC (a different β-globin mutation) from the other parent, the disease is called SC disease, which has many differences from homozygous sickle cell anaemia (see later). Where the child inherits HbS from one parent and a β-thalassaemia mutation from the other parent, the child suffers from the disease S-β-thalassaemia, which is also clinically distinct from homozygous sickle cell anaemia. In the UK, there are around 5000 children with sickle cell syndromes, with the numbers of

Table 6.6 Sickle cell syndromes		
Disease	**Abnormal globin gene**	**Haemoglobins present on electrophoresis**
Sickle cell anaemia	β-globin	HbS Small amounts of HbF No HbA
SC disease	β-globin	HbS 45–50% HbC 45–50% Small amounts of HbF No HbA
S-β-thalassaemia: two types of disease S-$β^0$-thalassaemia	β-globin	HbS 80% HbF 10–20% Raised HbA_2 (5%) No HbA
S-$β^+$-thalassaemia	β-globin	HbS 50–80% HbF 10–20% HbA 10–30% Raised HbA_2 (5%)

affected children born per year varying from <0.05 to >15 per 1000 live births in different parts of the country.

Immune and non-immune acquired haemolytic anaemias

The main cause of immune haemolytic anaemia in childhood is acquired auto-immune haemolytic anaemia (AIHA). This is relatively uncommon, with an incidence of 10 per million of the general population. AIHA is usually divided into 'warm' AIHA, in which the auto-antibodies are usually IgG and mediate red cell destruction only at around 37°C, and 'cold' AIHA, in which the antibodies are predominantly IgM and are able to mediate red cell destruction at lower temperatures. The distinction between 'warm' and 'cold' is clinically significant because it helps to identify the underlying cause of the AIHA and the management may be different.

Warm AIHA Most cases of warm AIHA in children are idiopathic and may be triggered by viral infections, including Epstein–Barr virus (EBV) and human immunodeficiency virus (HIV). Warm AIHA may also be secondary to other autoimmune diseases (e.g. systemic lupus erythematosus, SLE) or lymphomas, though this is usually only in older children. An important, and often severe, form of AIHA occurs in Evans' syndrome which is defined as acquired AIHA accompanied by immune thrombocytopenia.

Cold AIHA This is less common in children than warm AIHA. It may be idiopathic, secondary to infection (particularly EBV and *Mycoplasma pneumoniae*) or may present as paroxysmal cold haemoglobinuria, a self-limiting cold haemagglutinin disease seen mainly in children in the wake of viral infection.

Haemolytic anaemia may also occur in association with:

- infection – any severe infection (presumed 'immune' mechanism, but no auto-antibodies demonstrable);
- physical damage to red cells – for example, from heart valves or as part of microangio-

pathic haemolytic anaemia in disseminated intravascular coagulation (DIC) or Kasabach–Merritt syndrome;
- paroxysmal nocturnal haemoglobinuria (PNH), an acquired stem cell disorder, rare in children, due to acquired mutations in the *PIG-A* gene on the X-chromosome.

CLINICAL FEATURES

Presentation of neonatal anaemia

Anaemia in the neonate may present in the following ways:

- as an incidental finding on a blood count performed for other reasons (e.g. sepsis in a term baby or as a 'routine' in a preterm baby);
- with non-specific signs of pallor, tachypnoea and/or tachycardia;
- with failure to thrive;
- with evidence of bleeding;
- with jaundice if there is haemolysis;
- with physical anomalies suggestive of an inherited syndrome, e.g. abnormal thumbs in Fanconi anaemia and Diamond–Blackfan anaemia (see Chapter 7);
- with hydrops; the differential diagnosis of hydrops is shown in Table 6.7.

Table 6.7 Haematological causes of hydrops

A. Reduced red cell production
   Parvovirus
   Diamond–Blackfan anaemia
   Congenital dyserythropoietic
      anaemia
   Congenital leukaemia

B. Increased red cell destruction
   (haemolysis)
   Pyruvate kinase deficiency
   α-thalassaemia major
   Haemolytic disease of the newborn –
      Rhesus, Kell, ABO (rare)

C. Blood loss
   Twin–twin transfusion
   Feto-maternal haemorrhage

Anaemia due to blood loss   The presentation depends upon whether it is acute, in which case there are usually clinical signs of shock, or chronic, in which the presentation is more often with pallor or failure to thrive. Concealed blood loss may be difficult to identify since the most common cause is feto-maternal bleeding, which has no specific signs in the baby and requires a Kleihauer test on the mother's blood to make the diagnosis.

Clinical signs of internal blood loss in the baby depend upon its site:

- intracranial – may be asymptomatic, seizures, apnoeic spells or hypothermia;
- cephalhaematoma – usually extensive; often a history of Ventouse delivery;
- intra-abdominal – may be retroperitoneal or due to a ruptured liver or spleen, which give signs of abdominal swelling and/or shock.

Haemolytic anaemia   This almost always presents with jaundice. In haemolysis due to red cell membrane disorders, this is the only clinical sign in the first few days of life although splenomegaly may develop after a few weeks. Similarly, for the red cell enzymopathies, jaundice is the only clinical sign in the neonatal period. Jaundice due to G6PD deficiency is rarely associated with anaemia; indeed the jaundice is thought to be hepatic in origin rather than derived from red cell destruction. Most of the haemoglobinopathies, apart from α-thalassaemia major and HbH disease, do not cause neonatal jaundice. Infantile pyknocytosis typically presents with jaundice, mild hepatosplenomegaly and anaemia in a term baby within a few days or weeks of birth. The Hb level may fall as low as 4 g/dl and many neonates require one or two red cell transfusions before the condition resolves spontaneously around 4–6 weeks of age.

Immune haemolysis   This is easily diagnosed by the finding of a positive Coombs' test, and varies enormously in severity. In the worst cases of haemolytic disease of the newborn (usually due to anti-D, anti-c or anti-Kell), the baby is severely anaemic and hydropic at birth; there is also hepatosplenomegaly and, rarely, extramedullary haemopoiesis in the skin giving rise to large raised purplish papules (so-called

'blueberry muffin' baby). Purpura and petechiae due to thrombocytopenia with or without DIC may also be seen in severe cases. In milder cases, in those who have been treated with intra-uterine transfusions and in haemolytic disease of the newborn due to ABO incompatibility, jaundice rather than anaemia is usually the main clinical problem.

Anaemia of prematurity   This classically presents 4–8 weeks after birth; the Hb nadir may be as low as 6 g/dl, in comparison with term babies, who experience a physiological drop in Hb that is less marked (10–11 g/dl) and occurs a little later (8–12 weeks of age). Anaemia of prematurity is often asymptomatic but may cause poor weight gain, tachycardia and apnoeic attacks.

Presentation of anaemia in infants and children

Anaemia due to reduced red cell production

Nutritional deficiencies

Iron deficiency   The most commonly affected age groups are toddlers and adolescents. In toddlers, a good dietary history is important: there is often a history of drinking large amounts of cows milk. In adolescents, there is often a history of rapid growth together with a diet low in iron. Iron deficiency in younger school children is uncommon, and symptoms and signs of gastrointestinal causes of blood loss (Table 6.4) should be sought.

Deficiency of iron causes a number of other signs and symptoms apart from anaemia. These include:

- effects on epithelial function – koilonychia (spoon-shaped nails), angular stomatitis, painful glossitis, oesophageal web;
- effects on intellectual development: impaired cognitive function and slight reduction in predicted IQ correcting with iron supplementation have been widely, but not conclusively, reported;
- pica.

Folate and vitamin B_{12} deficiency   The commonest clinical presentations of folate and/or vitamin B_{12} deficiency apart from symptoms of anaemia are:

- gastrointestinal – failure to thrive, glossitis;
- neurological – paraesthesiae, subacute combined degeneration of the spinal cord;
- incidental finding of macrocytosis on a routine blood count.

There is also a well-recognized association between low maternal folate levels and fetal neural tube defects and between folate deficiency and raised homocysteine levels, which in turn have been shown to be associated with an increased risk of thrombosis in adults and children.

Bone marrow failure

The clinical features of bone marrow failure are detailed in Chapter 7, and only dyskeratosis congenita and dyshaemopoietic anaemias will be covered here.

Dyskeratosis congenita In this disorder, the diagnostic triad of skin pigmentation, nail dystrophy and leukoplakia is always present, although these features are rarely marked before the age of 7–8 years. Bone marrow failure in dyskeratosis congenita does not usually present until after the age of 10 years and its frequency increases with age so that >70% of young adults with the disease progress to severe pancytopenia if the other manifestations of the disease, such as pulmonary involvement, do not lead to premature death. Both Fanconi anaemia and dyskeratosis patients have an increased risk of malignancy, including acute leukaemia, which may present from adolescence onwards and increases with advancing age.

Dyshaemopoietic anaemias These disorders may present with gradual onset of anaemia and/or deficiencies in the other blood cell lineages. Children with myelodysplasia often have infections due to neutropenia and bleeding, purpura or bruising due to thrombocytopenia. Pearson's syndrome usually presents during the first 12 months of life with failure to thrive; these children have pancreatic insufficiency, anaemia and usually thrombocytopenia and neutropenia. In sideroblastic anaemia, anaemia is usually the only sign of

disease; since congenital sideroblastic anaemia is rare, acquired causes (particularly lead poisoning) should always be sought. Congenital dyserythropoietic anaemias vary in their presentation from mild anaemia discovered as an incidental finding to severe transfusion-dependent anaemia with splenomegaly; jaundice, pigment gallstones and iron overload due to increased iron absorption or transfusion are quite common; skeletal abnormalities similar to those in Fanconi anaemia are occasionally seen.

Bone marrow infiltration

In most cases, anaemia due to bone marrow infiltration is secondary to malignancy; the clinical features are those of the primary disease together with anaemia, thrombocytopenia and/or neutropenia due to reduced blood cell production. The main primary disorders causing bone marrow infiltration – myelofibrosis and osteopetrosis – present differently. The most common clinical features of myelofibrosis are splenomegaly with anaemia and a leukoerythroblastic blood film, but many patients are asymptomatic unless the pancytopenia is severe. Children with the autosomal recessive form of osteopetrosis present in infancy with hypocalcaemia, failure to thrive, anaemia, thrombocytopenia and a leukoerythroblastic blood film.

Anaemia due to increased red cell destruction

Red cell membrane disorders

Hereditary spherocytosis This disorder may present in the neonatal period with jaundice and spherocytes on the blood film; more often the diagnosis is made as a result of a family history or at the age of 6–8 years when children are noted to be pale, mildly jaundiced and not thriving. On examination; there is moderate anaemia and often mild splenomegaly; jaundice is usually mild but may be more apparent during upper respiratory tract infections. Chronic haemolysis leads to pigment gallstones in the majority of children, although these are usually asymptomatic. Mild forms of hereditary spherocytosis may be completely asymptomatic throughout life.

Hereditary elliptocytosis In its common autosomal dominant form, this condition is nearly always asymptomatic; anaemia is rare and jaundice unusual. If there is no anaemia due to hereditary elliptocytosis in the first few years of life, it will not develop later, and therefore these children do not need to be monitored.

Hereditary pyropoikilocytosis (HPP) In contrast to elliptocytosis, this presents with severe, transfusion-dependent microcytic anaemia and mild to moderate jaundice within the first few weeks of life. Most children also develop splenomegaly, and the transfusion dependence leads to iron overload, usually by the age of 2 years. Pigment gallstones also develop due to chronic haemolysis, although they may be prevented if the child undergoes splenectomy (see later).

Red blood cell enzymopathies

The commonest red cell enzymopathy, G6PD deficiency, can present in four main ways:

- positive family history
- neonatal jaundice
- acute haemolytic episodes, including favism
- chronic non-spherocytic haemolytic anaemia (uncommon).

The vast majority of children are completely well with no abnormal signs and symptoms. Acute haemolytic episodes are uncommon and present as sudden onset of marked jaundice, pallor, and haemoglobinuria (described as dark red/brown or 'Coca Cola') due to intravascular haemolysis. The anaemia in this situation is often severe (<3 g/dl), so affected children may be shocked on presentation. There is usually a history of viral illness, ingestion of broad beans (favism) or of certain drugs (Table 6.8) a few days or even hours beforehand. Nearly all affected children are boys; however, heterozygous females can sometimes develop haemolysis after exposure to the same triggers as affected boys. The much less common chronic non-spherocytic haemolytic anaemia occurs only in males; splenomegaly is

Table 6.8 Drugs and chemicals associated with haemolysis in patients who are G6PD-deficient

A. Antimalarials
   Primaquine
   Pamaquine
   (Quinine)[a]
   (Chloroquine)[a]

B. Antibiotics
   Nitrofurantoin
   Sulphones, e.g. dapsone
   Sulphonamides,[b]
      e.g. sulphamethoxazole
      (co-trimoxazole)
   Quinolones, e.g. nalidixic acid,
      ciprofloxacin
   (Chloramphenicol)[c]

C. Analgesics
   Aspirin (in high doses)
   Phenacetin

D. Chemicals
   Naphthalene (mothballs)
   Divicine (broad beans)
   Methylene blue

[a] Acceptable in acute malaria. [b] Some sulphonamides, e.g. sulfadiazene, do not cause haemolysis in most G6PD-deficient patients. [c] To be avoided in some types of G6PD deficiency (can be taken by patients with the common, Africa A− form of G6PD deficiency).

common but the anaemia varies in severity from transfusion dependence to mild anaemia. In contrast to G6PD deficiency, in PK deficiency chronic non-spherocytic haemolytic anaemia is common. The anaemia varies from severe (presenting with hydrops fetalis or neonatal anaemia) to mild chronic haemolysis. Pigment gallstones are common.

Haemoglobinopathies

α-thalassaemias The severity of α-thalassaemia depends on the number of deleted α-globin genes. Deficiency of all four α-globin genes causes α-thalassaemia major, which, unless treated in utero, is incompatible with life and presents as hydrops with intra-uterine or early neonatal death. There is massive hepatosplenomegaly, gross oedema and often pulmonary hypoplasia. Deletion of three genes causes HbH disease (so-named because of the precipitation of β-globin tetramers – HbH – within the red blood cells) in which the main clinical features are chronic, micro-cytic haemolytic anaemia (Hb usually 7–10 g/dl) with splenomegaly; most children are not transfusion-dependent. Deletion of one or two α-globin genes is asymptomatic and may be associated with mild anaemia in some cases; treatment is not required.

β-thalassaemia β-thalassaemia major usually presents in the first year of life with pallor and failure to thrive. After starting on regular red cell transfusions and iron chelation therapy, most patients are asymptomatic if fully compli-ant with treatment. For those with irregular compliance, complications due to iron overload usually become apparent during adolescence. These complications include cardiac failure, diabetes, liver disease (hepatitis, cirrhosis and, occasionally, hepatocellular carcinoma), poor growth, delayed sexual development hypothy-roidism and hypoparathyroidism. As patients approach their twenties, many are infertile and are already developing marked osteoporosis. Patients homozygous for milder β-thalas-saemia mutations have less severe disease, known as β-thalassaemia intermedia. Such patients have a lower transfusion requirement and may be transfusion-independent for many years; however, splenomegaly and iron over-load are frequently present even if the transfu-sion requirement is low. Children with β-thalassaemia trait are often mildly anaemic (9–11 g/dl) but treatment is neither necessary or available.

Sickle cell syndromes In many parts of the UK, these disorders are diagnosed as a result of neonatal screening programmes using Guthrie cards. Symptoms and/or signs of the disorders are unusual before 6 months of age because of persisting HbF. The most common clinical features in the first year of life are:

- dactylitis (swelling of the hands and/or feet or even a single digit due to sickling in the small bones);
- splenic sequestration (sudden onset of pallor, splenomegaly and often shock due

to sickling within the spleen; the Hb may drop below 3 g/dl within a few hours);
- infection (particularly septicaemia, pneu-monia or meningitis due to infection with capsulated organisms, such as *Pneumococ-cus*); in part, this increase in susceptibility is due to hyposplenism.

The most common clinical problems in pre-school and school children are:

- recurrent, painful bony crises (mainly in the limbs in younger children; also affect-ing the abdomen and lower back in older children);
- acute chest syndrome (sickling in the lungs can lead to severe hypoxia, sometimes accompanied by chest pain, and rapidly progressing bilateral pulmonary shadows on x-ray beginning in the lung bases; this is one of the commonest causes of death in all patients with sickle cell disorders);
- neurological complications (sickling in cerebral vessels may lead to infarction, haemorrhage, stroke, transient ischaemic attacks and fits; it is often occult and may present as learning difficulties);
- enuresis is common, affecting up to 50% of boys >8 years.

Sickle crises, whether in the bones or major organs such as the brain or lungs, may occur spontaneously or may be precipitated by certain well-recognized factors:

- cold
- dehydration
- fever/infection
- exercise
- hypoxia
- stress.

Infection is often the trigger; all patients with sickle cell disease are hyposplenic – probably as a result of splenic infarction due to sick-ling. The spleen tends to be enlarged in younger children with sickle cell disease and then, around the age of 3–4 years, the spleen becomes impalpable in almost all patients except those with S-β-thalassaemia.

By adolescence, many children with sickle cell disease have chronic organ damage in addition to the acute sickling episodes. The organs particularly affected by damage due to recurrent sickling are:

- lungs → chronic sickle lung disease
- kidneys → papillary necrosis and/or chronic renal failure
- brain → stroke, epilepsy, cognitive defects
- eyes → proliferative retinopathy
- heart → cardiomyopathy
- bones/joints → osteonecrosis
- liver/gallbladder → fibrosis/cirrhosis if iron-loaded; pigment gallstones
- priapism often starts in adolescence and if severe may lead to impotence.

All patients also suffer from chronic haemolytic anaemia and develop folate deficiency if prophylactic folic acid supplements are not given. The average Hb in homozygous sickle cell disease and S-β^0-thalassaemia is 6–8 g/dl, and in S-β^+-thalassaemia and SC disease it is generally higher at 9–12 g/dl. The severity and frequency of sickle cell crises and of organ damage also tend to be worse in patients with homozygous sickle cell disease and S-β^0-thalassaemia and rather less severe in S-β^+-thalassaemia and SC disease, but this varies from patient to patient. Patients with a genetically high HbF also tend to have milder disease. The overall mortality in children with sickle cell disease is around 3% in the first two decades of life and the median life expectancy is currently around 40 years for those with homozygous sickle cell disease; the overall life expectancy in milder disease, such as SC disease, is not reduced despite the crises and complications the patients endure. However, it is important to note that patients with SC disease have a particularly high risk (75%) of developing retinopathy and must undergo regular fundoscopy, since advanced retinopathy is a cause of blindness.

Immune and non-immune acquired haemolytic anaemias

Around 50% of children present with acute haemolysis, often several days after a viral infection. Such children are usually very pale with mild to moderate jaundice and may be febrile. In the remaining children, the haemolysis has a more gradual onset and is often secondary to chronic disorders, such as SLE. Children with Evans' syndrome usually present acutely and may be extremely unwell with pallor, shock, bleeding and sometimes infection as a result of severe anaemia, thrombocytopenia and, in 50% of cases, neutropenia.

Paroxysmal cold haemoglobinuria This disorder characteristically presents with acute abdominal pain, back pain, vomiting, diarrhoea and dark brown urine following exposure to cold. There is usually a history of preceding viral illness; symptoms and signs generally resolve spontaneously within a few weeks.

Paroxysmal nocturnal haemoglobinuria This condition may present in a number of ways, including with chronic intravascular haemolysis causing passage of dusky brown urine in the morning that clears during the day and sometimes associated abdominal/back pain; and/or with venous thrombosis, particularly of hepatic or portal veins; and/or with aplastic anaemia, which may develop at any time after onset of the disease.

Anaemia due to blood loss

Anaemia due to blood loss is relatively uncommon in childhood. It usually presents as occult gastrointestinal blood loss, which may be asymptomatic or associated with typical symptoms suggestive of peptic ulceration, oesophagitis or chronic inflammatory bowel disease. Many children present with iron deficiency, and blood loss should be considered in any child with iron deficiency despite a good dietary intake of iron (Table 6.4).

DIFFERENTIAL DIAGNOSIS

Neonatal anaemia

A suggested diagnostic algorithm for neonatal anaemia is shown in Fig. 6.1. The most useful parameters in identifying the likely diagnosis are:

- reticulocyte count
- mean cell volume (MCV)
- Coombs' test (direct antiglobulin test).

A low reticulocyte count is found in:

- anaemia of prematurity
- pure red cell aplasia – Diamond–Blackfan anaemia and transient erythroblastopenia of childhood

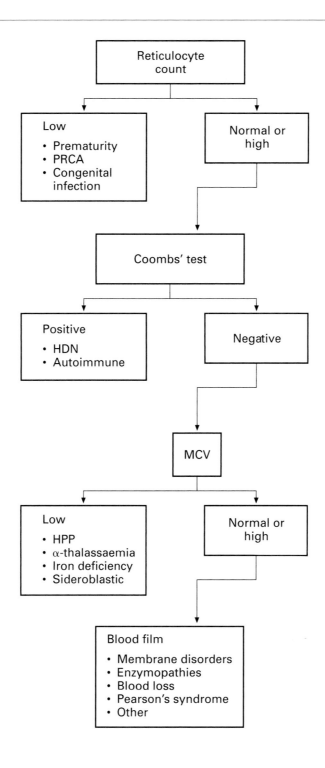

Figure 6.1

Suggested diagnostic algorithm for neonatal anaemia. PRCA, pure red cell aplasia; HDN, haemolytic disease of the newborn; MCV, mean cell volume; HPP, hereditary pyropoikilocytosis.

- congenital viral infection, e.g. CMV.

A raised reticulocyte count is found in:

- haemolytic disease of the newborn (allo-immune haemolysis)
- autoimmune haemolytic anaemia
- red cell membrane disorders
- PK deficiency (not usually in G6PD deficiency)
- α-thalassaemia major (*not* β-thalassaemia major or sickle cell syndromes)
- erythopoietin administration
- birth asphyxia
- placental insufficiency (intrauterine growth retardation, IUGR/maternal hypertension)
- acute blood loss.

A positive Coombs' test is usually seen in:

- haemolytic disease of the newborn
- autoimmune haemolytic anaemia.

The MCV is normal or raised in most cases of neonatal anaemia; a low MCV is therefore very useful diagnostically in the newborn. The MCV is low in:

- hereditary pyropoikilocytosis (HPP)
- sideroblastic anaemia
- α-thalassaemias – α-thalassaemia major, HbH disease, α-thalassaemia trait
- chronic intra-uterine blood loss (e.g. twin–twin transfusion)
- iron deficiency (rare except in babies given erythropoietin).

Further laboratory tests are usually necessary to establish an exact diagnosis. In anaemia due to reduced red cell production, the blood film is often helpful, but a bone marrow aspirate is required to make the diagnosis. (These disorders are discussed later.)

Haemolysis presenting as jaundice

Haemolysis in the neonate presenting as jaundice with or without anaemia is a more common diagnostic problem. The differential diagnosis of neonatal jaundice is shown in Table 6.9. Haemolytic disease of the newborn should be easily established by testing the

---

Table 6.9 Haematological causes of neonatal jaundice

A. Red cell membrane disorders
     Hereditary spherocytosis
     Hereditary pyropoikilocytosis
     Other: e.g. homozygous hereditary elliptocytosis

B. Red cell enzymopathies
     G6PD deficiency
     Pyruvate kinase deficiency
     Other: e.g. glucose phosphate isomerase deficiency

C. Haemoglobinopathies
     α-thalassaemias
     γ-thalassaemias
     Other: sickle cell syndromes (occasionally)

D. Immune
     Haemolytic disease of the newborn
     Maternal autoimmune haemolytic anaemia
     Drug-induced

E. Infection
     Bacterial
     Viral, e.g. CMV, rubella, herpes simplex
     Protozoal, e.g. toxoplasma, malaria, syphilis

blood group of the mother and baby together with the presence of maternal allo-antibodies and a positive Coombs' test. In haemolytic disease due to Rhesus antibodies, the number of circulating nucleated red cells is often very high (>100/100 white blood cells), leading to a spuriously elevated white cell count unless a manual differential count is carried out; the more severely affected babies also have thrombocytopenia. In haemolytic disease due to ABO incompatibility, the Hb is often normal and the nucleated red cell count is rarely elevated; however, there are very large numbers of spherocytes, in contrast to a relative paucity of spherocytes in Rhesus disease.

Haemolysis due to red cell membrane defects

This may be difficult to diagnose in the neonatal period. In hereditary spherocytosis, the blood film looks exactly the same as in ABO incompatibility. Other common causes of spherocytosis in the neonatal period include birth asphyxia, placental insufficiency and DIC. Therefore, to establish the diagnosis, further tests are required: osmotic fragility is increased, although the standard test of osmotic fragility may not be sensitive enough until around 6 months of age; examination of the parents' blood films is very useful since most cases are inherited, although de novo mutations do occur; gel electrophoresis of red cell membrane proteins may be necessary to confirm the diagnosis in difficult cases. Hereditary elliptocytosis is straightforward to diagnose just from the blood film. The film is usually suggestive too in HPP, as there are characteristic microspherocytes and extreme poikilocytosis with budding; in the latter, a useful test is to heat the sample, as red cell fragmentation occurs at 45–46°C whereas in normal cells it does not occur until the temperature is >48°C. Infantile pyknocytosis may resemble HPP, but the former condition is transient, the MCV is usually normal and the parents' blood films are normal, whereas in HPP at least one of the parents usually has elliptocytosis.

Diagnosis of haemoglobinopathies

This may also be difficult in the neonatal period because of the changes in globin chain synthesis that occur during fetal life and after birth. The investigations that help are (a) blood film and red cell indices and (b) Hb electrophoresis.

In α-thalassaemia major, the film shows huge numbers of nucleated red cells, hypochromia, microcytosis and target cells; Hb electrophoresis shows Hb Bart's and Hb Portland. In HbH disease, the film is also hypochromic/microcytic with target cells, but nucleated red cells are only slightly increased or normal and the anaemia is mild; Hb electrophoresis shows HbF, Hb Bart's, HbH and some HbA. In α-thalassaemia trait, the film shows only hypochromia/microcytosis without anaemia, and Hb electrophoresis shows mainly HbA and HbF plus a small amount of Hb Bart's. In β-thalassaemia major and trait, the blood film is normal at birth; Hb electrophoresis at birth in β-thalassaemia major shows only HbF (no HbA). In sickle cell syndromes, the film may show target cells but is often normal and the Hb is normal. Hb electrophoresis will always show HbF and (unless the baby is very preterm) HbS; in addition, babies with SC disease have HbC. Apart from those with S-β$^+$-thalassaemia, no babies with sickle cell syndromes have any HbA.

Red cell enzymopathies

These are usually straightforward to diagnose in the neonatal period. A G6PD assay should be performed in any cases of prolonged or severe jaundice unless there is an obvious alternative cause. PK deficiency is also diagnosed by assaying red cell enzyme levels; PK assays should be performed in cases of unexplained hydrops, those with haemolytic anaemia of unknown cause and where there is a family history.

Anaemia due to blood loss

This should be considered in any baby with unexplained anaemia at birth, particularly in otherwise well term babies and/or if the

Table 6.10 Microcytic hypochromic anaemia: diagnosis of iron deficiency and thalassaemia trait

	Iron deficiency	Thalassaemia trait	Chronic disease
Full blood count[a]			
MCV	Low	Low[b]	Normal/low
MCH	Low	Low	Low
MCHC	Low	Relatively preserved	Normal
Blood film	Targets +	Targets +	Normal
	Pencil cells +	Elliptocytes +	
	Anisocytosis ++	Basophilic stippling	
Serum iron studies			
Iron	Low	Normal[c]	Low
Transferrin[d]	High	Normal[c]	Low
Ferritin	Low	Normal[c]	Varies
Tf receptor[e]	High	High	Normal
Haemoglobinopathy screening			
Electrophoresis	Normal	No abnormal bands	Normal
HbA$_2$%	Normal	Raised in β-thalassaemia trait	Normal
		Normal in α-thalassaemi trait	

[a] MCV, mean cell volume; MCH, mean cell haemoglobin; MCHC, mean cell haemoglobin concentration;
[b] MCV often lower for the same Hb level in β-thalassaemia trait compared with iron deficiency;
[c] Infants and toddlers with thalassaemia trait often have concomitant iron deficiency;
[d] Serum transferrin is roughly equivalent to TIBC (total iron binding capacity);
[e] Serum transferrin receptor: not currently available in all laboratories, but gradually being introduced into many as a routine test.

blood film is hypochromic/microcytic. A Kleihauer test on maternal blood showing large numbers of HbF-containing cells is often the only clue that blood loss into the mother has occurred. Anaemia due to prematurity is usually a diagnosis of exclusion: the anaemia is normochromic/normocytic and reaches its nadir at 4–8 weeks of age.

Anaemia in infants and children

Anaemia due to reduced red cell production

Microcytic/hypochromic anaemias

The principal haematological manifestation of iron deficiency is microcytic, hypochromic anaemic. The most common differential diagnoses of a low MCV/low mean cell haemo- globin (MCH) are thalassaemia trait and anaemia of chronic disease. These can usually be readily distinguished by measuring serum iron, transferrin and ferritin and by Hb electrophoresis (see Table 6.10). In addition, there are differences in red cell morphology on the blood film: in iron deficiency, 'pencil-shaped' red cells are common; in thalassaemia trait, elliptocytes are more prominent and there is basophilic stippling in the red cells, whereas all of these features are usually absent in anaemia of chronic disease. Rarer causes of microcytic, hypochromic anaemia in childhood are inherited or acquired (e.g. lead poisoning) sideroblastic anaemia and HPP. Sideroblastic anaemia can only be diagnosed by looking for the presence of 'ring' sideroblasts on a bone marrow aspirate; serum iron and transferrin are also raised, in contrast to iron deficiency.

Table 6.11 Tests for folate and vitamin B_{12} deficiency		
	Folate deficiency	**Vitamin B_{12} deficiency**
Serum folate	Usually low (may be normal if recent folate intake)	Normal
Serum $B_{12}{}^a$	Slightly reduced in one-third of cases but corrects spontaneously when folate deficiency is treated	Low
Red cell folate[b] (EDTA sample)	Low	Slightly reduced in one-third of cases but spontaneously corrects when B_{12} deficiency is treated

[a] Most useful test to diagnose vitamin B_{12} deficiency.
[b] Most useful test to diagnose folate deficiency.

Macrocytic anaemias

The principal haematological manifestation of folate and/or vitamin B_{12} deficiency is macrocytic anaemia. Other causes of macrocytosis with or without anaemia include aplastic anaemias, red cell aplasias, dyshaemopoietic anaemias, liver disease, hypothyroidism, drugs and pregnancy. The diagnosis of folate or vitamin B_{12} deficiency is usually straightforward as the respective levels of folate and vitamin B_{12} are reduced in red cells and serum (Table 6.11). However, there may be pitfalls; for example, the red cell folate is low in one-third of cases of vitamin B_{12} deficiency, but this is not due to true folate deficiency since it corrects spontaneously once the B_{12} deficiency has been treated with vitamin B_{12} alone (Table 6.11).

Pancytopenias

Differential diagnosis of pancytopenias is covered in Chapter 7.

Anaemia due to increased red cell destruction

Diagnosis of the red cell membrane disorders and red cell enzymopathies in neonates has been discussed above. However, in infants and children, the diagnostic approach to haemolytic anaemia is slightly different. In any child with anaemia, haemolysis should be considered.

Tests for haemolysis

The first step is to establish whether there is any evidence of haemolysis using simple tests:

- serum unconjugated bilirubin (raised in haemolysis)
- reticulocyte count (raised in haemolysis)
- serum haptoglobins (low in haemolysis)
- blood film (will show polychromasia in all cases and spherocytes or other abnormal red cell morphology, depending on the underlying cause of the haemolysis).

Immune haemolysis

The next step is to examine whether or not the haemolysis is immune by doing a Coombs' test. In immune haemolysis, the Coombs' test is positive and usually no other diagnostic tests are necessary other than to ascertain whether the red cell antibody is 'warm' (IgG) or 'cold' (IgM) and identify the underlying cause, which is usually an infection (as discussed above).

Non-immune haemolysis

If the Coombs' test is negative, the blood film is the best guide to the likelihood of there being a red cell membrane disorder, enzymopathy or haemoglobinopathy. The presence of characteristic elliptocytes in hereditary elliptocytosis does not need further investigation unless there is moderate or severe anaemia, suggesting an unusually severe mutation. By contrast, it is usual to confirm the diagnosis of hereditary spherocytosis by showing that the osmotic fragility is increased. The diagnosis may be difficult in occasional cases in which the osmotic fragility is within normal limits, although nearly all cases show abnormal fragility after 24 hours' incubation, which is routinely carried out in most laboratories. In difficult cases of hereditary spherocytosis and for the diagnosis of other suspected membrane disorders, it is useful to send red cell samples from family members to specialized centres for electrophoresis and genetic analysis of red cell membrane proteins.

For the red cell enzymopathies, the diagnosis is usually suspected from the clinical history (G6PD deficiency) or the blood film (PK deficiency), and the appropriate enzyme assays are used to confirm the diagnosis. The autohaemolysis test may be useful to distinguish haemolysis due to red cell membrane disorders from a red cell enzyme deficiency; this identifies samples to be sent for tests of the rarer enzyme deficiencies in difficult cases. For the haemoglobinopathies, the diagnosis is often clear from the family history and blood film, and is usually confirmed by electrophoresis. The commonest differential diagnosis is that of a microcytic hypochromic anaemia (see Table 6.10). In difficult cases, and for prenatal diagnosis, molecular analysis of α- and/or β-globin genes is helpful and is necessary to confirm the presence of the α-thalassaemias.

Where haemolytic anaemia remains uncharacterized despite the above tests, a Ham's test should be performed to exclude paroxysmal nocturnal haemoglobinuria and a bone marrow aspirate examined to look for characteristic features of the dyserythropoietic anaemias.

Anaemia due to blood loss

The commonest causes of anaemia due to blood loss are gastrointestinal disorders, and referral to a paediatric gastroenterologist should be arranged. Other, generally rare, causes of anaemia that occasionally need to be considered are blood loss into the lung (pulmonary haemosiderosis), into the renal tract (haemosiderinuria, haemoglobinuria or haematuria), or from the female genital tract.

CLINICAL MANAGEMENT

Neonatal anaemia

Management of the inherited disorders is discussed later. For the acquired disorders, there are two principal approaches to management: treatment and prevention. In practice, the only treatment for severe or moderate neonatal anaemia is blood transfusion. The decision to transfuse is made on clinical grounds as well as the Hb, and established guidelines have been published by expert groups in many countries. Haemolytic disease of the newborn always resolves, although it may take up to 8 weeks to do so. In the first 1–2 weeks, haemolysis may be so severe that jaundice is the most prominent feature, so that exchange rather than top-up transfusion is required, together with phototherapy in order to prevent kernicterus. Blood transfusion may also be required for infantile pyknocytosis and for neonatal anaemia due to blood loss.

Anaemia of prematurity

The best approach is prevention. Blood transfusion is still often necessary in babies of <28 weeks' gestation or those requiring prolonged mechanical ventilation. However, the need for transfusion can be significantly reduced and sometimes abolished by:

- minimizing iatrogenic blood loss for laboratory tests
- prophylactic folic acid and iron to all preterm babies
- adherence to sensible, agreed transfusion guidelines

- judicious use of erythropoietin.

Doses for preterm babies:

- folic acid: 50 µg daily for the first 3 months of life
- iron: 5.5 mg (1 ml iron edetate) daily from 4 weeks to 12 months of age (may need to be increased, maximum 9 mg/kg/day, if on erythropoietin and blood film shows signs of iron deficiency)
- erythropoietin: 150–300 U/kg subcutaneously on alternate days from the first week of life for 6 weeks or until discharge from hospital.

Anaemia in infants and children

Anaemia due to reduced red cell production

Nutritional deficiencies

Iron deficiency The daily requirements for iron at different ages are shown in Table 6.12. Since the vast majority of children have iron deficiency due to their diet, the usual treatment is oral iron until the Hb returns to normal, followed by a further 3 months of oral iron to replenish iron stores. Dietary advice often prevents recurrence. Commonly used iron preparations in children are shown in Table 6.13.

Folate/vitamin B$_{12}$ deficiency Daily requirements for folate and vitamin B$_{12}$ are much lower (see Table 6.14) except in malabsorption or where there is increased demand as discussed above. For folate deficiency, treatment and prevention is with oral folic acid:

Table 6.12 Recommended dietary iron requirements for infants and children to prevent iron deficiency	
Age	**Amount of iron**
Term infant (<12 months)	1 mg/kg/day (maximum 15 mg/day)
Toddlers and prepubertal children (1–10 years)	10 mg daily
Adolescent boys (11–18 years)	12 mg daily
Adolescent girls (≥11 years)	15 mg daily

Table 6.13 Commonly used oral iron preparations				
Iron salt	**Preparation**	**Amount of iron**		**Daily dose to provide 3 mg/kg**
		per 100 mg[a]	**per ml[b]**	
Iron edetate	Elixir e.g. Sytron	14.5 mg	5.6 mg	0.5 ml/kg
Ferrous sulphate	Oral solution	20 mg	2.4 mg	1.25 ml/kg
Ferrous fumarate	Syrup	32.5 mg	9 mg	0.3 ml/kg
Ferrous gluconate	Tablets	11.7 mg (35 mg/300 mg tablet)	N/A	1 × 300 mg tablet/12 kg

[a] Amount of iron per 100 mg iron salt. [b] Amount of iron per ml of iron salt liquid.
N/A, not applicable

Table 6.14 Recommended dietary requirements of folate and vitamin B$_{12}$ for infants and children

Age	Folate (µg/kg/day)	Vitamin B$_{12}$ (cobalamin µg/day)
Infants (<12 months)	3.6	0.1
Toddlers, preschool and school children (age 1–16 years)	3.3	1.0
Adults	3.1	1.0

500 µg/kg (for children <12 months); 5 mg daily thereafter. Dietary vitamin B$_{12}$ deficiency in children is treated with oral cyanocobalamin 30–50 µg twice daily, and vitamin B$_{12}$ malabsorption is treated as for adults with intramuscular hydroxocobalamin.

Bone marrow failure syndromes

Clinical management of bone marrow failure syndromes is detailed in Chapter 7, so only dyshaemopoietic anaemias are covered here. These syndromes are very heterogeneous and often difficult to treat. The CDAs and sideroblastic anaemias vary from mild anaemia requiring no treatment to severe transfusion-dependent anaemia with iron overload, which is treated as for β-thalassaemia (see below). Children with sideroblastic anaemia should be given a trial of pyridoxine (100–400 mg/day), to which up to 50% will respond. The more severe cases of CDA may respond to splenectomy. For those who remain transfusion-dependent, bone marrow transplantation (BMT) is an option. The outlook with Pearson's syndrome is much worse and haematological support is usually all that can be offered, and most children die in the first few years of life owing to the combination of metabolic/nutritional problems and bone marrow failure (BMT is not indicated). Clinical management of myelodysplasia depends upon its severity and character. Where the principal problem is anaemia, treatment is transfusion with desferrioxamine for iron overload. Where there is progression to pre-leukaemia/leukaemia, BMT is normally the treatment of choice.

Bone marrow infiltration

Management of marrow infiltration by leukaemia/lymphoma is covered in Chapters 11–14. For myelofibrosis, treatment depends on the severity of pancytopenia; for asymptomatic children with no evidence of progression, no treatment is necessary, whereas for those who develop problems with severe pancytopenia, BMT is the only curative option. BMT is also the treatment of choice for children with the severe, autosomal recessive form of osteopetrosis.

Anaemia due to increased red cell destruction

Red cell membrane disorders

All children with hereditary spherocytosis should be given oral folic acid to minimize the degree of anaemia. Most will thereby maintain a Hb of 8–10 g/dl during childhood and will thrive. Splenectomy always leads to normalization of the Hb. The indications for splenectomy remain quite controversial. Most clinicians agree that it should be deferred until at least the age of 6 years except in very severe cases, and most now suggest that splenectomy only be carried out because of worsening chronic anaemia with failure to thrive and/or pigment gallstones. Children with HPP are transfusion-dependent and develop iron overload, which should be treated with desferrioxamine as for β-thalassaemia major; such children also respond very well to splenectomy. In HPP and transfusion-dependent hereditary spherocytosis, it may be reasonable to carry out splenectomy earlier, for example at the age of 4 years (balancing the risks of iron overload and transfusion versus those of post-splenectomy sepsis and thrombosis).

Red cell enzymopathies

Children with PK deficiency and with the uncommon forms of G6PD deficiency that cause chronic haemolysis are managed like those with the red cell membrane disorders; more often, the G6PD deficiency is asymptomatic and no treatment is required unless there is an acute haemolytic crisis.

Haemoglobinopathies

α-thalassaemias Although it is usually incompatible with life, children with α-thalassaemia major diagnosed early in fetal life have survived as a result of receiving intra-uterine transfusions, and are then managed as for β-thalassaemia major. Mild HbH disease manifests as chronic haemolytic anaemia, for which patients should receive regular folic acid. In more severe cases, regular or intermittent blood transfusion may be required and splenectomy may have a role in reducing or abolishing the transfusion requirement. α-thalassaemia trait requires no treatment.

β-thalassaemias By definition all patients are transfusion-dependent. Red cell transfusions are usually given every 4 weeks, and their frequency should be adjusted to maintain a pre-transfusion Hb of 9–9.5 g/dl, a level that permits good growth without unacceptable iron overload. All patients do develop iron overload. Chelation with subcutaneous desferrioxamine should be started after 10–15 units of blood or when the ferritin exceeds 1000 ng/ml, provided the child is at least 2 years of age (toxicity may be a problem in children <2 years). The ferritin should be maintained at 800–1500 ng/ml, varying the dose of desferrioxamine accordingly; the usual starting dose is 25 mg/kg 6 days per week by subcutaneous infusion over 8–12 hours; the maximum dose is usually 50 mg/kg except where administered in specialized centres. BMT is curative and should be offered to all children with an HLA-identical sibling since long-term cure is 90% where BMT is carried out before there is major organ damage; the risks of BMT-related mortality (5–10%) need to be balanced against those of transfusion/iron overload. The major factor predicting outcome with medical (non-BMT) treatment is compliance with desferrioxamine: 90% of good compliers survive into their thirties, in comparison with 20% of poor compliers. Oral iron chelators remain under development; current preparations have some value but are inferior to desferrioxamine in their ability to prevent iron-related organ damage. β-thalassaemia trait requires no treatment.

Sickle cell syndromes The most important aspect of management is strict adherence to measures to prevent sickle cell disease-related problems.

1. Prophylactic penicillin V should be started as soon as the diagnosis is made:
   <12 months: 62.5 mg twice daily
   1–6 years: 125 mg twice daily
   >6 years: 250 mg twice daily.
2. Folic acid is required by all patients to prevent megaloblastic anaemia due to haemolysis:
   <12 months: 500 µg/kg once daily
   >12 months: 2.5–5 mg once daily.
3. Education of children and parents about minimizing the risks of crises by avoiding cold, dehydration, hypoxia, overexertion, etc., and recognition of the signs of splenic sequestration and prompt treatment of infection.

Treatment in sickle cell disease is required either for acute sickle cell crises or for chronic organ damage. Painful crises are managed with copious fluids (intravenous or oral), and effective analgesia (including non-steroidal anti-inflammatory drugs and morphine if necessary); antibiotics and oxygen are given if there is evidence of infection or hypoxia, respectively.

Transfusion The usual indications for top-up transfusion are splenic or hepatic sequestration or aplastic crisis due to parvovirus infection. The usual indications for exchange transfusion are acute chest syndrome, stroke or prior to major surgery. In view of the high risk of recurrence of stroke, children with this complication receive monthly exchange transfusions for a minimum of 3 years; otherwise there are no good indications for regular transfusions. In occasional children with recurrent severe painful crises and frequent hospital admissions, a short-term (6–12 months) transfusion regimen may be the only way of returning the child to a normal home and school life.

Alternative approaches for severe sickle cell disease are allogeneic BMT and hydroxyurea. Hydroxyurea raises the HbF in 80–90% of cases, and preliminary results in children indicate that it is safe and reduces the frequency of painful crisis (hydroxyurea is myelosuppressive; blood counts must be frequently monitored and its long-term safety is unknown). BMT from HLA-identical sibling donors has a long-term cure rate of 80–90% but a transplant-related mortality rate of up to 10%; BMT is the only cure and is a reasonable option for children with major complications of their disease (e.g. stroke), who otherwise have a poor prognosis.

Immune and non-immune haemolytic anaemias

Many patients with acquired immune haemolytic anaemia require no treatment. Where the haemolysis is severe, 'front-line' treatment for immune haemolysis, including Evans' syndrome, is usually prednisolone (2 mg/kg). Intravenous immunoglobulin may be a useful adjunct in children with a poor or partial response to steroids, but it is rarely effective alone. Transfusion should be avoided (cross-matching is simple so long as blood for transfusion is issued as 'least incompatible') whenever possible, but it may be required as an emergency measure prior to steroid response, when it should be given slowly (5 ml/kg over 3–4 hours). In frequently relapsing cases or children requiring maintenance with high doses of prednisolone ($\geq$1 mg/kg), splenectomy should be considered depending upon the age of the child. In the most resistant cases, particularly those with Evans' syndrome, immune suppression with cyclosporin A, azathiaprine or

cyclophosphamide has been used successfully but requires very careful monitoring.

Management of paroxysmal nocturnal haemoglobinuria (PNH) depends upon its severity. For those with mild to moderate disease, anaemia due to a combination of haemolysis and iron deficiency (secondary to haemoglobinuria and haemosiderinuria) is usually the main problem; both folate and iron supplements are usually required. For children with PNH who progress to aplastic anaemia, the treatment is the same as for acquired aplastic anaemia (see Chapter 7).

CONCLUSIONS AND SUMMARY

The cause of anaemia in the majority of newborns, infants or children is easy to identify from first principles as being secondary to reduced red cell production, increased red cell destruction or blood loss. In most cases, simple tests (the reticulocyte count, MCV, blood film and Coombs' test) allow the most likely diagnosis to be identified. Since many of the anaemias are inherited, the ethnic origin, family history and a careful clinical examination are all crucial aspects of the diagnostic process.

In the neonatal period, transfusion remains the principal form of treatment, and current attention is focused on making transfusion safer by limiting the number of donors to which the baby is exposed and establishing strict but workable transfusion guidelines. In older infants and children, iron deficiency remains the most common cause of anaemia. However, increasing numbers of children with α- or β-thalassaemias and sickle cell syndromes are now being seen. Curative treatment for these, and other severe red cell disorders, is now possible (allogeneic BMT) but is restricted to the 30% of children with suitable sibling donors. Increasing knowledge about the molecular basis of severe inherited red cell disorders offers the prospect of innovative curative approaches, such as gene therapy, for all such severely affected children. However, a greater impact on anaemia worldwide requires attention to more fundamental problems of poverty, nutrition, education and infection.

FURTHER READING

Castro O. (1999) Management of sickle cell disease: recent advances and controversies. *Br J Haematol* **107:** 2–11.

Doyle JJ. (1997) The role of erythropoietin in the anaemia of prematurity. *Semin Perinatol* **21:** 20–7.

Olivieri N. (1998) Thalassaemia: clinical management. *Baillière's Clin Haematol* **11:** 147–62.

Wharton BA. (1999) Iron deficiency in children: detection and prevention. *Br J Haematol* **106:** 270–80.

7 Bone marrow failure

Owen P Smith

INTRODUCTION

In 1888, Paul Ehrlich described the first case of acquired bone marrow failure (aplastic anaemia) in a young woman who died after developing severe anaemia, bleeding into her skin and retinae, and high fever. The syndromes of inherited bone marrow failure only began to be characterized some 40 years later. By 1966, a crude classification was proposed by O'Gorman Hughes, entitled 'The Constitutional Aplastic Anaemias'. These were simplistically divided up into three groups: type I was Fanconi anaemia, which is aplastic anaemia with physical abnormalities; type II was Estren–Dameshek, familial aplastic anaemia without physical abnormalities; and type III was amegakaryocytic thrombocytopenia. Type II was subsequently shown to be a variant of Fanconi anaemia. Whilst this was the first real attempt to group and differentiate these so-called constitutional aplastic anaemias, in truth this classification added very little in terms of understanding disease aetiology and treatment.

Bone marrow failure results in blood cytopenias when the bone marrow fails to produce the haemopoietic lineages, platelets, neutrophils and red cells in sufficient quantities. The mechanism responsible for this impaired production can be divided into two broad categories: (i) where the defect is intrinsic to the bone marrow stem cells and/or stroma – the so-called inherited bone marrow failure syndromes; (ii) those where marrow failure results from an external insult such as viruses, toxins, drugs or more commonly where the extrinsic event is unknown. Clinically, patients with bone marrow failure can be sub-grouped into those in whom marrow failure is due to pluripotent stem cell damage or a lack of these cells and those who have a single cytopenia in which presumably committed progenitor cell development is defective. Over the past two decades, our understanding of the aetiology of these conditions has increased significantly, but, perhaps more importantly, during this same time period newer treatment strategies have been developed that have resulted in improved survival for children with these conditions.

ACQUIRED APLASTIC ANAEMIA

Acquired aplastic anaemia is characterized by peripheral blood pancytopenia, reduced bone marrow cellularity, increased marrow fat and the absence of morphological features suggestive of other disorders such as malignancy myelodysplastic syndrome (MDS) or myeloproliferative disease. The severe form (SAA) (Table 7.1) has the worst overall prognosis, with approximately 10% of patients being alive one year from diagnosis if only supportive therapy is given. Very severe aplastic anaemia (vSAA), defined by a neutrophil count of $<0.2 \times 10^9$/l, has a particularly bad outlook, the majority of patients succumbing to infection/haemorrhage early in the course of their disease if curative treatment is not initiated within a short period of time from presentation.

Aetiology/epidemiology

The annual European and North American incidence of aplastic anaemia in childhood is approximately 2 per 1 000 000 children, with approximately three-quarters having severe disease at the time of presentation. Boys seem to be more affected than girls and in the Far

Table 7.1 Criteria for severe aplastic anaemia (SAA)
Bone marrow hypocellularity: • <25% of normal, or   • 25–50% of normal and <30% residual haemopoietic cells   And two of the following peripheral blood parameters: • Absolute neutrophil count[a] $<0.5 \times 10^9/l$ • Platelet count $<20 \times 10^9/l$ • Reticulocyte count <1% corrected for haematocrit
[a] If the patient fulfils the above criteria and has an absolute neutrophil count $<0.2 \times 10^9/l$, the aplastic anaemia is termed very severe (vSAA).

are due to chloramphenicol, phenylbutazone and gold. Benzene and related aromatic hydrocarbons such as trinitrotoluene (TNT) and insecticides have also been implicated. Aplastic anaemia developing on the background of hepatitis occurs in approximately 5–10% of the cases reported in Europe and North America and is more commonly seen in the Far East. Bone marrow failure usually develops several weeks to months after liver function abnormalities appear, and these have usually returned to normal by the time the peripheral blood counts drop. The vast majority of hepatitis-associated aplasias are negative for hepatitis A, B and C viruses. Parvovirus B19 has been shown to cause SAA in immuno-compromised haemophiliacs, and indeed human immunodeficiency virus (HIV) can also cause marrow hypocellularity with pancytopenia.

The precise pathogenetic mechanisms responsible for SAA have not been fully worked out. Recent clinical and in vitro cellular and molecular studies indicate that stem cell damage or deficiency may be responsible for a significant number of cases, but it remains to be elucidated how the stem cell becomes damaged or indeed depleted in numbers in the marrow. It may be that in the majority of cases of acquired aplasia, this mechanism is immune-mediated, as the vast majority of these patients respond to

East the incidence appears to be 5- to 10-fold higher than in Western countries, which probably reflects environmental and not genetic factors.

The aetiology of SAA is varied, with greater than two-thirds of cases being idiopathic. The other known causes of SAA are listed in Table 7.2. As can be seen, many drugs have been implicated; however, the best documented cases of drug-induced SAA

Table 7.2 Aetiology of acquired aplastic anaemia
Idiopathic   • Viruses: hepatitis, herpes (Epstein–Barr virus, cytomegalovirus), parvovirus B19   • Toxins: benzene, insecticides   • Drugs: antibiotics (especially chloramphenicol), non-steroidal anti-inflammatory drugs (especially phenylbutazone), gold, D-penicillamine, anticonvulsants, antimalarials, antithyroids, antidepressants, carbonic anhydrase inhibitors, oral hypoglycaemics   **Immune**   • Drugs   • Viruses   • Autoimmune disease   • Graft-versus-host disease   • Chemotherapy (busulphan)   • Radiation

immunosuppression. In patients with inherited bone marrow failure, the mechanism of stem cell damage will probably be different and involve pre-existing genetic damage.

Clinical features

The majority of children with aplastic anaemia present with symptoms and signs related to the cytopenias. The commonest presentation is where the child is feeling completely well when easy bruising and/or bleeding is noticed by the parents, and this is particularly true for the idiopathic form. The presence of enlarged liver, spleen and lymph nodes should trigger a search for another cause of the cytopenia(s).

Routine investigation of a child suspected of having bone marrow failure is shown in Table 7.3. A full blood count with mean cell volume (MCV) and reticulocyte count and a blood film examination is mandatory to exclude any evidence of dysplastic neutrophils and circulating blasts, and should be the first investigation. Bone marrow aspirate and trephine biopsy are essential to access cellularity and cellular detail and to exclude

the presence of dysplasia and any infiltrative process. On the same marrow sample, chromosomal analysis should be performed to exclude a clonal cytogenetic lesion. Culture of peripheral blood lymphocytes looking for spontaneous or diepoxybutane-stress chromosome breakages will exclude Fanconi anaemia, and a Ham's acidified serum test, and urinary haemosiderin will exclude paroxysmal nocturnal haemoglobinuria (PNH). Serum vitamin B_{12}, folate and auto-antibodies should also be assessed. Virological testing for hepatitis A, B and C, cytomegalovirus, Epstein–Barr virus and parvovirus B_{19} should also be part of routine testing in patients with evidence of marrow failure. Pancreatic function testing should be carried out in children presenting with short stature and a history suggestive of steatorrhoea, to screen for Shwachman–Diamond syndrome.

Differential diagnosis

The differential diagnosis of blood pancytopenias is legion. However, when it is associated with marrow hypocellularity (aplastic anaemia) the possible diagnoses usually

---

Table 7.3 Routine work-up of bone marrow failure[a]

FBC, film and reticulocyte count	
Marrow aspirate and biopsy	Cellularity, infiltration
Cytogenetics	Clonality (?MDS, ?leukaemia)
Clastogen stress assay	Exclude Fanconi anaemia
Hams (acidified serum) test and urinary haemosiderin	Exclude PNH
Haematinics	Exclude vitamin B_{12}, folate deficiency
Auto-antibodies (ANA, dsDNA)	Exclude SLE and other autoimmune disorders
Virology	Exclude hepatitis (A, B, C), EBV, CMV, parvovirus B19, HIV
Pancreatic function	Exclude SDS

[a] FBC, full blood count; MDS, myelodysplastic syndrome; PNH, paroxysmal nocturnal haemoglobinuria; ANA, antinuclear antibodies; dsDNA, double-stranded DNA; SLE, systemic lupus erythematosus; EBV, Epstein–Barr virus; CMV, cytomegalovirus; HIV, human immunodeficiency virus; SDS, Shwachman–Diamond syndrome.

include inherited causes such as Fanconi anaemia, Shwachman–Diamond syndrome, hypoplastic MDS, aplastic presentation of acute leukaemia (myeloid and lymphoid) and overwhelming sepsis.

Clinical management

Once a diagnosis of SAA is made, the treatment strategy will involve an initial supportive treatment protocol followed by a more definitive treatment plan in the form of allogeneic bone marrow transplantation (BMT) or immunosuppression.

Supportive therapy

Supportive treatment involves packed red cell transfusions to be given as per standard indications for red cell transfusion, that is the patient should be transfused when the haemoglobin level is causing symptomatic anaemia. Troublesome haemorrhage is usually only seen when the platelet count falls below $15 \times 10^9/l$ and therefore the transfusion trigger is usually around this level, but it should be remembered that platelet requirements will usually increase when the patient is infected and when the patient is also receiving red cell transfusions. As platelet transfusions are usually contaminated with white cells, which express class I and class II histocompatibility antigens, and as these provide a very potent stimulus in sensitizing the recipient, all platelet and indeed all blood products should be filtered. If the patient is CMV-negative, all red cell and platelet concentrates should also be CMV-negative. Whenever possible, apheresis platelet products (i.e. single donor) should be used, as this will significantly decrease allo-sensitization, and those patients who are sensitized should receive HLA-matched platelets. Infection and neutropenic fevers in patients with severe aplastic anaemia should be managed in an identical fashion to those in patients with acute leukaemia (see Chapter 4).

Bone marrow transplantation

Once the diagnosis of SAA is made, the child and immediate family members should be tissue-typed, as BMT is now considered the treatment of choice for these patients providing an HLA-identical related donor is available, as the overall survival rate exceeds 80%. It is now well established that a more favourable outcome is seen in those children who have had (i) few transfusions prior to BMT, (ii) a shorter interval from diagnosis to BMT, and (iii) no infection going into BMT. The two major complications seen in patients undergoing transplantation for SAA are graft failure rejection and graft-versus-host disease (GVHD). The main factors influencing engraftment/rejection are shown in Table 7.4. Preparative treatment with cyclophosphamide alone is not as effective as

Table 7.4 Predictors of engraftment/graft failure[a]	
Preparative regimen	CyP + ATG better than CyP alone
	CyP + ATG better than CyP alone
GVHD prophylaxis	CyA better than no CyA
Number of donor cells infused	$<2\text{--}3 \times 10^8/\text{kg}$ recipient body weight incurs a greater risk of graft failure
Alloimmunization	The greater the number of pre-BMT transfusions, the more likely is graft failure

[a] GVHD, graft-versus-host disease; CyA, cyclosporin A; CyP, cyclophosphamide; ATG, antithymocyte globulin; BMT, bone marrow transplantation.

when it is combined with further immuno-suppression with antithymocyte globulin (ATG) or radiation (total body, total lymphoid, or thoraco-abdominal); however, it should be remembered that the main drawback of radiation is the significant increase in GVHD, interstitial pneumonitis and late tumours, the latter being particularly relevant in children. The withdrawal of cyclosporin A too early in the post-BMT period has been associated with an increased risk of rejection – so much so that a number of BMT groups have advocated its use for one year post transplant. A further important predictor of graft rejection is the number of blood products transfused prior to the BMT, as more than 40 units of platelets correlates with a significantly increased risk of graft rejection. Thus, the decision to transplant should be made as quickly as possible after the diagnosis of SAA, as this will reduce the number of transfusions that the child will receive. The total donor bone marrow cell dose is also predictive, as <2–3 × 10^8 mononuclear cells per kilogram recipient body weight has been associated with an increased probability of graft rejection.

GVHD continues to leave significant problems for children undergoing a matched sibling transplant, with approximately 10% and 30% developing acute and chronic forms respectively despite GVHD prophylaxis with cyclosporin A and methotrexate. The most important risk factor for GVHD in HLA-matched sibling BMT is the recipient age; that is, the lower the age the less likely the development of GVHD. Clearly, the risk of GVHD is increased with marrow from an allo-immunized donor, in particular when the donor is female and has been pregnant in the past.

Immunosuppressive therapy

BMT from an HLA-matched sibling is only available to approximately one-third of patients with SAA. Recent trials using immunosuppressive therapy (IST) with anti-lymphocyte globulin (ALG) and cyclosporin A have produced very encouraging results, almost equivalent to those undergoing matched sibling BMT. However, several important disadvantages of IST remain; for example, the haematological response tends to be slow, taking 1–4 months of treatment before counts improve. Recovery is less complete than with BMT, relapse is not uncommon, and there would appear to be a significant risk of developing second tumours and clonal haematological disorders such as myelodysplasia, acute leukaemia and PNH – at least in adults with SAA who have undergone IST.

Those patients who do not have an HLA-matched sibling and who fail IST are candidates for a transplant from a related HLA single-antigen-mismatch donor or from an unrelated phenotypically matched donor using cyclophospha- mide and radiation as a conditioning regimen, as the risk of graft rejection in this group is much higher.

INHERITED BONE MARROW FAILURE (Table 7.5)

The inherited bone marrow failure syndromes account for approximately one-third of all cases of childhood aplastic anaemia. Whilst these syndromes almost always present in childhood with symptoms related to the predominant cytopenia, some patients may present as late as the fifth decade of life. Physical abnormalities may or may not be obvious at presentation, and in the majority of cases a single cytopenia is usually the most common haematological feature, which in time may evolve into hypoplastic anaemia or bone marrow aplasia. The syndromes that continue predominantly as single cytopenias include Kostmann's disease (neutropenia), Diamond–Blackfan anaemia (anaemia), and thrombocytopenia with absent radii (thrombocytopenia), whilst patients with Fanconi anaemia, dyskeratosis congenita, Shwachman–Diamond syndrome or amega-karyocytic thrombocytopenia usually go on to develop bone marrow aplasia. Common to all of these syndromes is a predisposition to malignant change, particularly leukaemia, and epithelial tumours are not uncommon in Fanconi anaemia and dyskeratosis congenita, especially in the older patient. In the recent past, the inheritance patterns of these

Table 7.5 Inherited bone marrow failure syndromes			
Syndrome	Inheritence[a]	Malignancy	Year described
Pancytopenias			
Fanconi anaemia	AR	Leukaemia and cancer	1927
Shwachman–Diamond syndrome	AR	Leukaemia	1964
Dyskeratosis congenita	XLR, AR, AD	Leukaemia and cancer	1910
Amegakaryocytic thrombocytopenia	AR, XLR	Leukaemia	1974
Cytopenias			
Diamond–Blackfan anaemia	AR, AD, sporadic	Leukaemia	1938
Kostmann's disease	AR	Leukaemia	1956
Thrombocytopenia with absent radii	AR	Leukaemia	1969

[a] AR, autosomal recessive; AD, autosomal dominant; XLR, X-linked recessive.

syndromes have begun to be delineated and we now know that all types of inheritance have been documented in these syndromes. Indeed, both X-linked and autosomal inheritance may be seen in dyskeratosis congenita, with two-thirds of patients having X-linked recessive inheritance, whilst 10% of patients with Diamond–Blackfan anaemia demonstrate autosomal dominant inheritance.

Fanconi anaemia (FA)

Guido Fanconi first described this syndrome in 1927 in a family in which three male children between the ages of 5 and 7 years had pancytopenia and birth defects. The observations he made in this family and in future families led him to assign chief criteria for making the diagnosis of Fanconi anaemia (FA), which included pancytopenia, hyperpigmentation, skeletal malformations, small stature, urogenital abnormalities and familial occurrence – all phenotypic correlations that we still use today. Interestingly, Fanconi called the anaemia 'perniziosiforme' because the anaemia was macrocytic.

Although FA is a rare autosomal recessive disease characterized by multiple congenital abnormalities, bone marrow failure and cancer susceptibility (including leukaemia), over 1000 cases have now been reported.

Thrombocytopenia is usually the first cytopenia to appear, with aplasia occurring between the ages of 5 and 10 years in typical cases. Less commonly recognized is the risk for the development of myelodysplasia, which is said to occur in 1 in 20 FA patients. The mean survival is approximately 16 years, with complications of bone marrow failure being the major cause of death. It should be remembered that because FA patients are living longer due to advances in the therapy of bone marrow failure, they are at increased risk of developing solid tumours, with approximately 5% reported to have liver tumours and an equal number of other cancers that are considered secondary, especially head and neck squamous cell carcinomas of poor prognosis.

FA is a DNA-repair syndrome, and is diagnosed by finding chromosomal aberrations in cells treated with clastogenic agents such as diepoxybutane or mitomycin C, and in some centres gene mutation analysis or mapping is now becoming the gold standard in cases where the FA gene has been cloned. FA is genetically heterogenous, as complementation studies to date have identified eight separate genes (FA-A to FA-H) that produce the FA phenotype. The genes corresponding to complementation groups FA-A, FA-C and FA-G have been cloned, and the FA-D and

FA-E genes have been localized to chromosomes 3p22–26 and 6p21–22 respectively. The FA-C gene accounts for approximately 15% of cases studied but the incidence would appear to differ between populations. Carrier detection is now beginning to be offered to families at risk for FA-C mutations. How the FA gene products interfere with chromosomal stability is not clear, but defects causing increased apoptosis may be operating.

The mainstay of treatment is supportive, using leukodepleted, irradiated red cell and platelet transfusions. Aggressive iron chelation should be instigated when the ferritin rises above 1000 ng/l. Androgen therapy should be considered, especially when a suitable bone marrow donor is not available. A starting dose of 0.5–2 mg/kg/day should show a response within 2 months. Those who do respond have a better overall prognosis, with a median survival of up to 20 years compared with 12 years for those who fail to respond.

BMT is the treatment of choice when an HLA-identical sibling donor has been identified. The use of low-dose cyclophosphamide (5 mg/kg/day for 4 days) with thoracoabdominal irradiation (500–6000 cGy) for the preparative regimen of FA patients has led to a dramatic improvement in survival, with a long-term survival rate in excess of 80% in some centres. Before a family member is used as a donor, he or she should undergo clastogenic stress testing or mutational analysis to exclude FA. When a sibling donor is not available, a search for either a mismatched related or unrelated donor should be initiated, especially when the patient is showing signs of significant failure or when clonal change (MDS or leukaemia) has occurred. Results of transplants using these alternative donors are encouraging, especially when T-cell-depleted grafts are used and when the donor is a very good match, as determined via high-resolution HLA class II matching. Safer transplantation therapies will come over the next decade from umbilical cord and nonmyeloablative stem cell procedures.

Dyskeratosis congenita (DC)

Dyskeratosis congenita (DC), also known as the Zinsser–Cole–Engman syndrome, is a rare, predominately X-linked recessive multisystem disorder. There is a wide spectrum of clinical manifestations and it typically presents at a later age than FA, although there is great overlap between the two. The predominant manifestation is dermatological, and symptoms usually appear within the first decade of life; these are reticulated hyperpigmentation of the face, the neck and shoulders, and mucosal membranes, leukoplakia, and dystrophic nails. In most cases, inheritance of DC is X-linked recessive, in contrast to the autosomal recessive inheritance in FA, although some cases of autosomal recessive and dominant inheritance have been well described in DC. FA is associated with a high incidence of haemopoietic clonal disorders, and recently patients with DC have gone on to develop acute leukaemia. The genetics of DC is now beginning to be understood, as positional cloning strategy studies have shown the DKC1 gene responsible for the X-linked form of DC to be located at Xq28, and indeed the gene has now been cloned.

The treatment of DC is unsatisfactory at the present time, androgens with or without corticosteroids having an unpredictable success rate. Allogeneic BMT can reverse the bone marrow aplasia; however, it has little impact on the other systemic manifestations of the syndrome. It should also be remembered that there is high morbidity and mortality, with a significant number of patients dying from respiratory failure secondary to pulmonary fibrosis. Approximately one in ten patients with DC will go on to develop a squamous cell or adenocarcinoma of the oropharynx and gastrointestinal tract.

Severe chronic neutropenia

Severe chronic neutropenia includes a heterogeneous group of diseases characterized by a neutrophil count chronically less than 0.5×10^9/l. The group comprises Kostmann's disease, Shwachman–Diamond syndrome, cyclical neutropenia and glycogen storage disease type 1B. These children tend to suffer from numerous pyogenic infections, and approximately ten years ago recombinant granulocyte colony stimulating factor (G-CSF) was given to this group, which resulted in a total reduction in the number of pyogenic infections, significant reductions in the need for intravenous antibiotics and a dramatic improvement in the quality of life. Over 700 children worldwide have been treated with G-CSF; documented adverse effects included the development of acute myeloid leukaemia (AML) in approximately 5% of the patients in the cohort with Kost-mann's disease, suggesting that congenital neutropenia is a preleukaemic syndrome. None of the patients with cyclical or idio-pathic neutropenia developed leukaemia, suggesting that G-CSF was not involved in the development of leukaemia. It is the Kost-mann group and the Shwachman–Diamond group that would appear to be at risk of developing MDS and/or AML.

Kostmann's disease (KD)

Kostmann's disease (KD), originally described as infantile genetic agranulocytosis in 1956, is one of the group of severe congeni-tal neutropenias. Both autosomal dominant and autosomal recessive patterns of inheri-tance have been described. Whilst bone marrow cellularity and culture studies vary from patient to patient, a maturational arrest of neutrophil precursors at the promyelo-cyte/myelocyte stage with normal eosinophil and monocyte maturation patterns is seen in the majority of cases. KD is the severest form of congenital neutropenia, and usually pre-sents shortly after birth with life-threatening pyogenic infections, severe persistent neu-tropenia (neutrophil count $<0.2 \times 10^9$/l), and allied haematological abnormalities such as anaemia, monocytosis and eosinophilia.

Immunological abnormalities such as ele-vated serum immunoglobulins are associated with chronic infection and are usually seen at some stage during the course of the illness. Perhaps the most exciting advance in the treatment of KD over the past 10 years has been the use of G-CSF. The vast majority of these children require daily dosing with G-CSF; however, it should be pointed out that

there is great individual variation in the amount and also the frequency of growth factor administration. It should be remem-bered that the total dose of G-CSF adminis-tered should be titrated against not only the neutrophil response but also the clinical response.

Following the success of recent trials using recombinant G-CSF in severe congenital neu-tropenia, the natural history of KD is now becoming apparent. Prior to G-CSF treatment, the vast majority of these children succumbed to recurrent pyogenic infections, and it is only in the past 5–10 years that these patients are being kept alive with G-CSF administration. It would appear that a significant proportion of patients with KD are predisposed to acquired mutations of the G-CSF receptor, causing karyotypic abnormalities, MDS and AML. It is imperative now that patients with KD should be monitored closely for such bone marrow changes, and once they develop them, a search for an allogeneic bone marrow donor, preferably a matched sibling, should be undertaken with a view to transplantation.

KD is probably a heterogeneous group of disorders. Recent evidence suggests that point mutations in the gene for the G-CSF receptor, that is in the critical region of the intracellular part of the G-CSF receptor, occur only in a subgroup of severe congenital neutropenia patients, the vast majority of whom are KD patients. Screening for this and other mutations involving the G-CSF recep-tor, and indeed looking for clonal cytogenetic abnormalities on a regular basis, may be helpful with management decisions vis-à-vis BMT in these patients.

Side-effects of long-term G-CSF treatment include osteoporosis, vasculitis, spleno-megaly and bone marrow fibrosis. Regarding malignant transformation, it was felt initially that a myelodysplastic/leukaemic picture may develop secondary to long-term G-CSF treatment, but review of the literature reveals no evidence for this.

Cyclical neutropenia

Although cyclical neutropenia is not an inher-ited bone marrow failure syndrome, it is worth mentioning in the context of KD as sometimes it can be mistakenly called the latter. Cyclical neutropenia is a rare disease manifested by a transient neutropenia with a periodicity of 15–35 days, more classically every 21 days. Fluctuation is not confined to the neutrophil counts, but also occurs in the rest of the haemopoietic compartment, and therefore it should be considered as cyclical haemopoiesis. The diagnosis is usually made with a familiar history of recurring infections every 3 or 6 weeks. Clinical diagnosis is confirmed by carrying out a twice-weekly neutrophil count for at least 6–8 weeks. Bone marrow examination usually shows a paucity of mature polymorphonuclear leukocytes with no obvious maturation arrests.

The management of cyclical neutropenia has been revolutionized by the introduction of recombinant G-CSF therapy, which shortens the neutrophil nadir and reduces the frequency of infections. It should be remembered, however, that G-CSF does nothing to affect cycling of the other blood elements. The overall prognosis is excellent with G-CSF therapy and in a significant number of patients the severity and clinical manifestations tend to diminish with age.

Shwachman–Diamond syndrome (SDS)

Shwachman–Diamond syndrome (SDS) was described over 30 years ago, and is a rare autosomal recessive disorder that usually manifests in infancy and is characterized by pancreatic insufficiency, short stature and bone marrow dysfunction. Numerous additional features have been described, including metaphyseal dysostosis, epiphyseal dysplasia, immune dysfunction, liver disease, growth failure, renal tubular defects, insulin-dependent diabetes mellitus and psychomotor retardation. Although neutropenia is one of the required diagnostic criteria for SDS, other haematological manifestations have been associated with this disorder. These include anaemia, raised fetal haemoglobin, thrombocytopenia, intermittent neutropenia, impaired neutrophil chemotaxis and aplastic anaemia. Like other constitutional bone marrow failure syndromes, there is a predilection to leukaemic transformation. The

precise pathogenetic defect responsible for the haematological abnormalities seen in SDS is not known. Similar to the other inherited bone marrow failure syndromes, in particular FA, a stem cell abnormality has been proposed to be the most likely contender, because bone marrow progenitors from patients with SDS have a decreased CFU-GM and CFU-E growth potential on culture. Recent work also points to abnormalities within the stroma.

Leukaemic transformation in patients with SDS may be as high as 15–20%, providing that these patients live long enough and the natural history declares itself. The predominant leukaemic form is myeloid, which is usually associated with the development of clonal cytogenetic abnormalities, in particular monosomy 7. It would appear therefore that children with SDS and evidence of myelodysplasia are more likely to have structural abnormalities of chromosome 7 than expected.

Numerous therapeutic interventions directed at bone marrow dysfunction have been used in a small number of patients with varying success. They have included cyclosporin A for associated severe aplasia, G-CSF for profound neutropenia and lithium to improve cytoskeletally mediated neutrophil dysfunction. At present, the only definitive treatment for bone marrow dysfunction seen in SDS is allogeneic BMT. It should be pointed out, however, that experience with allogeneic BMT is limited to a handful of cases.

Pearson's syndrome (PS)

Pearson's syndrome (PS), first described in 1979, is a rare, often fatal, congenital disorder of unknown aetiology characterized by refractory sideroblastic anaemia, vacuolation of bone marrow precursors and exocrine pancreatic insufficiency. The anaemia is usually severe, transfusion-dependent and macrocytic, and appears early in infancy with variable degrees of neutropenia and thrombocytopenia. The pathogenesis and underlying molecular defect were elucidated 10 years later and ascribed to mitochondrial respiratory changes in function occurring secondary to rearrangements of mitochondrial DNA (mtDNA). Subsequently it was discovered that mtDNA abnormalities were not confined to the bone marrow but were also present in fibroblasts, gut and muscle, making PS a multisystem mitochondrial disorder of early childhood. The cases of PS that present to haematologists are those with refractory anaemia that is found to be sideroblastic in origin following bone marrow examination. It is therefore prudent to screen for rearrangements of mtDNA in all infants presenting with sideroblastic anaemia. This anaemia, as stated above, is usually a macrocytic sideroblastic anaemia that is refractory to pyridoxine, and is usually seen within the first three months of life. Bone marrow culture studies usually show a marked inhibition of erythroid colony growth but preserved granulocyte–macrophage colony growth. Elevations of fetal haemoglobin have been observed in numerous patients with PS, and in one case there was an associated positive erythrocyte i-antigen.

From the haematological point of view, treatment is aimed at keeping the haemoglobin level around 10 g/l. Defects within the respiratory chain cause lactic acidosis, and indeed this is the main cause of death in these children early on. If they can be kept alive, it is not unusual that the mitochondrial defect within the erythroid cells in the bone marrow removes and the haemoglobin corrects. However, it should be stressed that the majority of these children do badly in the first few years of life.

Diamond–Blackfan anaemia

Diamond–Blackfan anaemia is a rare, inherited disorder manifested as failure of erythropoiesis in the neonatal period or in infancy. Clinical diagnostic criteria include reticulocytopenia with macrocytic and normocytic anaemia, along with overall normal marrow cellularity and isolated erythroid hypoplasia. Other lineages are usually normal and the white blood cell count tends to be within the normal range. The majority of cases are considered to be sporadic, although autosomal recessive and autosomal dominant patterns of inheritance have been documented. Approxi-

mately one-third of cases are associated with a wide variety of congenital abnormalities and malformations. The typical presentation is anaemia documented in the first 6 months of life, with an incidence of around 5 per million live births.

The mainstay of treatment is corticosteroids, and greater than half of the patients will respond, especially if they are macrocytic at the commencement of steroids. However, many may require prolonged treatment. Long-term transfusional support for those refractory to steroid treatment is indicated, with concomitant long-term intravenous or subcutaneous iron chelation therapy. One in six patients with Diamond–Blackfan anaemia will ultimately go through spontaneous remission. Treatment with stem cell factor, interleukin-3 (IL-3), combinations of these, cyclosporin A, androgens and splenectomy have been mainly disappointing. Recent work has shown that the gene responsible for Diamond–Blackfan anaemia may be located on chromosome 19q13. The underlying defect for Diamond–Blackfan anaemia would appear to be in the stem cell progenitor cell compartment located at the erythroid progenitor level (CFU-GEMM, BFU-E, CFU-E).

Thrombocytopenia with absent radii (TAR)

Thrombocytopenia with absent radii (TAR) is a rare, autosomal recessive disorder that is usually diagnosed at birth, as the vast majority of these patients are thrombocytopenic and have the pathognomonic physical sign of bilateral absent radii. Other skeletal abnormalities involving the ulnae, fingers and lower limbs are also seen but are much less common. TAR differs from FA in several ways: the absent radii are accompanied by the presence of thumbs; the thrombocytopenia is the only cytopenia; there is absence of spontaneous or clastogenic stress-induced chromosomal breakage; and evolution to aplastic anaemia or leukaemia has not been reported. It is not uncommon for these children to be anaemic and have transient, high white cell counts at presentation (the former is felt to be secondary to bleeding as it is always accompanied by a reticulocytosis, and the latter usually subsides by 6 months of age). The striking morphological feature within the bone marrow is the absence or greatly reduced numbers of megakaryocytes, with normal granulopoietic and erythroid compartments. The precise pathophysiological defect responsible for TAR is not known; however, the restoration of platelet count seen following sibling allogeneic BMT supports the idea that the thrombopoietic defect lies within the haematopoietic stem cell compartment rather than being a deficiency of thrombopoietin or some other platelet humoral factor.

The majority of children with TAR have recurrent significant bleeding episodes in the first 6 months of life. Intracerebral and gastrointestinal haemorrhage are the usual causes of mortality, with previously 1 in 4 of these children dying by 4 years of age. The majority of these deaths, however, occur in the first year of life. The severity of the bleeding problem is related to the degree of the thrombocytopenia, which in the majority of children is usually below $20 \times 10^9/l$, and in some there has been evidence of qualitative platelet defects (storage pool and abnormal aggregation profiles). The mainstay of treatment is judicious use of single-donor platelet concentrates, aiming to keep the platelet count above $20 \times 10^9/l$, especially in the first year of life, as this is the time of maximum morbidity and mortality. With this more aggressive platelet transfusion protocol approach, the unacceptable haemorrhagic mortality and morbidity rate should dramatically decline. If the patient survives the first year of life, survival appears to be normal. All elective reconstructive orthopaedic surgery should be postponed during the first few years of life. Prenatal diagnosis of TAR is possible, with absent radii easily visualized with radiography and/or ultrasound and thrombocytopenia diagnosed following fetal blood sampling obtained by fetoscopy or cordocentesis. This relatively recent advance in obstetric care allows for the possibility of prophylactic antenatal management.

Amegakaryocytic thrombocytopenia (AMEGA)

Amegakaryocytic thrombocytopenia (AMEGA) is an extremely rare disorder of infancy and early childhood. The thrombocytopenia is non-immune and usually severe, and early bone marrow examination shows a normal karyotype, absent or greatly reduced numbers of megakaryocytes but normal granulopoietic and erythroid elements. Some patients have macrocytic red cells with increased expression of i-antigen and elevated haemoglobin F levels, implying that the pathophysiological trigger occurs at the stem cell level. The inheritance pattern in the majority of cases is X-linked, the remainder being autosomal recessive. AMEGA patients can be broadly divided into two groups: those with physical anomalies and those without. The pattern of somatic anomalies is not unlike that seen with FA; however in those children tested there was no evidence of a DNA-repair abnormality. The presence of anomalies influences the outcome; the projected median survivals are 6 years for those with no anomalies and 2 years when anomalies are present. Those with isolated thrombocytopenia usually die from haemorrhagic complications whilst those with aplasia, which usually occurs after a relatively long period of thrombocytopenia, succumb to infection and bleeding. AMEGA is considered to be a leukaemia-predisposition syndrome.

Platelet transfusions are the main therapeutic intervention from diagnosis. Treatment with corticosteroids alone or in combination with androgens has been disappointing and splenectomy has no role. Encouraging platelet responses following the administration of IL-3 have been reported and clinical trial results with thrombopoietin are eagerly awaited. Allogeneic BMT offers the only probable chance of cure.

Other syndromes associated with marrow failure

Rarer syndromes associated with inherited marrow failure include: reticular dysgenesis, Down's syndrome, Dubowitz's syndrome,

Seckel's syndrome, congenital triosomy-8 mosaicism, and familial ataxia–pancytopenia syndrome (see Young and Alter, 1994).

FURTHER READING

Schrezenmeieir H, Bacigalupo A, eds. (2000) *Aplastic Anaemia: Pathophysiology and Treatment.* Cambridge: Cambridge University Press.

Smith OP, Cox J. (1999) Inherited bone marrow failure: the men behind the empty space. *Br J Haematol* **107**: 242–6.

Smith OP, Hann I, Reeves B, Milla P, Chessells JM. (1996) Haematologic abnormalities in Shwachmann–Diamond syndrome: a review of twenty-one cases. *Br J Haematol* **94**: 279–84.

Vulliamy TJ, Knight SW, Heiss NS et al. (1999) Dyskeratosis congenita caused by a 3′ deletion: germ line and somatic mosaicism in a female carrier. *Blood* **94**: 1254–60.

Young NS, Alter BP. (1994) *Aplastic Anaemia: Acquired and Inherited.* Philadelphia: WB Saunders.

8 Primary haemostatic defects

Owen P Smith

INTRODUCTION

Damage to the vascular endothelium usually leads to exposure of the subendothelial matrix, which encourages adherence of platelets through various receptors but primarily GPIb–V–IX complex via the ligand, von Willebrand factor (vWF); see Chapter 2. These adherent platelets in turn become activated and release their contents and thus recruit other platelets from the circulation to aggregate via the platelet receptor, GPIIb–IIIa, through the ligands fibrinogen and vWF. Platelets also cooperate with blood coagulation proteins by providing an ideal environment to increase their enzymatic catalytic efficiency in generating thrombin (secondary haemostasis). Inherited and acquired defects of vWF, platelets and collagen (subendothelial matrix) give rise to the commonest cause of bleeding disorders in man, namely primary haemostatic defects. von Willebrand's disease is now regarded as the most common of the inherited bleeding disorders, with a worldwide prevalence estimated as being as high as 1%. Despite its relatively high prevalence, many features of the disease have only recently been elucidated, allowing for a clear classification and thus more appropriate forms of therapy. The same can be said of the inherited platelet disorders – both quantitative and qualitative. However, we are still very much in the dark in relation to the pathophysiology of collagen vascular disorders that give rise to primary haemostatic bleeding.

VON WILLEBRAND'S DISEASE (vWD)

In 1926, the Finnish physician Erik von Willebrand published the first account of an inherited bleeding disorder affecting consanguineous families from the Åland archipelago, which lies in the gulf separating Sweden and Finland. The proband, Hjordid S, a 5-year-old girl with severe bleeding since birth, had had four of her sisters die between the ages of 2 and 4 with uncontrollable bleeding from the nose and gut. In addition, there was a family history, in both parents and relatives of both sexes, of milder bleeding problems, suggesting autosomal dominant transmission of a mild disorder that became more severe in the homozygous or compound heterozygous state. Bleeding was usually from skin or mucous membranes, with haemorrhage into joints or deep tissues being rare. In his original paper, von Willebrand reported that at the age of 3, Hjordis S sustained a deep lip laceration from which she bled profusely for 3 days, thereafter becoming unconscious. At the age of 13, she bled to death during her fourth menstrual period. von Willebrand did not succeed in determining where the primary defect lay in this bleeding diathesis, and it is only in the last 25 years that our understanding of the molecular pathophysiology of this condition has advanced significantly.

von Willebrand's disease (vWD) is the commonest inherited bleeding disorder in man, with a gene prevalence of approximately 1% of the population. There is significant phenotypic heterogeneity even among members of the same family. The majority of individuals have type 1 vWD, with type 3 vWD being seen in 1–2 per million of the population. Bleeding tends to be predominantly mucocutaneous, so-called 'wet purpura', the commonest type being epistaxis, easy bruising, gum bleeding following tooth brushing and, in adolescent girls, heavy menses. Bleeding into joints is rare and typically only seen in individuals with severe type 3 disease where the circulating plasma factor VIII levels are usually around 2%. The considerable variation in clinical phenotype is most likely to be due in part to the effect that ABO blood group antigens have on circulating plasma vWF levels, for example the mean vWF levels for individuals of blood group O are approximately 75%, while for type AB individuals they are 123% when compared with a pool of normal donor plasma. Age and stress also result in increases in plasma vWF levels.

Laboratory confirmation of vWD comprises screening tests and specific investigations to confirm the diagnosis and allow correct classification. Unfortunately, to date the majority of routine tests used in the diagnosis of vWD have low sensitivity and specificity, and in the presence of bleeding symptoms or a positive family history these should be preformed repeatedly along with other more specific tests. Since vWF and factor VIII:C are both acute phase proteins, their levels may be transiently elevated into the normal range by any form of stress. The tests commonly used for the biochemical evaluation of possible vWD are factor VIII:C, vWF antigen (vWF:Ag), vWF:ristocetin cofactor (vWF:Ricof), vWF multimer analysis, and the bleeding time. VWd is subdivided into partial quantitative deficiency (type 1), qualitative deficiency (type 2) and total deficiency (type 3) of vWF.

Type 1 vWD accounts for approximately 70% of cases and is inherited in an autosomal dominant fashion. Biochemically, it is characterized by a 30–50% level in circulating vWF:Ag, factor VIII:C and vWF:Ricof. A full range of vWF multimers are usually seen on agarose gel analysis.

Type 2 vWD now includes subtypes 2A, 2B, 2M and 2N. Penetrance is more complete than for type 1 and it probably comprises 20–30% of all vWD cases.

Type 2A vWD, the most common qualitative vWD variant, is typically inherited in an autosomal dominant fashion, although reces-sive inheritance has also been described. Biochemically it is characterized by a disproportionately low vWF:Ricof relative to the vWF:Ag level and decreased circulating intermediate- and high-molecular-weight vWF multimers. As large vWF multimers have significant haemostatic activity, the selective absence of these multimers predictably results in bleeding. To date, more than 25 different point mutations, all resulting in single amino acid substitutions, have been identified in individuals with type 2A vWD.

Type 2B vWD is clinically and biochemically very similar to pseudo-vWD (see below). It is usually diagnosed by the increased platelet agglutination induced by low concentrations of ristocetin. However, it should be remembered that in some cases defects can be delineated in the absence of ristocetin. Like type 2A vWD, the mutations causing type 2B are clustered within exon 28 of the *vWF* gene. These mutations result in 'gain-of-function', that is, there is spontaneous binding of the mutant vWF to GPIb, with the consequential loss of high-molecular-weight multimers from the plasma and a tendency to thrombocytopenia. The thrombocytopenia may be intermittent and exacerbated by conditions such as infection, pregnancy, DDAVP (desmopressin) or advanced age.

Type 2M vWD is characterized by impaired vWf–platelet adhesion, but with associated normal sized circulating vWF multimers ('M' for multimer). Several variants are associated with decreased ristocetin-induced binding to platelets due to mutations in the GPIb binding domain of vWF. These patients may have significant bleeding symptoms despite normal factor VIII:C levels.

Type 2N vWD ('N' for Normandy) is an autosomal recessive disorder characterized by reduced binding of vWF to factor VIII:C and consequently low circulating factor VIII:C levels. The platelet-dependent functions and multimer patterns of vWF appear normal. This condition therefore mimics haemophilia A. Over ten separate mutations, all at the N-terminus of vWF protein in the region of the factor VIII:C binding domain, have been identified in individuals with this type of vWD. In addition, some individuals with type

1 vWD have been shown to co-inherit type 1 and type 2N alleles, resulting in disproportionately low factor VIII:C as compared with vWF:Ag and vWF:Ricof.

Type 3 vWD is the severest form of the disease, with patients presenting with potentially life-threatening episodes of bleeding typically seen in severe secondary haemostatic defects. It is autosomal recessive, and heterozygotes are often phenotypically normal, although biochemically significant heterogeneity can be seen, with some individuals having decreased plasma and/or platelets vWF:Ag and vWF:Ricof levels. Type 3 vWD is a quantitative disorder in which there is virtually no detectable vWF, resulting in moderately severe factor VIII deficiency as well. The commonest mutation causing type 3 vWD is a frameshift mutation in exon 18 of the gene, and indeed this is the mechanism responsible for the disease originally described by Erik von Willebrand.

The main objective of treatment is to correct the two laboratory hallmarks of the disease, namely, the prolonged bleeding time, and the low factor VIII:C level. For practical purposes, it is important to distinguish among type 1, type 2B, other types of 2 and type 3 disease before commencing treatment. As most patients have a quantitative defect, it is pos-sible to stimulate endogenous release with DDAVP either by intravenous, subcutaneous or nasal routes. While this treatment is inexpensive and infection-free, it does have a number of rare side-effects, notably, hyponatraemia and seizures, especially in young children. Failure to respond occurs in approximately 10–15% of patients, and in those who do not respond a significant number become refractory when the drug is given over an extended period (tachyphylaxis). DDAVP is not recommended when major surgery is planned, in type 3 and type 2B, or in situations where DDAVP has failed to correct the bleeding time and when it is imperative to achieve adequate mucosal haemostasis. For these patients, blood products, in the form of factor VIII concentrate or the newer vWF concentrate are usually given, as no specific concentrate is available for vWD (Table 8.1). Patients should be advised against the use of aspirin-containing compounds and nonsteroidal anti-inflammatory drugs.

THROMBOCYTOPENIA

In this section, the causes of thrombocytopenia are divided into two broad categories: those arising on a background of an estab-

---

Table 8.1 Therapeutic intervention in children with von Willebrand's disease

	Haemate P[a]	DDAVP[b]	Tranexamic acid[c]	Platelets
Type 1	−/+	+	+	−
Type 2A	−/+	+	+	−
Type 2B	+	−	+	−
Type 2N	+	−	+	−
Type 2M	+		+	−
Type 3	+	−	+	−
Pseudo vWD	−	−	−	+

Following diagnosis of type 1 and 2a vWD, the majority of children should undergo a dose–response trial of DDAVP (desmopressin) in order to establish those patients who do not respond favourably and hence would be offered a vWF concentrate.
[a] <30% dosage 40–50 IU/kg bolus, followed by 20 IU/kg twice daily; >30% dosage 20–40 IU/kg daily;
[b] 0.3 µg/kg intravenously;
[c] Especially when there is oral cavity bleeding.

lished genetic defect (inherited thrombocy-topenia) and those that are acquired either around the time of birth (congenital thrombo-cytopenia) and those that occur later in child-hood.

Inherited thrombocytopenia

The inherited thrombocytopenias comprise a group of platelet formation abnormalities in which platelet numbers are reduced (Table 8.2). In the vast majority of patients, the platelet count is only mild to moderately reduced $(50 \times 10^9/l$ and $100 \times 10^9/l)$ and therefore significant spontaneous haemor-rhage tends not to be problematical. There are, however, a small number of notable exceptions where spontaneous bleeding is a prominent clinical feature of the syndrome. These include Wiskott–Aldrich syndrome, amegakaryocytic thrombocytopenia and thrombocytopenia with absent radii (TAR), where the platelet count is usually very low, and the Bernard–Soulier and Chediak–Higashi syndromes, where there is also a marked platelet dysfunction. Immune-mediated throm-bocytopenia is a major differential diagnosis in children with low platelet counts, and therefore making the correct diagnosis of these conditions is important, as it usually prevents the useless and potentially danger-ous prescribing of immunosuppressants such as corticosteroids. Although the inherited nature of these conditions has been known for the past 30 years, the molecular basis for the thrombocytopenia has only been fully elu-

Table 8.2 Inherited thrombocytopenias

Disorder	Inheritance	Platelet feature
With dysfunctional platelets		
Bernard–Soulier syndrome	AR	↓ Aggregation to ristocetin
Pseudo-von Willebrand's disease	AD	↑ Aggregation to ristocetin
Type 2b von Willebrand's disease	AD	↑ Aggregation to ristocetin
Montreal syndrome	AD	Spontaneous aggregation
Gray platelet syndrome	AR	α-granule defect
Paris–Trousseau syndrome	AD	Giant α-granules
Wiskott–Aldrich syndrome	X-linked	↓ Dense granules in some
X-linked thrombocytopenia	X-linked	↓ Dense granules in some
Chediak–Higashi syndrome	AD	↓ Aggregation to Ep and Co
Factor V Quebec	AD	↓ Aggregation to Ep
Without dysfunctional platelets		
May–Hegglin anomaly	AD	Function studies vary
Alport's syndrome variants		
Epstein's syndrome	AD	↓ Aggregation to Ep and Co
Eckstein's syndrome	AD	Normal platelet function
Fechtner's syndrome	AD	Function studies vary
Sebastian's syndrome	AD	Normal platelet function
Thrombocytopenia with absent radii	AR	↓ Aggregation to Ep and Co
Pure genetic thrombocytopenia	AD	Not known
Mediterranean thrombocytopenia	AD	Not known

AR, autosomal recessive; AD, autosomal dominant; Ep, epinephrine (adrenaline); Co, collagen.

cidated in a very small number of these conditions, in particular those arising from defects in vWF and its platelet receptor, the GPIb–V–IX complex.

GPIb–V–IX complex

The GPIb–V–IX complex forms one of the major adhesion receptors on the platelet surface and plays a pivotal role in primary haemostasis in mediating vWF attachment after collagen exposure on the damaged vessel wall (see Chapter 2). Three inherited bleeding disorders associated with gene defects within this complex are described below.

Bernard–Soulier syndrome (BSS)

The Bernard–Soulier syndrome (BSS) is the best characterized inherited thrombocytopenia, which has in association an abnormal platelet function. Typically, there is moderate to severe thrombocytopenia and a prolonged bleeding time; platelet morphology usually reveals 'giant' forms. The platelets in this condition are incapable of interacting with vWF, and hence the bleeding seen is typical of a primary haemostatic defect. Whilst BSS platelets show normal shape change, secretion, signal transduction and aggregation in response to ADP, adrenalin, collagen and arachidonic acid, they do not aggregate with ristocetin in the presence of vWF. BSS is inherited in an autosomal recessive manner with the underlying molecular defects being due to quantitative or qualitative defects in the GPIb–V–IX complex. Numerous variants of BSS have been described at the molecular level. Treatment is with HLA-matched platelets.

Pseudo-vWD

Pseudo-von Willebrand's disease is an autosomal dominant disorder characterized by mild intermittent thrombocytopenia, mild bleeding, absence of high-molecular-weight vWF multimers, and increased ristocetin-induced platelet aggregation. It is caused by a mutation(s) in GPIbα causing a conformational change in the receptor that in turn leads to enhanced vWF binding and hence

spontaneous platelet aggregation and thrombocytopenia. It can be differentiated from type 2B vWD, where the mutation resides in the vWF protein, by spontaneous aggregation of the patient's platelets with normal plasma.

Montreal platelet syndrome

The Montreal platelet syndrome is characterized by thrombocytopenia, large platelets, spontaneous platelet aggregation and a reduced response to thrombin-induced aggregation. It can be distinguished from BSS by its autosomal dominant inheritance and a normal platelet agglutinability response to ristocetin. The platelets have a quantitative and qualitative reduction of the calcium-dependent proteinase calpain that prevents them from returning to a normal volume after agonist stimulation.

Gray platelet syndrome

The Gray platelet is an extremely rare autosomally inherited syndrome characterized by a markedly reduced platelet α-granule content but normal dense bodies and lysosomes. Other features include a prolonged skin bleeding time, morphologically large platelets and highly variable platelet aggregation profiles. The platelet α-granules that are present, in reduced numbers, are deficient in the storage proteins, coagulation factor V, vWF, platelet factor 4, β-thromboglobulin, fibrinogen, platelet-derived growth factor (PDGF) and thrombospondin. Concomitant elevations in plasma levels of platelet factor 4 and β-thromboglobulin are seen. Myellofibrosis is not an uncommon finding in these patients and the continuous premature release of α-granule proteins such as PDGF into the bone marrow microenvironment may be key to its development. The accompanying thrombocytopenia and bleeding symptoms are usually mild. In patients with the Gray platelet syndrome, the appropriate on-demand or prophylactic treatment needs to be individualized. For example, those patients with moderate thrombocytopenia and evidence of abnormal platelet aggregation would be most likely to benefit from a combination of platelet transfusion and

DDAVP, whilst in those with very mild thrombocytopenia and a prolonged bleeding time, DDAVP alone is all that is needed.

Paris–Trousseau syndrome

The Paris–Trousseau syndrome is a recently described autosomal dominant syndrome comprising mild thrombocytopenia, a moderate haemorrhagic tendency, giant α-granules in a subpopulation of platelets, bone marrow micromegakaryocytes with enhanced megakaryocyte apoptosis and a deletion of the distal part of chromosome 11 at position 11q23. The giant α-granules fail to release their content following thrombin exposure and perhaps this may explain the moderate bleeding events seen in this disorder.

Wiskott–Aldrich syndrome (WAS)

The Wiskott–Aldrich syndrome (WAS) is inherited as an X-linked recessive trait and is characterized by eczema, microthrombocytopenia and combined immunodeficiency. It is often fatal by the early teens because of infection, lymphoma or bleeding. Haemorrhagic events in this syndrome are common during the first two years of life and the reason for this is multifactorial. For example, platelet survival is modestly reduced to half normal; ineffective megakaryocytopoiesis is prominent, as reflected by a platelet turnover of 25% that of normal with a normal megakaryocyte mass, and there is evidence of platelet functional abnormalities related to abnormal storage of adenine nucleotides and impaired platelet energy metabolism. Allogeneic bone marrow transplantation is the treatment of choice when there is a fully matched donor available, as this corrects the abnormal stem cell compartment. When there is no suitable donor available then splenectomy is the therapeutic first choice, as this usually raises the platelet count into the normal range and improves platelet survival and there is normalization of platelet size. It should be remembered that splenectomy is not advocated for the other hereditary thrombocytopenic disorders as little benefit is usually seen.

Wiskott–Aldrich syndrome variants (X-linked thrombocytopenia)

This is a heterogeneous group of thrombocytopenic disorders with X-linked inheritance. Some families have microthrombocytopenia and no associated abnormalities, while others have mild eczema and impaired immune responses. The thrombocytopenia is usually less severe in WAS variants and requires no treatment, but in the rare case with severe thrombocytopenia splenectomy has been shown to be effective. Both WAS and WAS variants appear to be caused by different mutations of the same gene on the short arm of the X-chromosome (Xp11.2).

Oculocutaneous albinism: Hermansky–Pudlak and Chediak–Higashi syndromes

Oculocutaneous albinism denotes a group of inherited disorders characterized by reduced or absent pigmentation of the skin, hair and eyes. Whilst the majority of these patients have an isolated platelet storage pool defect, in some an accompanying low platelet count can occur.

The Hermansky–Pudlak syndrome is an autosomal recessive disorder with the classic triad of oculocutaneous albinism (tyrosinase-positive), platelet dense-body or combined dense-body and α-granule storage pool deficiency, and depositions of ceroid-like material in the monocyte–macrophage system. The bleeding tendency is usually mild (related to the storage pool defect and not thrombocytopenia, as the latter is not a feature syndrome); however, excessive bleeding following tooth extractions and tonsillectomy is the rule.

The features of the Chediak–Higashi syndrome include partial oculocutaneous albinism, the presence of giant granules in all granule-containing cells, neutropenia, peripheral neuropathy, and platelet storage pool deficiency which usually involves the dense bodies. Thrombocytopenia usually occurs during the accelerated phase of the disease, which involves the development of pancytopenia, hepatosplenomegaly, lymphadenopathy, and extensive tissue infiltration with lymphoid cells. The precise molecular basis of Chediak–Higashi syndrome has not been fully elucidated and the only curable therapeutic modality is allogeneic bone marrow transplantation.

Factor V Quebec

This condition is characterized by an autosomal dominant inheritance pattern, mild thrombocytopenia, quantitative and qualitative defects in platelet factor V, an adrenaline platelet aggregation defect, and a severe post-traumatic bleeding tendency. Defects in multimerin, a large complex multimeric protein expressed in platelet α-granules, and endothelial cell Weibel–Palade bodies are most likely to be responsible for the low platelet factor V level, but its deficiency also plays a role in the reduced levels of the other α-granule proteins, fibrinogen, vWF, thrombospondin and osteonectin.

May–Hegglin anomaly

This is an autosomal dominant disorder, characterized by giant platelets, variable thrombocytopenia and Dohle-like inclusions within granulocytic cells, including monocytes. A small percentage of patients have persistent leukopenia that has been associated with occasional infections, and in one case neutrophil chemotaxis and chemokinetic responses were impaired. Platelet function has been reported to be normal in some and impaired in others. Troublesome primary haemostatic bleeding that is seen in approximately 40% of these patients is felt to be most likely secondary to the degree of thrombocytopenia at the time of haemorrhage.

Alport variants

Alport's syndrome is associated with the findings of sensorineural deafness (usually high tone deafness), haematuria, cataracts and progressive renal failure. The disorder is a heterogeneous group with the majority having autosomal dominant inheritance. Many variants of Alport's syndrome have been described, the most common being associated with hyperprolinaemia. The genetic

basis of this syndrome is believed to involve deletions and/or rearrangements in the α5(IV) collagen gene located on Xq22. Three variants have been described with associated thrombocytopenia.

Epstein's syndrome was first described in 1972 in a family with features of Alport's syndrome, macrothrombocytopenia and defective platelet aggregation and secretion in response to ADP and collagen. Three years later *Eckstein's syndrome* was reported and described to have all the features that characterized Epstein's syndrome but, by contrast, had normal platelet function.

Fechtner's syndrome is characterized by the same morphological features as those seen in the Sebastian platelet syndrome but, unlike the latter, Fechtner's syndrome is associated with deafness, cataract and renal failure. The white cell inclusion bodies (Fechtner inclusions) that are characteristic of the syndrome resemble toxic Dohle bodies (seen with infection and malignancies) and May–Hegglin granulocyte inclusions.

Whilst these syndromes are associated with mild to moderate bleeding tendency, significant haemorrhagic morbidity is usually encountered following trauma, dental extraction and other forms of surgery, and platelet concentrates are the main therapeutic intervention. It should be remembered that the progressive renal failure seen in these patients usually adds to the haemorrhagic tendency but also it is the main aetiological factor contributing to overall morbidity and indeed mortality.

Sebastian platelet syndrome

The Sebastian platelet syndrome resembles the May–Hegglin anomaly but the Dohle-body-like inclusions seen in granulocytes are different, in that they are smaller, and ultrastructural analysis shows them to consist of ribosomes and dispersed filaments without an enclosing membrane. They are detected by light microscopy only if the blood smears are stained within 4 hours after venipuncture which implies that this syndrome is a more frequent cause of hereditary thrombocytopenia, since a number of cases may go undetected. This syndrome is felt to be a variant of Fechtner's syndrome without the associated Alport's syndrome features. It is inherited in an autosomal dominant manner and whilst the bleeding tendency is considered to be mild to moderate, haemorrhagic deaths have been reported.

Inherited bone marrow failure syndromes

Thrombocytopenia with absent radii and amegakaryocytic thrombocytopenia are also included in the differential, diagnosis, and the reader is referred to Chapter 7 for further discussion.

Trisomy syndromes

Moderately severe thrombocytopenia is seen in some cases of trisomy-18 syndrome, trisomy-13 syndrome and to a lesser extent in trisomy 21. Both trisomy 13 and 18 are usually diagnosed at birth as the associated abnormalities are usually quite striking. The majority of these cases die in the neonatal period from non-haemorrhagic sequelae.

Pure genetic thrombocytopenia

This is an autosomal dominant macrothrombocytopenic disorder characterized by a chronic low platelet count, a normal platelet half-life, normal platelet function (aggregation and adhesion), normal skin bleeding time, absent platelet-associated immunoglobulins and a morphologically normal bone marrow megakaryocyte compartment. Although the molecular lesion causing the thrombocytopenia has not been elucidated, platelet isotope studies using homologous and autologous platelets are highly suggestive that there is a pure production defect within the bone marrow. The majority of cases are picked up following routine blood tests that are carried out for non-haematological indications. As the majority of these patients will have platelet counts in the region of 50 to $100 \times 10^9/l$ with normal skin bleeding times, the haemorrhagic potential for spontaneous bleeding is low and only rises at menses, following trauma or surgery.

Mediterranean macrothrombocytopenia

This type of macrothrombocytopenia was initially reported from Australia in blood donors with Greek and Italian ancestry and has subsequently been shown to be present in the North African immigrant population in France. The thrombocytopenia is mild with platelet counts running between $100 \times 10^9/l$ and $150 \times 10^9/l$ and platelet morphology showing only a mild increase in platelet size. Inheritance is autosomal dominant and the low platelet count is very rarely if ever associated with troublesome bleeding.

Acquired thrombocytopenia

Immune (idiopathic) thrombocytopenic purpura (ITP) of childhood

Idiopathic or immune thrombocytopenic purpura (ITP) is defined as thrombocytopenic purpura without any other associated condition. Two different forms of ITP can be distinguished: the acute and the chronic forms. Acute ITP is predominantly seen in young children aged between 2 and 5 years, and is usually preceded by a viral illness or prodrome that has a higher incidence in the autumn and winter months. Bleeding is uncommon when the platelet count is above $50 \times 10^9/l$; however, when the platelet count decreases below this concentration there is a proportional increase in bleeding manifestations. Spontaneous bleeding is frequent when the platelet count is below $15 \times 10^9/l$ and may be life-threatening when it falls below $10 \times 10^9/l$. Along with thrombocytopenia, an elevated mean platelet volume can be present as a sign of increased platelet production. Normal or elevated numbers of megakaryocytes are usually seen on bone marrow examination; however, it should be stressed that examination of the bone marrow is not required to make the diagnosis in the vast majority of cases. The diagnosis is one of exclusion in that the vast majority of children will have had a preceding viral infection or will have been vaccinated in the previous month. Physical examination is usually normal with the exception of cutaneous bleeding.

Acute ITP of childhood is most likely a heterogeneous group of disorders whose cardinal clinical feature is a low circulating platelet count with bruising. It is most likely caused by an inappropriate immune response to several different stimuli. The antibody produced by the immune response is cross-reacting activity to platelet surface protein, the most likely contender being GPIIb–IIIa. Subsequently these antibody-coated platelets then bind to the Fc receptors on macrophages based in the reticuloendothelial system. Greater than 90% of children who develop acute ITP respond spontaneously, and why approximately 10% go on to develop a chronic course is not known. Recent evidence suggests that platelet FcγRII receptor polymorphism may be predictive of chronicity.

Laboratory tests that help exclude other causes of thrombocytopenia include blood film, looking for the presence of micro-angiopathic haemolytic anaemia, platelet clumping (pseudo-thrombocytopenia), or blasts. Bone marrow examination is not required in the vast majority of children with acute ITP; however, it is the author's practice that if corticosteroids are to be used as first-line treatment then a bone marrow examination should be done to exclude acute leukaemia. The majority of children will respond spontaneously and if treatment is required then intravenous immunoglobulin (1 g per kg $\times$ 2 days) and/or prednisolone (2 mg per kg per day $\times$ 7 days with taper) are front-line treatment. The vast majority of children will respond; however, it should always be remembered that corticosteroids and immunoglobulins do indeed have side-effects. In those children who fail to respond with severe thrombocytopenia then anti-D antibody, danazol, cyclosporin A and azathioprine have also been used with varying success.

In the small number of patients who develop chronic ITP and remain symptomatic, treatment is problematical and splenectomy is probably the most effective. It should be remembered, however, that splenectomy is not always successful and indeed has immediate medium- and long-term side-effects.

Congenital thrombocytopenia

Congenital thrombocytopenia is defined as a low platelet count at birth not resulting from the association of a specific gene defect, and accounts for the majority of cases of neonatal thrombocytopenia. Thrombocytopenia is a common finding in sick neonates, however, and since the introduction of automated cell counters it is now considered a relatively common (approximately 1%) finding in apparently normal infants. In the vast majority of cases the thrombocytopenia results from increased platelet destruction, which can arise by several mechanisms, the majority of which are not known. It is helpful to consider aetiological factors contributing to neonatal thrombocytopenia in terms of whether the insult is maternally, infant or placentally based (Table 8.3). Immune-mediated thrombocytopenia is usually seen in term babies that are clinically well and may be responsible for one third of cases of thrombocytopenia seen in the general neonate population. There are two broad groups of conditions: those mediated by an alloimmune mechanism and those with associated auto-immune phenomena.

Neonatal alloimmune thrombocytopenia (NAIT)

This arises following maternal sensitization to paternal antigens present on fetal platelets. It occurs in approximately 1 in 1500 to 1 in 2000 births, with the mother having a normal platelet count and a negative history for bleeding. The maternal allo-antibody produced does not react with the mother's platelets but crosses the placenta and destroys fetal platelets. The paternally-derived fetal platelet antigen target against which the maternal allo-antibody is directed is usually HPA-1a (also called PLA-1 or Zw^a), which is present on platelets of 98% of the population and is responsible for NAIT in approximately 80% of cases. The second most common platelet antigen involved in NAIT is HPA-5b (also called Br^a, Zav^a or Hc^a). Whilst NAIT is in other ways analogous to haemolytic disease of the newborn due to Rhesus or ABO incompatibility, in NAIT, the first child

Table 8.3 Congenital thrombocytopenias

Material factors
Immune thrombocytopenia
  Neonatal alloimmune thrombocytopenia
  Maternal autoimmune thrombocytopenia

Intrauterine infections (TORCH syndromes)
  Toxoplasmosis
  Rubella
  Cytomegalovirus
  Herpes simplex
  Other (including HIV and parvovirus B19)

Pre-eclampsia/hypertension

Drugs

Infant factors
Disseminated intravascular coagulation

Primary microangiopathic haemolytic anaemias
  Haemolytic uremic syndrome
  Thrombotic thrombocytopenic purpura

Giant haemangioma syndrome (Kasabach–Merritt syndrome)

Hypercoagulable states
  Birth asphyxia
  Cyanotic congenital heart disease
  Respiratory distress syndrome
  Necrotizing enterocolitis
  Bacterial infection
  Rhesus haemolytic disease
  Anticoagulant deficiency (homozygous antithrombin, protein C and S deficiency)
  Heparin-induced thrombocytopenia

Rare bone marrow diseases
  Transient abnormal myelopoiesis
  Haemophagocytic lymphohistiocytosis
  Osteopetrosis
  Congenital leukaemia
  Metastatic neuroblastoma

Placental factors
Infarction

Angiomas (chorioangiomas)
Lupus anticoagulants/anticardiolipin antibodies

is usually affected with thrombocytopenia. Given that 2% of the population is HPA-1a-negative, it is somewhat surprising that the frequency of NAIT is lower than what would be predicted from the prevalence of this allo-antigen.

NAIT typically presents as an isolated severe thrombocytopenia in an otherwise healthy child at birth. Severe thrombocytopenia may be present early in gestation, and at least 20% of cases suffer intracranial haemorrhage (ICH), some sustaining it in utero, which usually results in long-term severe neurological sequelae such as porencephalic cysts and optic hypoplasia. Widespread petechial haemorrhage is present in more than 90% of cases, while cephalo-haematomata, haematuria and gastrointestinal bleeding occur in a significantly smaller number of children. Typically, the platelet count spontaneously returns into the normal range within 3 weeks after birth.

Neonates with alloimmune thrombocytopenia usually have platelet counts below $20 \times 10^9/l$. The diagnosis of NAIT is usually confirmed by platelet antigen typing of the parents, showing the antigen to be absent on the father's platelets and present on the mother's platelets, or by demonstrating in the mother's serum antibody activity to the antigen using indirect immunofluorescence assay or enzyme-linked immunoassay.

The mainstay of treatment for affected infants is washed, irradiated, maternal platelet concentrates. Both unrelated matched and maternal platelets can be administered; however, maternal platelets are preferred because of their certain compatibility, availability and, perhaps more importantly, safety. With de novo cases of NAIT, platelets can be rapidly procured from the mother and following washing and γ-irradiation given to the infant in a matter of a few hours. Random donor platelets should be given to infants who are actively bleeding while awaiting maternal platelets. In less severe cases, high-dose (1 g/kg) immunoglobulin therapy on two consecutive days will usually increase the platelet count within 2 days of administration. In those cases of known NAIT, where elective Caesarean section is the preferred route of delivery, platelets are usually collected from the mother a few days before surgery and if this is deemed logistically problematical then platelets can be collected early in the pregnancy or indeed when the mother is not expecting and frozen for use at a later stage. Alternatively, non-maternal HPA-1a-negative platelets can be ordered in advance from the blood bank.

All children born to fathers homozygous for the implicated antigen will harbour the antigen and half of the children will have it if there is paternal heterozygosity. This has important implications for future pregnancies, as imaging with ultrasound early in pregnancy will allow intervention should it be required. Sampling fetal blood at 20 weeks allows an accurate assessment of the platelet count, but also fetal allo-antigen genotyping can be carried out on the same sample. Knowing the fetal platelet count and whether there is intracranial bleeding present usually dictates the type of therapeutic intervention that is most appropriate. For example, a fetus with severe thrombocytopenia and evidence of ICH will probably benefit from antigen-negative platelets transfused weekly. At the other end of the clinical spectrum, a fetus who is at risk of NAIT and who has mild thrombocytopenia and a normal cranial ultrasound may equally benefit from infused maternal immunoglobulin therapy alone. It should be remembered, however, that to date there is no published randomized trial comparing the more aggressive approach of intra-uterine platelet transfusion with the least aggressive therapeutic modality of maternal immunoglobulin. Elective Caesarean section is recommended for all affected mature fetuses as this will allow postnatal management to be optimal.

Maternal autoimmune thrombocytopenia (AIT)

Autoimmune thrombocytopenia is due to the passive transfer of auto-antibodies from mothers with isolated ITP or it may be seen in association with conditions that have immune-dysregulatory features such as maternal systemic lupus erythematosus, hypothyroidism and lymphoproliferative states. Unlike NAIT, the specificity of the platelet antibody seen in AIT is towards antigen(s) common to maternal and fetal platelets. Approximately 1 in 10 000 pregnancies are complicated by maternal ITP. The risk of significant infant morbidity and mortality is minimal, as the infant platelet count is rarely less than $50 \times 10^9/l$, ICH rarely if ever happens and when it does occur it is not related to birth trauma. It is also clear that there is no correlation between the platelet count and level of auto-antibody seen in the mother and the severity of thrombocytopenia observed in the infant; in fact, it has been well documented that women with normal platelet counts following splenectomy for ITP still deliver babies who are thrombocytopenic. Autoimmune thrombocytopenia needs to be distinguished from incidental or 'gestational' thrombocytopenia where the thrombocytopenia is usually mild ($70–100 \times 10^9/l$) with no bleeding history; there is no history of thrombocytopenia outside pregnancy and the platelet count swiftly returns to normal following delivery. Infants born to mothers with 'gestational' thrombocytopenia never have or extremely rarely have a low platelet count.

The bleeding manifestations, including the risk of ICH, in children of mothers with AIT are significantly less than in children with NAIT. These infants are usually very well and born at term. The neonatal platelet count often falls after birth to a nadir on days 1–3 and it is during this time frame that bleeding occurs. Spontaneous recovery of the infant platelet count is usually observed within 3 weeks after birth. However, if the platelet count is below $20 \times 10^9/l$ or if there is significant bleeding then intravenous immunoglobulin (1 g/kg) should be given on two consecutive days, and if this fails to raise the platelet count then a short course of oral prednisolone (2–4 mg/kg/day) for 7–14 days should be added. The mother's immune thrombocytopenia should be treated in accordance with the severity of her platelet count and not for a theoretical risk estimate of bleeding in the baby. As there are no reliable maternal predictors of severe thrombocytopenia in the infant, prenatal treatment of the mother with immunoglobulin and/or steroids does not make therapeutic sense. The

birth is usually by spontaneous vaginal delivery and only in those pregnancies where problems are anticipated or if there is a history of a previous complicated delivery is Caesarian section contemplated.

Intrauterine infections (TORCH syndromes)

Intrauterine viral infections rarely produce severe thrombocytopenia ($<20 \times 10^9/l$), and therefore therapeutic intervention in the form of platelet concentrate and/or antiviral therapy is only indicated when active bleeding or surgical intervention is being considered. The mechanism(s) responsible for thrombocytopenia secondary to intrauterine infection is not fully understood. In the vast majority of cases the platelet count returns into the normal range within 2–4 weeks after birth but may persist to 4 months of age. The well-established intrauterine infections that cause congenital thrombocytopenia are outlined below.

Toxoplasmosis. Thrombocytopenia is seen in a quarter of cases of congenital toxoplasmosis and in approximately 20% of these cases the platelet count is below $50 \times 10^9/l$.

Congenital rubella. Mild to moderate thrombocytopenia is seen in approximately 20% of affected cases. Haemolytic anaemia and dermal extramedullary haemopoiesis that resembles the skin manifestation seen in congenital leukaemia, so-called 'blueberry muffin', are other haematological abnormalities seen.

Cytomegalovirus (CMV). Like the other herpesviruses, especially herpes simplex (type I and II), CMV can cause thrombocytopenia in the fetus and newborn. In two published studies thrombocytopenia was observed in 36% and 77% of infants infected with CMV, and in the former the platelet count was below $50 \times 10^9/l$ in greater than one-third of the infants.

Herpes simplex. Infection with herpes simplex only causes problems to the fetus when the mother has a primary infection prior to 20 weeks' gestation, and thrombocytopenia is a well-established haematological abnormality associated with this infection.

Other causes of intrauterine viral-induced neonatal thrombocytopenia include human immunodeficiency virus (HIV) and parvovirus B19. Estimates of the rates of HIV viral transmission from mother to newborn are variable, between 20% and 60% depending on the study. The risk is reduced significantly when the mother is asymptomatic but increases with the length of time that she is seropositive. Thrombocytopenia is rarely if ever the first clinical manifestation of congenital HIV and, like parvovirus B19 infection, thrombocytopenia seems to be less frequently seen than with the other well-established causes of intrauterine viral-induced thrombocytopenia.

Other causes of congenital thrombocytopenia are shown in Table 8.3.

FUNCTIONAL PLATELET DISORDERS

Platelet function defects can result from a diminished platelet response to weak agonists (storage pool defects and release defects or aspirin-like syndromes) or where there is an absence of platelet aggregation to all agonists such as is seen in Glanzmann's thrombasthenia, dysfibrinogenaemia or afibrinogenaemia (Table 8.4). These disorders cause primary haemostatic bleeding ranging from mild to severe.

Glanzmann's thrombasthenia

This is an inherited disorder resulting from a quantitative or qualitative defect within the GPIIb–IIIa receptor complex. The diagnostic features are absent platelet aggregation to ADP, collagen, adrenaline and thrombin, but they do agglutinate in the presence of ristocetin. The only available curative treatment for these patients is bone marrow transplantation, which to date has been performed successfully in a number of patients. Because of the risk of platelet antibody formation, platelet transfusion should be given judiciously, and also when dental work is being performed the use of tranexamic acid and/or DDAVP may be worthwhile.

STORAGE POOL DISORDERS

These include patients with deficiencies of dense granules, α-granules and both types of granules – so-called storage pool diseases. A number of inherited thrombocytopenic conditions have associated storage pool disease and have been mentioned above, such as Chediak–Higashi, Wiskott–Aldrich, and TAR syndromes as well as the May–Hegglin anomaly and Gray platelet syndrome. Inherited abnormalities in platelet metabolism such as cycloxygenase deficiency, thromboxane synthetase deficiency and thromboxane A_2 receptor defects can give rise to impairment of platelet content release.

Classically, storage pool disorders and release defects are associated with an abnormal second wave of aggregation, secondary to abnormal release of nucleotides from the

Table 8.4 Platelet function disorders
Storage pool disorders (SPD)
Dense granule storage pool disease (δ-SPD)
Hermansky–Pudlak
Chediak–Higashi
Wiskott–Aldrich
TAR
May–Hegglin
α-granule storage pool disease
Gray platelet syndrome
α,δ-storage pool disease
Release defects
Aspirin-like syndromes
Cyclooxygenase deficiency
Thromboxane synthetase deficiency
Thromboxane A_2 receptor defects
Drug-induced
Aspirin
Other non-steroidal anti-inflammatory agents
Furosemide
Nitrofurantoin

storage granules. Platelet aggregation studies may not always identify these patients and therefore it is prudent to measure the contents of the adenine nucleotides in the α-granules as a measure of release. It should be remembered that renal and liver failure; aspirin and non-steroidal anti-inflammatory drugs are relatively common causes of acquired defects in platelet function in children. Treatment is aimed at removing a potential cause, and in those with inherited defects the use of DDAVP, cryoprecipitate and/or platelet infusions is the mainstay of treating severe haemorrhagic diseases.

Inherited collagen–vascular disorders that can cause primary haemostatic bleeding include Ehlers–Danlos syndrome, pseudoxanchoma elasticum, Marfan's syndrome, oestogenesis imperfecta and hereditary haemorrhagic telangectasia (HHT).

FURTHER READING

Christensen RD, ed. (2000) *Haematological Problems of the Neonate*. Philadelphia: WB Saunders.

Hoffman R, Benz EJ, Shattil SJ, Furie B, Cohen HT, Silberstein LE, McGlave P, eds. (2000) *Haematology Basic Principles and Practice*, 3rd edn. Edinburgh: Churchill Livingstone.

Lilleyman J, Hann I, Blanchette V, eds. (1999) *Paediatric Haematology*, 2nd edn. Edinburgh: Churchill Livingstone.

Loscalzo J, Schafer A, eds. (1998) *Thrombosis and Haemorrhage*, 2nd edn. Baltimore: Williams and Wilkins.

Williams Y, Lynch S, McCann S, Smith O, Feighery C, Whelan A. (1998) *Br J Haematol* **101**: 779–82.

9 Secondary haemostatic defects

Owen P Smith

INTRODUCTION

Haemophilia A (factor VIII deficiency) is the second commonest inherited bleeding disorder in man, with a frequency of approximately 1 in 5000 male births. Haemophilia B (factor IX deficiency) is approximately one-sixth as common as haemophilia A. When there is a family history of haemophilia, newborns are usually picked up early, as the condition is usually suspected. However, in one-third to one-half of all affected individuals, the haemophilia A or B arises from de novo mutations and it may be some time before a firm diagnosis is made, as a significant number of these children will be seen in the general paediatric setting. Haemophilia has a worldwide distribution, and affects all racial groups. Haemophilia A and B are clinically indistinguishable. In the severe form, the phenotype is characterized by bleeding into the joints and soft tissues. Both the factor VIII and factor IX genes were cloned over 15 years ago and as a result recombinant factor VIII and factor IX are the treatment of choice, at least in the western world, as we begin the new millennium. Cure with gene therapy may also be realized in the first decade of the first century of the new millennium.

INHERITED SECONDARY HAEMOSTATIC DEFECTS

The first documented account of an inherited bleeding disorder was in the second century AD. The Babylonian Talmud describes the decision of Rabbi Juddah that the son of a woman whose three previous sons had bled to death following circumcision be excused from the rite. Although further descriptions by Arabic physicians appear in the twelfth century, it was not until the eighteenth century that the first reports on a possible genetic basis and effective treatment with blood transfusion appeared. By the 1950s, fresh frozen plasma was the main treatment, and then in the late 1960s Poole and Shannon made the first major advance in haemophilia treatment with the discovery that factor VIII was concentrated in cryoprecipitate. This discovery made it possible for blood banks to prepare a potent 'wet' concentrate, and together with the plasma industry's advances in coagulation factor concentrate preparation, haemophilia care was dramatically altered from being a solely hospital-based management to one where treatment could be home-administered immediately following trauma or the first sign of bleeding. This major innovation in prophylaxis markedly reduced hospitalizations and the incidence of crippling deformities in children and adolescents with haemophilia A and B. Advances in recombinant DNA technology led to the cloning of the factor VIII and factor IX genes in the early 1980s. Today, we have two recombinant factor VIII gene products and both have been shown to be safe, effective and extremely well tolerated in both children and adults. The next milestone in the history of haemophilia treatment clearly will be curing the disease, with gene therapeutics.

Haemophilia A and B

The term 'haemophilia' originally applied to a life-long haemorrhagic disorder; however, by the early 1950s the disease was classified into two types based on specific plasma protein deficiencies. Factor VIII deficiency (haemophilia A) and factor IX deficiency (haemophilia B) are both inherited as sex-linked recessive disorders and together occur with an approximate frequency of 1 in 10 000 of the population.

Factor VIII deficiency

Haemophilia A is the most severe and (after von Willebrand's disease – see Chapter 8) the second commonest congenital bleeding disorder. Its relatively high incidence is in part due to the high mutation rate and the X-linked pattern of inheritance. A large number of mutations in the genes encoding factor VIII and factor IX have been found. In approximately one-third of newly diagnosed infants with haemophilia, there is no family history of the disorder and the haemophilia has resulted from spontaneous (de novo) mutations. The gene encoding factor VIII is large, comprising 186 kilobases and 26 exons. The commonest genetic defect causing factor VIII deficiency is the so-called inversion 22, which can be detected by Southern blot analysis (see Chapter 3). Other types of genetic defects within the factor VIII gene causing factor VIII deficiency are shown in Table 9.1.

The normal factor VIII molecule is a glycoprotein, synthesized mainly in the hepatocyte, which circulates in a stable complex with von Willebrand factor protein. Coagulant activity is termed factor VIII activity (factor VIII:C) while the immunological quantitation of factor VIII is factor VIII antigen (VIII:C Ag). Following activation by factor Xa and thrombin, factor VIIIa acts as a cofactor for factor IXa in the formation of factor Xa. It is not surprising therefore that the clinical

syndromes associated with haemophilia A and B are phenotypically identical.

Haemorrhagic complications in moderate and severe haemophilia may become obvious after birth, especially if the child is circumcised. Severity and type of bleeding are related to the absolute level of circulating plasma factor VIII:C (Table 9.2). A minimal effective level for haemostasis is about 25–30 U/dl for haemophilia A and 20–25 U/dl for haemophilia B. Those with severe deficiency (<1 U/dl) usually experience repeated and often spontaneous haemorrhages, most commonly haemarthroses, and if they are not treated adequately will develop chronic synovitis resulting in target joint formation with eventual crippling arthropathy. While musculoskeletal bleeding is by far the commonest clinical event, other spontaneous haemorrhagic manifestations frequently occur and may be life-threatening (Table 9.2). Significant reductions in the number of bleeds and overall morbidity, especially in children with severe haemophilia A and B, can be achieved by the early introduction between 1 and 2 years of age of thrice weekly (30–35 U/kg each infusion) or alternate daily prophylactic factor replacement therapy. While long-term studies are needed to assess the overall cost-effectiveness of prophylaxis, it is clear that prevention of chronic joint damage and other long-term side-effects of recurrent bleeding can be achieved with such an approach.

Successful treatment in acute or potentially acute (pre-surgery) bleeding is usually achieved with adequate and prompt factor replacement therapy (Table 9.3). The level of factor concentrate required to achieve adequate haemostasis will depend on the type of bleeding. It should be remembered that the initial plasma half-life of infused factor VIII:C is 3–6 hours during equilibration with the extravascular space; thereafter the plasma half-life will be approximately 12 hours. As stated above, the amount of factor concentrate given will depend on the type of bleed and also on the weight of the child.

One unit of factor VIII:C/kg body weight raises the factor VIII:C level by 2% (2 U/dl), or: units of factor VIII:C equals body weight (kg) $\times$ the desired level (U/dl) $\times$ 0.5. For the

Table 9.1 Documented haemophilia A mutations	
• Gross deletions	• Frameshift
• Insertions	• Nonsense
• Duplications	• Splice site
• Intron 22	consensuses
inversion	• Missense

Table 9.2 Bleeding manifestations in haemophilia A and B in relation to absolute level of circulating plasma factor VIII: C

	Severe (<1 U/dl)	Moderate (1–4 U/dl)	Mild (5–40 U/dl)
Age of onset:	<1 year	<2 years	>2 years
Type of bleeding			
Haemarthroses:			
Spontaneous	+ + + +	+ +	−
Following minor trauma	+ + + +	+ + +	−
Muscle haematoma	+ + + +	+ +	−
Central nervous system	+ +[a]	+	−
Haematuria	+ + + +	+ +	−
Surgery	+ + + +	+ + +	+ +
Dental extraction	+ + + +	+ + +	+ +
Trauma to soft tissue:			
Mild	+ + + +	+ +	−
Significant	+ + + +	+ + +	+

[a] Prevalence approximately 3% (mean age 14 years).
+ + + +, usual, + + +, common, + +, less common, +, rare, −, very rare.

majority of early superficial soft tissue bleeds and haemarthroses, factor VIII levels of 25–30 U/dl are usually adequate. If the bleed is more severe and a longer period of treatment is anticipated, then the desired level should be between 30 and 50 U/dl. Increasing the level above 50 U/dl is sufficient to treat major soft tissue or visceral bleeds and minor surgical procedures. With major surgery, a pre-operative level of 100 U/dl is considered mandatory by most physicians treating haemophilia, and therefore daily trough levels of 50–100 U/dl for approximately 7–12 days are sufficient to facilitate wound healing. With severe or pharyngeal and CNS bleeding, 100 U/dl correction is also required, and treatment is usually more protracted. Indeed, in patients with an intracerebral bleed, it may be necessary to continue treatment until imaging reveals that the brain lesion has fully resolved.

Factor IX deficiency

Haemophilia B is the third commonest inherited bleeding disorder following von Wille-brand's disease and haemophilia A, with a prevalence of 10–15% that of haemophilia A. As with factor VIII treatment the dosage and frequency of administration of factor IX is governed by the type of bleeding and its plasma half-life (18–24 hours) (Table 9.3). Unlike factor VIII, recovery of infused factor IX is lower than expected – presumably because factor IX is absorbed to sites in the vascular endothelium, recently shown to be collagen IV. Thus these patients require approximately twice the amount per dose once daily to treat bleeding. The exception is on the first day of surgery, when a twice-daily dose is usually administered to achieve the desired level.

Factor IX concentrates are also known as prothrombin complex concentrates (PCCs) because they contain a lot of vitamin K-dependent factors II and X and occasionally factor VII. They have been the mainstay of replacement therapy in haemophilia B patients with haemorrhagic episodes requiring prophylaxis for surgery. Their usage over the past few years, however, has been in decline because of the associated risk of thrombosis and disseminated intravascular

Table 9.3 Guidelines for factor replacement therapy for haemorrhage in haemophilia A and B

Site of bleed	Haemostatic factor level	Factor dosing		Comment
		Haemophilia A	Haemophilia B	
Joint	30–50 U/dl minimum	20–40 U/kg qd as needed	30–40 U/kg qd as needed	Rest/immobilization/physical therapy rehabilitation following bleed. Several doses may be necessary to prevent or treat target joint.
Muscle	40–50 U/dl minimum	20–40 U/kg qd as needed	40–60 U/kg qd as needed	Calf/forearm bleed is limb-threatening, significant blood loss with femoral/ retroperitoneal bleed.
Oral mucosa	Initially 50 U/dl; then antifibrinolytic coverage usually suffices	25 U/kg	50 U/kg	Antifibrinolytic therapy is critical. Do not use PCCs or APCCs.
Epistaxis	Initially 80–100 U/dl; then 30 U/dl until healing occurs	40–50 U/kg; then 30–40 U/kg qd	80–100 U/kg; then 70–80 U/kg qd	Local measures: Pressure/packing/cautery useful for severe or recurrent bleed
Gastrointestinal	Initially 100 U/dl, then 30 U/dl until healing occurs	40–50 U/kg; then 30–40 U/kg qd	80–100 U/kg; then 70–80 U/kg qd	Lesion is usually found – endoscopy highly recommended. Antifibrinolytic therapy may be useful.
Genitourinary	Initially 100 U/dl, then 30 U/dl until healing occurs	40–50 U/kg; then 30–40 U/kg qd	80–100 U/kg; then 70–80 U/kg qd	Evaluate for stones or urinary tract infection. Lesion usually not found. Prednisolone 1–2 mg/kg/d × 5–7 days may be useful.
Central nervous system	Initially 100 U/dl, then 50–100 U/dl for 14 days	50 U/kg; then 25 U/kg q 12 hours or by continuous infusion	100 U/kg; then 50 U/kg q 24 hours. Continuous infusion or HPPs may be possible	Anticonvulsants frequently used preventatively, neuro follow-up. Lumbar puncture requires prophylactic factor coverage.
Trauma or surgery	Initially 100 U/dl; then 50 U/dl until wound healing begins; then 30 U/dl until wound healing complete	50 U/kg; then dose q 12 hours or by continuous infusion	100 U/kg; then dose q 24 hours or as above	Perioperative and postoperative management plan must be in place pre-op; evaluation for inhibitors crucial prior to elective surgery.

HPP, high-purity product; PCC, prothrombin complex concentrates; APCC, activated prothrombin complex concentrates.
Reprinted with permission from DiMichele D. (1996) *Pediatric Clinics of North America* **43**(3): 709–36.

coagulation due to the presence of activated factors such as factor Xa, VIIa and trace amounts of thrombin. More recently, the vast majority of patients with haemophilia B are being treated with high-purity factor IX products produced by monoclonal antibody immuno-affinity purification techniques. These products have been shown to be less likely than PCCs to produce thromboembolic side-effects. Recently, recombinant factor IX (Benefix, Genetics Institute–Baxter Hyland) has been introduced. Recovery of recombinant factor IX is less than that of plasma-derived factor IX. Thus, to raise a given individual's plasma concentration by 1% the recombinant product should be given in doses of 1.2 U/kg rather than 1.0 U/kg for the plasma-derived products.

Factor VIII and factor IX inhibitors

Inhibitors have been documented against all coagulation factors, but they are most frequently directed against factor VIII. The development of inhibitors to factor VIII in patients with haemophilia significantly complicates effective replacement therapy. The precise incidence of inhibitor development is not known. However, with factor VIII it is said to occur in approximately 20% of patients and with factor IX in 5% of patients. There is no evidence that pure products, that is monoclonally purified and recombinant factor VIII or factor IX, induce more inhibitor formation than the earlier intermediate-purity products.

The inhibitors themselves are all allo-antibodies, usually of the IgG class 4, kappa light-chain type with varying abilities to neutralize the procoagulant action of factor VIII. Once induced, these antibodies rarely disappear spontaneously, unlike auto-antibodies to factor VIII. They are usually first suspected when the patient responds suboptimally to factor VIII therapy, and the presence of an antibody is then quantified using an in vitro assay measuring the inhibitory effect expressed in Bethesda units (BU) or New Oxford units (OU). One Bethesda unit (BU) is equal to the amount of patient plasma that inactivates half of the factor VIII in an equal mixture (50:50 mix) of normal pooled reference plasma and patient plasma incubated at 37°C for 2 hours. The Oxford method uses lyophilized factor VIII concentrate instead of normal plasma with an incubation time of 4 hours at the same temperature. One BU is equal to 1.2 OU.

The inhibitor status can be classified as high response or low response, depending on the rise in plasma inhibitory activity following infusions of factor VIII. This rise usually begins 3–5 days after infusion of factor VIII and peaks approximately 3 weeks thereafter. If the antibody increment is more than 5 BU, the patient is said to be a 'high responder' having an anamnestic response and is unlikely to respond to factor VIII, whereas 'low responders' may have a favourable response to standard or higher doses of factor VIII infusions. Unfortunately, the majority of patients with inhibitors are 'high responders'.

It is not always possible to predict favourable clinical response in patients with inhibitors following infusions of factor VIII, as no two patients with similar levels of antibodies behave in the same way. Likewise it is almost impossible to predict those patients who will develop inhibitors in the first instance; however, age, severity, exposure days, race and family history of inhibitors appear to be more important predictors.

The management of patients with factor VIII inhibitors continues to be a challenging clinical problem. Because of the small number of patients with inhibitors, no randomized trials had been carried out as of 2001. The various therapeutic approaches that are currently used are based on the type and severity of haemorrhage, antibody titre, anamnestic response and the availability of therapeutic options (Table 9.4). Clearly, the treatment of choice would result in a persistently raised factor VIII coagulant activity, but this may not always be possible and other treatments that bypass factor VIII may be required to achieve adequate haemostasis. If the antibodies are in high titre, it is important to consider other therapies that may reduce the inhibitor level and allow greater efficacy of infused factor VIII.

Table 9.4 Therapeutic modalities for patients with factor VIII inhibitors

Increasing factor VIII levels
    Desmopressin (DDAVP)
    Human factor VIII
    Porcine factor VIII

Bypassing agents
    Prothrombin complex concentrates
    Activated prothrombin complex
        concentrates
    Recombinant human factor VIIa

Reducing inhibitor levels
    Immune tolerance therapy
    Immunoglobulin infusion
    Plasma exchange
    Protein A sepharose affinity column
    Immunosuppression (cytotoxics)

Treatment of the acute bleeding

In general, the amount of inhibitor(s) circulating is roughly inversely related to the success of most treatment options. When present in low titre (<5 BU) it may be possible to saturate the antibody using high doses of factor VIII, followed by lower-dose schedules to raise the plasma factor VIII concentration into a range promoting haemostasis. While the main objective of this approach is to achieve a measurable factor VIII level, preferably between 30 and 50 U/dl, it must be remembered that the clinical response does not always correlate with the plasma level. Once bleeding is controlled, a maintenance treatment programme is undertaken that reflects the type and severity of haemorrhage. In applying this approach, all currently available factor VIII concentrates can be used, as no one preparation has been shown to have a clear advantage over others. If an inhibitor is present in low amounts in a patient with mild haemophilia who has sustained minor bleeding, it may be worth administering desmopressin (DDAVP, 0.3 µg/kg) to release any endogenous stores of factor VIII, thus inactivating the inhibitor and allowing the normal circulating factor VIII to become effective. Desmopressin is contraindicated in severe haemophilia and/or severe bleeds. In the relatively recent past, porcine factor VIII (Hyate:C, Porton-Speywood, UK) was used in the treatment of patients with factor VIII as the porcine factor VIII had a lower degree of cross-reactivity to anti-human factor VIII but retained a measurable activity in the human coagulation system. As more effective treatments have become available, mainly the bypassing agents, porcine factor VIII has fallen out of favour with most physicians treating haemophilia.

Bypassing agents

The treatment of choice for patients with high-responding factor VIII inhibitors are bypassing agents, mainly recombinant human factor VIIa (rhVIIa) and the PCCs. It is becoming more apparent that the former is now the treatment of choice. Development of rhVIIa represents an exciting new advance in bypassing-agent therapy in the treatment of haemophiliacs with antibodies against factor VIIIc and factor IX. Because rhVIIa requires tissue factor to complex with it before it can achieve its full proteolytic potential, it will only activate factor X and factor IX at those sites where tissue factor is generated. This 'site-specific' activation greatly reduces the systemic coagulopathy that is seen with other bypassing agents. Additional advantages using this agent are that it can be given independent of antibody titre and used in haemophilia B patients, it is not inactivated by antithrombin and possible viral contamination is eliminated. It is administered every 2–3 hours initially in the case of severe bleeding at doses of 70–100 µg/kg. The duration of treatment is governed by the clinical response and type of bleed. While good to excellent results have been reported, the optimal dose scheduling for efficacy and cost are only beginning to be fully realized.

The activated PCCs (Hyland's Autoplex and Immuno's FEIBA) are the best known plasma-derived bypassing agents. The main problem in the past has been that there were some side-effects of systemic coagulopathy (thrombosis and bleeding) and myocardial infarction when given in repeated doses. However, despite these side-effects, these bypassing agents have until very recently been the mainstay of treatment of bleeding in inhibitor patients.

Reducing inhibitor levels

A number of methodologies have been tried and tested in children with high-responding factor VIII inhibitors. The most successful of these has been immune tolerance treatment (ITT) using a variety of different protocols. Common to all of these protocols are the main drawbacks of this therapy: its cost, the length of time to achieve tolerance being months to years and the fact that it is labour-intensive. Furthermore, like all available treatments for factor VIII inhibitors, response is not guaranteed. What is clear, however, is that the earlier that treatment starts and the lower the inhibitor level at commencement of ITT, the greater the chance that the child will be tolerized. A randomized trial looking at high-dose factor VIII will hopefully occur in North America, Europe and Australasia in 2002.

In haemophilia B the development of antibodies is significantly lower than in haemophilia A. One complication of factor IX replacement therapy is anaphylactic shock, which is more likely to occur in those without detectable factor IX antigen, and this anaphylaxis occurs in approximately half of the children severely affected with antibodies against factor IX. The treatment of choice for these high-risk children is rhVIIa. Children without a history of anaphylaxis can receive rhVIIa or FEIBA. Immune tolerance therapy has also been successfully used in patients with factor IX allo-antibodies. Nephrotic syndrome has been a complication in some of these patients.

Carrier detection

A woman is an obligate carrier of haemophilia if one of the following conditions is met:

1. Her father has haemophilia.

2. She has given birth to two or more sons with haemophilia.
3. She has given birth to one son with haemophilia and there is a well-documented family history of haemophilia on the maternal side of her pedigree.

Therefore, carrier testing is unnecessary if the individual is an obligate carrier. It must be remembered, however, that a detailed history is imperative and can provide considerable insight into the likelihood of carriership. Laboratory confirmation that a woman is carrying a faulty factor VIII or factor IX gene is divided into two kinds of analysis, namely clotting factor assays and DNA-based techniques. If the woman's factor VIII (or factor IX) level is very low, it is reasonably certain that she is a carrier. The ratio of factor VIII (or factor IX) activity and factor VIII (or factor IX) antigen in her plasma can also be determined. If she has considerably less factor VIII (or factor IX) activity than antigen, this indicates that one of her factor VIII (or factor IX) genes is directing production of an abnormal (and non-functional) form of factor VIII (or factor IX); that is, she is a carrier for haemophilia. It must be remembered, however, that such testing only gives a probability, which is not helpful in approximately one-sixth of cases. Therefore, genetic diagnosis by analysis of factor VIII or factor IX genes within families by either polymorphism-based gene tracking (linkage analysis) or mutational detection are the preferred methods of carrier detection and prenatal diagnosis of haemophilia. Polymorphism-based gene tracking, although having several limitations, is much simpler and more widely available than mutation detection. Its use permits accurate and rapid determination of female carrier status and prenatal diagnosis in a large proportion of families analysed to date. It must be remembered that carrier detection in prenatal diagnosis has become increasingly an integral part of the care of a patient and family with haemophilia.

Other coagulation factor deficiencies

Deficiencies of all coagulation factors have been described (Table 9.5). However, it should

Table 9.5 Laboratory diagnosis, therapeutic options, genetics and original descriptions of the inherited secondary haemostatic disorders

Deficiency	PT	APTT	TT	Factor assay (U/dl)	Half-life (hours)	Levels needed for haemostasis (U/dl)	Treatment choice	Genetics	Original description (name/year)
Factor VIII	N	↑	N	<50	12	100	FVIII (pd/rh)	X-R	
Factor IX	N	↑	N	<50	24	100	FIX (pd/rh)	X-R	
Fibrinogen	↑	↑	↑	<50	120	100 mg/dl	FI (pd) or cryo	AR/Ch 4	Raba/1920
Prothrombin	↑	↑	N	<50	50–80	25–35	PCC	AR/Ch 11	Morawitz/1905
Factor V	↑	↑	N	<50	36	20–35	FFP	AR/Ch 1	Owren/1947
Factor VII	↑	N	N	<50	6	15	FVII (pd/rh)	AR/Ch 13	Alexander/1951
Factor X	↑	↑	N	<50	25–60	10–20	PCC	AR/Ch 13	Hougie/1957
Factor XI	N	↑	N	<35	40–80	40–60	FIX (pd) or FFP	AR/Ch 4	Rosenthal/1953
Factor XII	N	↑	N	<50	–	–	–	AR/Ch 4	Ratnoff/1955
PK	N	↑	N	–	–	–	–	AR/Ch 4	Hathaway/1965
HMWK	N	↑	N	–	–	–	–	AR/Ch 3	Saito/1975
Factor XIII	N	N	N	<5	150	1–3	FXIII (pd) or FFP	AR/α,Ch 6, β,Ch 1	Duckert/1960

PT, prothrombin time; APTT, activated partial thromboplastin time; TT, thrombin time; ↑, increased; N, normal; AR, autosomal recessive; X-R, X-linked recessive-PK, prekallikrein; HMWK, high-molecular-weight kininogen; pd, plasma-derived; Ch, chromosome; rh, recombinant human; FFP, fresh frozen plasma; PCC, prothrombin complex concentrate; cryo, cryoprecipitate; α, alpha chain of factor XIII; β, beta chain of factor XIII.

be remembered that the number of patients with haemophilia A greatly outnumbers all of these put together. Common features of these rarer forms of coagulation factor deficiencies include variable bleeding and autosomal recessive inheritance. Below are brief descriptions of the salient features of these deficiencies.

Fibrinogen

Fibrinogen deficiencies can be grouped into those where there is a quantitative defect (hypo- and afibrinogenaemia) and those with qualitative defects (dysfibrinogenaemia). Afibrinogenaemia is associated with moderate to severe bleeding, which can occur spontaneously or following minimal trauma. Some patients develop haemarthroses, and vital organ haemorrhage is not uncommon. Prothrombin time, activated partial thromboplastin time and thrombin time (PT, APTT and TT) are all prolonged, as there is an inability to form a clot. On testing, the bleeding time is also prolonged and there is usually abnormal platelet aggregation to all agonists, resembling Glanzmann's thrombasthenia (see Chapter 8). Patients with hypofibrinogenaemia have a very mild bleeding tendency, but in the majority of patients no bleeding is documented whatsoever. The treatment of symptomatic patients is with fibrinogen concentrate, and when this is not available cryoprecipitate is the second best option. It should be remembered that patients with afibrinogenaemia run the risk of developing allo-antibodies and a number of patients are reported to have developed anaphylaxis following infusions of fibrinogen concentrate.

Dysfibrinogenaemia can present with bleeding, thrombosis or both. The PT and APTT are usually normal until the fibrinogen levels fall below 80 mg/dl. The TT is elevated, but it should be remembered that in a small minority of cases the TT can be shortened and these individuals may have thrombotic complications. The fibrinogen concentration can be normal or low. Most patients with dysfibrinogenaemia have a fibrinogen antigen that is markedly elevated above the fibrinogen activity levels.

The treatment of choice for patients with a quantitative defect in fibrinogen is fibrinogen concentrate or cryoprecipitate. It should be remembered that prophylactic therapy is generally not recommended because of the serious risk of developing antibodies with associated anaphylaxis. Most individuals with dysfibrinogenaemia, on the other hand, do not require therapy. However, in those who have a history of bleeding and are at high risk of bleeding, for example following major surgery, fibrinogen concentrate or cryoprecipitate can be given. In those individuals with a history of thrombotic events, oral anticoagulation therapy is the treatment of choice.

Prothrombin

Prothrombin deficiency is an extremely rare bleeding disorder characterized by markedly elevated PT and APTT, with the former being elevated to a greater extent. The disorder is autosomal recessive. The patients bleed soon after birth. The diagnosis is confirmed by factor II assay, which is reduced whilst the other vitamin K-dependent factors are within the normal range. Patients should be treated with PCCs or plasma to achieve a prothrombin level of between 25 and 35 U/dl. Given the long half-life of prothrombin, repeated infusions are usually not necessary for isolated bleeding episodes.

Factor V

Factor V deficiency is an autosomal recessive bleeding disorder and the levels of factor V tend not to correlate, with the bleeding tendency. Plasma and platelet levels of factor V do not necessarily correlate, and the clinical tendency may depend more on the level of platelet factor V. It should be remembered that approximately one-fifth of the body mass of factor V is found in platelet α-granules. PT and APTT are prolonged and it is necessary to check the factor VIII levels in these patients, as combined factor V and factor VIII deficiency has now been described in over 50 families. The gene causing this combined deficiency has been mapped to 18q21, the gene product of which is an intermediate Golgi department protein (ERGKP53). As there is no factor V concentrate available, patients are treated with viral-inactivated plasma aiming to bring the factor V clotting activity to approximately 20–25 U/dl. An initial plasma dose to raise the level to 15–20 U/dl, followed by 3–6 U/dl every 24 hours, is appropriate, since the half-life of factor V is 36 hours. Platelets containing factor V can also be given in cases of severe bleeding. It should be remembered, however, that patients may develop platelet antibodies and therefore this treatment should be withheld unless the clinical situation dictates that platelets should be given.

Factor VII

This condition is again autosomal recessive and is associated with severe bleeding similar to that seen in haemophilia A and B. Interestingly, some patients with very low levels of factor VII do not have any bleeding problems while some patients with low levels have developed thrombotic events. It is clear, however, that the majority of patients with levels in excess of 2 U/dl do not have major bleeding problems. The precise explanation for this remains to be fully elucidated. Patients have an isolated prolonged PT and the diagnosis is confirmed by factor assay. Treatment is with specific factor VII concentrate, and because factor VII has a short half-life it must be infused frequently, that is every two to three hours. Plasma-derived and recombinant factor VIIa are commercially available.

Factor X

Individuals who have severe factor X deficiency (<1%) usually have a phenotype identical to that of individuals with severe haemophilia A or B. A small number of patients will bleed extensively, exhibiting both primary and haemostatic-type bleeding. These patients run a high risk of spontaneous intracerebral bleeds. The precise mechanism responsible for this very severe phenotype is not fully understood but probably reflects the role that factor Xa plays in the prothrombinase complex. Menorrhagia is frequent in adolescent females, and oestrogens may be of help in raising the factor X level in such individuals. Factor X activity levels of 10–15 U/dl are adequate to control minor bleeding such as haemarthroses and soft tissue bleeds. Prothrombin complex concentrates are rich in factor X, and these can be given to the severe patient on a prophylactic basis. Patients with factor X deficiency rarely develop alloantibodies.

Factor XI

Factor XI deficiency is an uncommon coagulopathy with an autosomal recessive inheritance and is particularly prevalent among Ashkenazi Jews of Eastern European descent. It is somewhat unique in showing a poor correlation in both the heterozygote and the homozygote between circulating factor XI level and bleeding tendency. Patients who are symptomatic tend to have a mild to moderate bleeding disorder with an isolated elevated APTT. Bleeding usually occurs late in life or after surgical or dental procedures. Factor XI concentrate is available, but because of a number of reported thrombotic complications with its use caution is required in ensuring that the level of factor XI does not exceed 100 U/dl. Patients undergoing minor surgical/dental procedures usually respond favourably to antifibrinolytic agents such as tranexamic acid.

Contact factor proteins

Deficiencies in factor XII, prekallikrein and high-molecular-weight kininogen, although giving a prolongation of the APTT, are not in the main associated with a bleeding diathesis. They are usually picked up following investigation of a prolonged APTT in a patient going for surgery. Once diagnosed, the patient and surgical colleagues can be reassured that these deficiencies are not associated with an increase predisposition to bleeding.

Factor XIII

Individuals clinically affected with factor XIII deficiency have plasma levels of less than 1 U/dl. The deficiency is usually associated with a high risk of intracranial haemorrhage and umbilical stump haemorrhage. Other bleeding manifestations include soft tissue haemorrhages, haemarthroses and haematomata. Surgery is usually complicated by poor wound healing and abnormal scar formation. Affected male individuals may have aligospermia, and females commonly have repeated spontaneous abortions. Since factor XIII deficiency does not prolong the PT, APTT or TT, specific testing must be carried out, such as quantitative assay showing fibrinoligase (factor XIII) activity. If this test is unavailable then solubility of a fibrin clot in 5 M urea is useful as a screening test.

As only small amounts of factor XIII are required for normal haemostasis and because the half-life of factor XIII is approximately 150 hours, prophylactic treatment for severely affected individuals can be given on a three- to four-weekly basis with factor XIII concentrate. Virally inactive plasma could also be used.

ACQUIRED SECONDARY HAEMOSTATIC DEFECTS

The acquired secondary haemostatic coagulation disorders are far more common than the inherited disorders and are usually associated with multiple coagulation factor deficiencies. These usually present with either prolongation of routine coagulation laboratory values such as PT, APTT or TT or indeed clinical bleeding. Table 9.6 outlines some of the commoner causes of acquired secondary haemostatic defects.

Extracorporeal membrane oxygenation (ECMO), metabolic disorders, disseminated intravascular coagulation (DIC) and massive transfusion syndromes are covered elsewhere in this book.

Vitamin K

Vitamin K is a fat-soluble vitamin, which is obtained predominantly from green vegetables and bacterial gut flora. It is crucial for the procoagulant factors II, VII, IX and X and the natural anticoagulants protein C and protein S. Its main function is as a cofactor in γ-carboxylation of these proteins. Vitamin K itself is recycled, and when this process is blocked as with warfarin administration, these vitamin K-dependent factors are not produced in adequate amounts.

Haemorrhagic disease of the newborn

This syndrome usually occurs on the second to fourth day of life as a result of decreased synthesis of vitamin K-dependent factors. The aetiology of vitamin K deficiency in newborns is multifactorial and includes reduction of vitamin K stored in the fetus and neonate, functional immaturity of the liver, lack of bacterial synthesis of vitamin K in the gut and low amounts of vitamin K in breast milk. Most children now are given vitamin K at birth. Exceptions to the rule are those children with known glucose-6-phosphate dehydrogenase (G6PD) deficiency in the family, as a significant number of these patients will develop frank haemolysis. In those children who present with frank bleeding, vitamin K and infusions of fresh frozen plasma can be given to arrest the blood loss.

Because vitamin K is fat-soluble and therefore depends on pancreatic lipases, bile and a normal intact intestinal anatomy, it is not surprising therefore that biliary obstruction, malabsorption and antibiotic usage can all give rise to vitamin K deficiency. Treatment is either oral or intravenous replacement; however, it should be remembered that the intravenous route is

Table 9.6 Acquired secondary haemostatic defects

• Vitamin K deficiency
    Haemorrhagic disease of the newborn
    Antagonism to vitamin K (warfarin)
    Malabsorption
    Biliary obstruction
    Antibiotics
• Liver disease
• Cardiopulmonary bypass surgery
• Extracorporeal membrane oxygenation
• Congenital heart disease
• Metabolic disorders (Gaucher's disease)
• Inhibitors of coagulation proteins
• Disseminated intravascular coagulation
• Massive transfusion syndrome

associated with an increased risk of anaphylaxis. As in haemorrhage disease of the newborn, haemostasis needs to be corrected rapidly, and fresh frozen plasma or indeed a cocktail of concentrates that contain factors VII, II, IX and X can be given instead.

Liver disease

The coagulopathy associated with liver disease is complex, involving reduced synthesis of vitamin K-dependent procoagulant factors, non-vitamin K-dependent procoagulant factors, structurally abnormal coagulation proteins such as seen in dysfibrinogenaemia, as well as a reduced amount of natural anticoagulants, protein C, protein S and increased fibrinolytic activity with elevated levels of tissue plasminogen activator (t-PA) and reduced α_2-antiplasmin. A significant number of these patients are also vitamin K-deficient because of associated malabsorption. It should also be noted that these children may have quantitative and qualitative platelet defects. Correcting the coagulopathy usually involves replacement of vitamin K and addition of fresh frozen plasma. When volume restriction is imperative, factor concentrates such as factor VII concentrate and PCC can be given along with platelets and DDAVP.

Cardiopulmonary bypass

Children undergoing cardiac pulmonary bypass may have significant haemorrhage either during the procedure or afterwards. The coagulopathy associated with cardiopulmonary bypass is multifactorial, involving activation of the contact pathway, fibrinolytic pathway, tissue factor pathway and platelets; also these children can suffer from significant platelet function defects. Paradoxically, some will develop heparin-induced thrombocytopenia, and this is discussed in greater detail, both in terms of pathogenesis and treatment in Chapter 10.

Congenital heart disease

A significant number of patients with congenital heart disease will have defects in primary haemostasis, but some will also have prolonged PT and APTT. A number of studies have shown that these are secondary to procoagulant factor deficiencies. It should be remembered, however, that in children with cyanotic heart disease with associated polycythaemia, the elevation in PT/APTT may be spurious, that is may be secondary to a sampling defect, as there will be an alteration in the plasma anticoagulant ratio, especially when the haematocrit is greater than 60%. This should always be remembered when interpreting coagulation results in these patients.

Acquired inhibitors in non-haemophiliac patients

These are usually directed against factor VIII. In children, they are extremely rare and are usually seen with the background of autoimmune disease. Bleeding manifestations are usually those seen in haemophilia A and B, and the treatment usually consists of bypassing-agent therapy (see above). Prompt recognition and treatment may be life-saving. Newborns born to mothers with a history of acquired factor VIII deficiency should be screened for factor VIII activity, as transplacental transfer of the inhibitor may occur. Inhibitors to all of the other coagulation factors have been reported but are extremely rare.

FURTHER READING

Berntorp E. (1996) The treatment of haemophilia: including prophylaxis, constant infusion and DDAVP. *Baillière's Clin Haematol* **9**: 259–71.

DiMichele D. (1996) Haemophilia. New approaches to an old disease. *Paediatr Clin North Am* **43**: 709–36.

Hathaway WE, Goodney SH. (1993) *Disorders of Haemostasis and Thrombosis: A Clinical Guide.* New York: McGraw-Hill.

Feinstein DI. (1994) Acquired disorders of Haemostasis. In: Coman RW, Hirsch J, Marder VJ, Salzman EW, eds. *Haemostasis and Thrombosis: Basic Principles in Clinical Practice*, 3rd edn. Philadelphia: JP Lippincott: 881–905.

Staudinger T, Locker GJ, Frass M. (1996) Management of acquired coagulation disorders in emergency and intensive care medicine. *Semin Thrombosis Haemostasis* **22**: 93–104.

10 Thrombotic disorders

Owen P Smith

INTRODUCTION

The rapid transformation of fluid blood to a gel-like substance (clot) has been recognized since antiquity. Around 2650 BC in China, Huang Ti wrote 'when it coagulates within the pulse the blood ceases to circulate beneficially; when the blood coagulates within the feet it causes pains and chills'. Early in the eighteenth century (1731), Petit appreciated that blood clotting was a means to stem blood loss from wounds, and indeed John Hunter some 80 years later ruled 'where there is full power of life, the vessels are capable of keeping the blood in the fluid state'. By 1852, Rokitansky differentiated one type of venous thrombosis that arises as a consequence of primary inflammatory or chemical changes in the blood. This idea was later developed and stated in a more specific fashion by Virchow (1856) in his classic triad of describing the causes of thrombosis: 'abnormalities of the blood vessels, alterations in the constituents of the blood and aberrations of blood flow'. In 1874, Osler helped describe platelet aggregation, and six years later Hayem sited the importance of platelet plugs in preventing blood loss after tissue injury. Howell and Holt's landmark paper in 1918 described the isolation of the first physiological anticoagulant molecule, antithrombin. They suggested that antithrombin and heparin are normal constituents of blood and together act as a safeguard against inappropriate intravascular clotting. We had to wait until 1965 for the first hereditary basis of thrombosis ('thrombophilia') to be established by Egberg, reporting antithrombin III deficiency as an autosomal disorder associated with recurrent familial venous thromboembolic phenomenon. By 1938, Silberberg had stated that the endothelial layer of blood vessels was most likely acting as a negative regulator of procoagulation. Since then, significant advances, especially in the past 10–15 years, have taken place in relation to understanding the clinical and molecular mechanisms of hypercoagulable states, both acquired and inherited.

Plasma levels of many of the haemostatic coagulation factors are lower in newborns than in older children and adults. At the end of gestation, a healthy normal newborn should have approximately half the adult values of the vitamin K-dependent coagulant factors (factors II, VII, IX and X) and contact factors (factors XII and XI, prekalikrein and high-molecular-weight kininogen). In preterm infants, these levels are even lower. The natural anticoagulants, antithrombin and protein S, are also approximately 50% of adult values at term, with a similar relationship to gestational age. The plasma levels of the procoagulant cofactors, factors V and VIII and fibrinogen, are the same in term infants as in adults. Like the coagulation system, the fibrinolytic system is also physiologically immature in the neonate. Overall, the fetus and neonate are less efficient in generating thrombin, and as a result thrombotic disease in early childhood is rare; when thrombotic disease is seen, either it is secondary to an acquired prothrombic state or the child has inherited gene defects predisposing to clot formation. However, when it does occur in childhood, it can be fatal or associated with several sequelae such as amputation, organ dysfunction and post-phlebitic syndrome. The peak incidence for these thrombotic events is undoubtedly the neonatal period, where the use of indwelling catheters in the tertiary-care paediatrics is almost the norm.

ACQUIRED THROMBOTIC TENDENCY (Table 10.1)

Central venous catheter devices

Central venous catheter devices have revolutionized the medical management of paediatric patients with a variety of different illnesses, ranging from neonates requiring indwelling vein or artery catheterization to older children undergoing bone marrow transplantation and high-dose chemotherapy, which is usually short-term. Patients requiring a more permanent fixed device include children receiving total parenteral nutrition for gastrointestinal pathology, small children requiring haemodialysis, children with cystic fibrosis requiring regular antibiotics and nutritional support, those with immuno-deficiency requiring antibiotics and immunoglobulin therapy, and children with inherited coagulation disorders such as haemophilia who require regular prophylactic concentrate administration.

Unfortunately, thrombosis related to the placement of such catheters continues to be a therapeutically challenging complication in terms of diagnosis, prophylaxis against thrombosis and also treatment of established thrombosis within the catheter. Regarding suspected thrombosis within the catheter or within the vessel, venography continues to be the gold standard investigation, and performance of linograms should be discouraged as these will give a high false-negative value. Once diagnosed, the line should be treated with heparin to prevent subsequent venous embolic events, and the very troublesome post-phlebitic syndrome. The vast majority of venous thromboembolic events in children occur in the upper limbs, as most catheters in young children are placed there. Once the catheter is in place, prevention of clot formation can be achieved using regular flushes of either unfractionated heparin or low-molecular-weight heparin into the catheter device. Removal of the catheter may be required, depending on the severity of symptoms and also what the future clinical needs for the child are. Once clot formation occurs, the catheter may be salvaged using either antithrombotic or antifibrinolytic agents; however, it should always be remembered that these therapeutics pose special risks in the paediatric age group compared with the adult age group in relation to haemorrhage.

Prophylactic anticoagulation against vessel thrombosis with warfarin has been shown to decrease the incidence of thrombosis from approximately 40% to 10% in one study of children receiving standard doses of chemotherapy. Low-molecular-weight heparin given subcutaneously has also been shown to reduce statistically significantly the incidence of thrombosis in children undergoing chemotherapy for cancer. Once catheter occlusions occur, these can be treated success-

---

Table 10.1 Acquired thrombotic tendency

- Indwelling vascular catheters

- Renal artery and vein thrombosis

- Acquired natural anticoagulant deficiency
  A. Nephrotic syndrome → antithrombin deficiency
  B. Purpura fulminans
     Varicella → protein S deficiency
     Meningococcaemia → protein C deficiency

- Necrotizing enterocolitis (NEC)

- Respiratory distress syndrome

- Heparin-induced thrombocytopenia/thrombosis syndrome (HIT/HITTs)

- Maternal anticardiolipin antibodies/lupus anticoagulant

- Extracorporeal membrane oxygenation (ECMO)

- Haemolytic uraemic syndrome/thrombotic thrombocytopenia purpura HUS/TTP

- Birth asphyxia

fully with the installation of intraluminal urokinase. It should also be remembered that, whilst very uncommon, death from venous thromboembolic disease in children does occur. Therefore, early detection of such thrombotic events and adequate treatment are absolutely mandatory in this group of children.

Renal artery and vein thrombosis

Renal artery thrombosis, especially in the neonatal period, is commonly associated with umbilical artery indwelling of umbilical artery catheters. It may be difficult to diagnose, and hypertension and heart failure may be the presenting clinical features. There is usually extension of the thrombus to other vascular beds such as the aorta. Its incidence can be as high as 1 in 6 neonates. Factors that can reduce its incidence include prophylactic anticoagulants, using a smaller catheter, and also concentration of fluids infused. Both medical and surgical approaches have been used, with variable outcome.

Renal vein thrombosis is more common than renal artery thrombosis in the neonatal period. It is associated with birth asphyxia, dehydration, hypotension, cyanotic heart disease, polycythaemia, and babies born to diabetic mothers. The commonest presenting features are flank swelling followed by haematuria, microscopic haematuria, renal dysfunction and thrombocytopenia. Usually ultrasound will reveal renal enlargement with or without evidence of venous thrombosis. The use of anticoagulants and thrombolytic agents in this condition continue to be evaluated. Survival rates in babies are as high as 80% and renal status after recovery ranges from normal function to renal atrophy, hypertension and chronic renal failure.

Natural anticoagulant deficiency

Purpura fulminans is a term used to describe an acute, often lethal, syndrome of disseminated intravascular coagulation (DIC) and purpuric skin. The skin lesion is rapidly progressive, characterized by microvascular thrombosis in the dermis, which ultimately results in perivascular haemorrhage and necrosis with minimal inflammation. Clinically, the lesion can be distinguished from simple haemorrhage into the skin, in that the lesions in purpura fulminans are usually raised and indurated and have a circumferential area of redness, and over time the lesions blister and break down, reflecting skin necrosis.

Inherited and acquired abnormalities of the protein C pathway are now believed to be responsible for the majority of patients with this clinical syndrome. The three commonest situations where purpura fulminans is seen are (i) severe bacterial infections, especially meningococcal disease, (ii) homozygous protein C or protein S deficiency, and (iii) autoimmune protein S deficiency. Rarer clinical conditions associated with purpura fulminans include warfarin-induced skin necrosis, cholestasis and antiphospholipid syndrome. In patients with severe meningococcaemia and purpura fulminans, these require immediate and intensive management. Early recognition, aggressive resuscitation and specific therapy are often required in the accident and emergency room, and this initial intervention is probably the single most important factor responsible for those who achieve a favourable outcome.

It is now known that the significant morbidity encountered in severe meningococcaemia is secondary to widespread microvascular thrombosis, resulting in tissue necrosis, which eventually leads to organ failure; in the majority of patients this leads to significant complications including skin grafting, amputation and renal dialysis. It is increasingly apparent that acquired protein C deficiency plays a crucial role in the pathophysiology of this syndrome. Protein C concentrate infusions have been used successfully in patients with severe acquired protein C deficiency secondary to meningococcaemia, resulting in a reduced mortality and morbidity. It must be emphasized, however, that protein C is used in this syndrome as an adjuvant haemostatic agent and perhaps also as an inflammatory modulator.

Autoimmune protein S deficiency has been reported in a number of patients with so-called idiopathic purpura fulminans and also in children with extensive thromboembolism. It is occasionally seen in infants and children in the convalescent period following varicella or streptococcal infection. The protein S levels are usually very low or undetectable at presentation, and auto-antibodies are usually IgG or IgM, which can be monoclonal or polyclonal in nature. These antibodies are transient, resulting occasionally in the inhibition of protein S activity, but more consistently they bind to protein S, resulting in increased protein S clearance from the circulation. The clinical picture is similar to that seen with severe acquired protein C deficiency induced by meningococcal sepsis, namely DIC, progressive purpura (which in time leads to extensive areas of skin necrosis), impaired perfusion of the limbs or digits, peripheral gangrene with limb amputation, and multiorgan dysfunction secondary to thromboembolic events. Sensible therapeutic outcome is dependent on early recognition of the underlying pattern of physiological mechanism responsible for the purpura lesions. Currently, protein S concentrates are not available and therefore replacement with plasma is the best alternative strategy, although it should be remembered that bringing the plasma protein S level into the normal range with infusions of plasma is rarely, if ever, achieved because of the small amount of protein S in fresh frozen plasma and the ability of the antibody to bind protein S, thus enhancing its clearance from the circulation. One of the best therapeutic options is to perform large-volume plasma exchange. Additionally, intravenous immunoglobulin may be of benefit as well. Antibodies directed against protein C are much less common.

Antithrombin deficiency

Acquired deficiencies of antithrombin have been associated with a large number of diseases, which in turn have an increased rate of venous and arterial thrombosis. As antithrombin is synthesized and secreted by the liver, it is not surprising that protein synthesis inhibition causes antithrombin deficiency. Antithrombin deficiency is more commonly seen in children with nephrotic

syndrome or inflammatory bowel disease and in those undergoing plasmapheresis. It should also be remembered that plasma turnover of antithrombin is increased by approximately one-quarter during heparin therapy and reverses on removal of the drug, that is there is a rebound state. Antithrombin concentrates are available for acquired and inherited deficiency states.

Necrotizing enterocolitis (NEC)

The majority of infants with necrotizing enterocolitis (NEC) have evidence of thrombocytopenia. In one study, 90% of infants studied had a platelet count of $<150 \times 10^9/l$ and over half had a platelet count of $<50 \times 10^9/l$. In the severe thrombocytopenic group, the majority had bleeding complications. A number of patients with NEC have evidence of DIC, and these usually show low functional and immunological evidence of antithrombin. Thrombosis in this condition is less of a problem than bleeding.

Respiratory distress syndrome

A significant number of infants with respiratory distress syndrome develop DIC. Postmortem findings in some of these infants who die from respiratory distress syndrome show pulmonary microvascular thrombosis. Increased levels of pro-inflammatory cytokines and concomitant downregulation of the protein C pathway, including low levels of circulating protein C as well as low levels of antithrombin, are most likely to be implicated in the thrombotic disease seen in this syndrome.

Heparin-induced thrombocytopenia/thrombosis syndrome (HIT/HITTS)

Heparin-induced thrombocytopenia (HIT) constitutes the severest adverse effect of heparin therapy. It has a highly variable incidence, depending on the type of heparin used and whether the patient was infected/inflamed at the time of heparin administration. The incidence generally varies between greater than 1% and less than 15% of adults receiving unfractionated heparin. The true incidence in children is not known. There are two types of HIT: type 1 occurs within 1–2 days of heparin administration, is non-immune and is usually totally benign; type 2 usually occurs after a later period of 7–14 days, is immune-mediated and is associated with paradoxical thrombosis–thromboembolism (HITTS). Fortunately, HITTS is extremely rare in neonates as well as children; nevertheless, when a child is receiving heparin, no matter how small the dose to keep a catheter patent or if having total parenteral nutrition, a watchful eye should always be kept on daily platelet counts. Accurate diagnosis is difficult and optimal treatment modalities are still to be established, especially in children. HITTS remains a devastating complication of the use of unfractionated heparin. Low-molecular-weight heparin induces less HIT/HITTS and as it becomes more used in paediatrics, less HIT/HITTS will be seen. Once established, HITTS should be treated by removing the heparin and administering either a heparinoid or recombinant hirudin.

The mechanism of HIT/HITTS is now known and is due to the development of antibodies to heparin–platelet factor 4 (PF4) complex. Platelet activation is mediated by the immune complex binding to the FcγRIIa receptor on the platelets, causing platelets to aggregate and produce thrombotic occlusion.

Antiphospholipid antibodies and lupus anticoagulant

Antiphospholipid antibodies are a heterogeneous group of antibodies that include lupus anticoagulant (LA) and anticardiolipin antibodies (ACLAs). Lupus anticoagulants are immunoglobulins that prolong the clotting time of in vitro phospholipid-dependent coagulation assays. Anticardiolipin antibodies are immunoglobulins that can be assessed by ELISA assay using cardiolipin as a target antigen. Although they are commonly associated with systemic lupus erythematosus, they are also seen in otherwise healthy individuals. There is a strong association between their presence and venous thromboembolic disease, both in adults and in children. In the asymptomatic child with positive ACLAs and/or LA who is undergoing surgery, it is difficult to know whether or not to give heparin prophylaxis. Anti-β_2-glycoprotein 1 status may help in this scenario, in that if the anti-β_2-glycoprotein 1 level is high then the thrombogenic potential is greater and therefore prophylactic anticoagulation may be prudent. To date no prospective clinical trials have been carried out. Both venous and arterial disease can occur in children with ACLAs, especially those who have concomitant thrombocytopenia, that is antiphospholipid syndrome.

Extracorporeal membrane oxygenation (ECMO)

Another procedure associated with thrombotic disease is extracorporeal membrane oxygenation (ECMO). This technique allows for artificial oxygenation in patients in whom cardiovascular respiratory failure has occurred. Whilst haemorrhage is more common in children on ECMO, in particular intracranial haemorrhage, thrombotic disease also occurs. Markers of coagulation activation and thrombin generation are usually present in these patients, and in one series of neonatal surgical patients treated with ECMO, 7% developed thrombosis during treatment. Other studies have suggested the incidence to be higher, and superior venocaval and inferior venocaval clotting is the commonest documented.

Haemolytic uraemic syndrome (HUS)

Haemolytic uraemic syndrome (HUS) is a severe clinical disease characterized by thrombocytopenia, micro-angiopathic haemolytic anaemia and renal failure. Whilst the pathobiology of the syndrome has not been fully elucidated, the fibrin–platelet thrombus in the microcirculation is initiated in the majority of patients by bacterial toxins that can induce endothelial damage in some renal and extrarenal arteries, arterioles and capillaries. It is one of the commonest causes of childhood renal failure. The other important contributing factor to its pathogenesis may be elevated levels of abnormal von Willebrand factor protein, most of which is released into the circulation by damaged endothelium and in turn enhances platelet aggregation and adhesion. Treatment is essentially supportive, with early renal dialysis allowing for better control of fluid and electrolyte balance. Unlike the situation in thrombotic thrombocytopenic purpura, the role of plasma infusions and plasma exchange remain to be proven.

Thrombotic thrombocytopenic purpura (TTP)

Thrombotic thrombocytopenic purpura (TTP) is a syndrome characterized by micro-angiopathic haemolytic anaemia, thrombocytopenia, fever, neurological syndrome and renal dysfunction. TTP has a fundamental pathological lesion that is similar to HUS, namely, thrombotic micro-angiopathy, and is caused by many factors, all of which initially induce endothelial damage. In the past, some authors believed that they should be considered a single condition, that is HUS-TTP; however, the vast majority of cases of HUS have now been shown to be due to verotoxin. Again the pathophysiological events in TTP like HUS have not been fully elucidated, but endothelial damage and von Willebrand factor multimer composition, in particular the presence of unusually high von Willebrand factor multimers in the circulation, causes platelet activation and thrombus formation.

TTP should not be considered as a single disorder but as a heterogeneous group of at least four subtypes: (i) a single episode of TTP that seldom if ever recurs; (ii) intermittent TTP (characterized by occasional relapses and infrequent intervals); (iii) secondary TTP (usually seen in association with recognized clinical scenarios such as bone marrow transplantation, chemotherapy, pregnancy, and infections, e.g. HIV); (iv) chronic relapsing TTP (frequent episodes occurring at regular intervals). The commonest form seen in infancy and children is the chronic relapsing variety, which may be different from its adult counterpart as there is no end organ damage and only very small quantities of plasma (without plasma exchange) are needed to reverse the anaemia and thrombocytopenia.

However, the multimeric profiles characterized by the presence of unusually high von Willebrand factor multimers seen in both chronic relapsing types are similar, making it most likely that they are indeed the same disease state.

The mainstay of treatment is plasma exchange with plasma or cryosupernatant. Plasma infusions have also been shown to work, but, following therapeutic controlled clinical trials, plasma exchange is now considered to have superior efficacy. Plasma exchanges should be continued until the platelet and lactic dehydrogenase levels return into the normal range. For those patients who do not respond to first-line treatment, a variety of other therapeutic approaches can be considered. These include corticosteroids, immunosuppression (vincristine, azathioprine), immunoglobulins, antiplatelet aggregating agents (aspirin, dypridamole) and splenectomy. It should also be stated that all of these approaches have been reported to be successful anecdotally and not in a controlled clinical setting.

Birth asphyxia

Birth asphyxia reflected by low Apgar score is strongly associated with thrombosis in neonates. It is usually accompanied by a low platelet count, the mechanism of which is not entirely clear, but consumption secondary to thrombin generation and DIC is probably the key event, as hypoxia is known to upregulate tissue factor expression, reduce thrombomodulin activity and enhance plasminogen activator inhibitor 1 production by endothelial cells.

INHERITED THROMBOPHILIC TENDENCY

Genetic defects predisposing to thrombosis are outlined in Table 10.2. Until recently, the vast majority of inherited defects, accounting for 5–10% of patients, were protein C, protein S and antithrombin deficiency. Over the past five years, understanding of the molecular pathogenesis of inherited thrombotic disease has increased greatly, especially concerning the protein C anticoagulant pathway. This

> **Table 10.2 Inherited thrombotic tendency**
>
> - Defects within the protein C pathway
>   - A. APCR and FV^{R506Q} (factor V Leiden)
>   - B. Protein C deficiency
>   - C. Protein S deficiency
>   - D. $FII^{G20210A}$ (prothrombin gene variant)
>   - E. High circulating levels of factor VIII
>
> - Antithrombin deficiency
>
> - Hyperhomocysteinaemia
>   - A. Cystathionine B-synthase
>   - B. Methionine synthase
>   - C. Thermolabile
>   methylenetetrahydrofolate reductase
>
> - Fibrinolytic pathway
>   - A. ↑PAI-1 (4G/5G polymorphic status)
>   - B. Plasminogenaemia
>
> - Dysfibrinogenaemia
>
> - Haemoglobinopathy
>
> - Platelet defects

pathway accounts for the majority of genetic defects associated with venous thromboembolic disease, namely, protein C deficiency, protein S deficiency, prothrombin gene variant, factor V Leiden and high levels of factor VIII (see below). The efficiency of this pathway to anticoagulate an individual is also influenced by external factors such as inflammation and endotoxaemia (see below).

Protein C and protein S deficiencies

Hereditary protein C and protein S deficiencies (homozygosity or compound heterozygosity) are associated with a high venous thromboembolic risk at birth or in the first few months of life. The first clinical manifestation is usually skin purpura (clotting within the small vessels of the dermis) mainly affecting extremities, and in some cases massive large-vessel thrombosis (renal venocaval and iliac veins) can also be a presenting feature. Laboratory markers of DIC are usually present in the first week of life. Low levels of

protein C and protein S are also seen. DIC is associated with other aetiologies, especially infection, and therefore it is important to make the correct diagnosis of hereditary protein C or protein S deficiency, since optimum therapy involves factor replacement (protein C concentrate in protein C deficiency or fresh frozen plasma in protein S deficiency) and heparin in the acute phase and oral anticoagulation in the long term. Within hours of factor replacement, restoration of plasma coagulation proteins and platelet levels is seen. The usual starting dose is 50–100 units/kg as a loading dose and thereafter at 10–15 units/kg per hour, titrating against the plasma concentration of protein C. Once a steady state is achieved, protein C can be administered subcutaneously, as venous access in small babies may prove a major problem that includes the risk of catheter thrombosis. Most of these children end up on long-term oral anticoagulation therapy.

The phenotype associated with hereditary protein S deficiency is very similar to that of hereditary protein C deficiency, namely, heterozygotes generally develop thrombosis during adulthood but in the neonatal period homozygotes develop purpura fulminans. There is no protein S concentrate available, and fresh frozen plasma is used in the acute phase, with a switch to oral anticoagulation thereafter.

Activated protein C resistance (APCR) and factor V^{R506Q}/factor V Leiden

The diagnosis of activated protein C resistance (APCR) is demonstrated by an abnormally low activated protein C sensitivity ratio. In the vast majority of patients, APCR is associated in greater than 90% of cases with a unique single-point mutation (G1691A) of the factor V gene. This gives rise to substitution of glutamine for arginine at position 506 of the factor V molecule (FV^{R506Q}), which is the site of primary cleavage of factor Va by activated protein C, thus promoting procoagulant activity through thrombin generation and clot formation. The mutation is commonly referred to as factor V Leiden, after the Dutch city where the mutation was identified. There is a prevalence of approximately 4% in the UK and Ireland, rising to 15% in Scandinavian countries and being as low as 0% in Australian Aboriginals and Asian and Japanese populations. APCR represents greater than 50% of all inherited thrombophilias and is seen in approximately 25% of patients with recurrent venous thromboembolic disease. The significance of APCR in patients who lack FV^{R506Q} is unclear, but may be explained by non-specificity of the simple functional assay.

Prothrombin (factor II) gene variant (FII^{G20210A})

This is the second most commonly described inherited mutation resulting in a prothrombotic state. The mutation in the 3'-untranslated region of the gene has prevalence rates varying from 0.7% to 4% with an overall gene frequency of 2%. Homozygosity has been described, and the vast majority of these patients have had severe venous thrombotic complications. The precise mechanism by which this mutation causes an increased propensity to develop clot formation is unknown; however, there is increased circulating prothrombin plasma concentration in these patients, and therefore the presumption is that thrombin generation is over-efficient. There is no functional assay for the screening of this defect and PCR analysis is by far the commonest way to screen at the present time.

Antithrombin III deficiency

Reducing functional defects are also associated with a high risk of venous thromboembolic disease. The homozygous state is extremely rare and appears to be incompatible with life. Presentations of antithrombin deficiency in neonates include myocardial infarction at birth, aortic thrombosis, sagittal sinus thrombosis and cerebral thrombosis.

Hyperhomocysteinaemia

Homocysteine most likely promotes clotting through upregulation of tissue factor (TF) expression on TF-bearing cells. Numerous studies over the past decade have shown that an elevated level of homocysteine is associated with arteriovascular and venous thrombolic disease. Deficiencies in vitamins B_6 and B_{12} and folic acid give rise to elevated levels in homocysteine. The commonest inherited predisposition to mild to moderate hyperhomocysteinaemia is the polymorphism in the gene for 5,10-methylenetetrahydrofolate reductase, MTHFR^{C677T}. This translates to an alanine-to-valine substitution and results in a thermolabile form of the enzyme, with 38% enzyme activity in the homozygous form and 65% in the heterozygous form versus 100% in the wild type. To date, there does not appear to be a significant association between the heterozygous MTHFR polymorphism and either elevated homocysteine or thrombotic risk. Homozygotes for this mutation occur in approximately 10% of European and North American Caucasian populations.

Other inherited thrombophilias

Several other inherited gene defects affecting the fibrinolytic, anticoagulant and procoagulant pathways and causing defects in haemoglobin and platelets have been shown to associate with inappropriate clotting (Table 10.2).

MANAGEMENT

The indications for use of anticoagulants in infants and children have changed dramatically over the past 20 years, with major advances in tertiary paediatric care such as ECMO, cardio-pulmonary bypass, haemodialysis and the use of intra-arterial and intravenous indwelling catheters. The choice of anticoagulant is dependent upon the duration of anticoagulation; therefore, in the acute phase, heparins, either unfractionated or low-molecular-weight forms, are used, whilst in the longer term, oral anticoagulants are the treatment of choice. In more specific disease states such as inherited or acquired protein C or antithrombin deficiencies, factor concentrate replacement as an adjuvant haemostatic support is used more and more. In children who develop heparin-induced thrombocytopenia, recombinant hirudin or a heparinoid should be considered (Table 10.3).

Table 10.3 Anticoagulants used in clinical paediatrics
Heparin:
Unfractionated
Low-molecular-weight
Warfarin/other vitamin K antagonists
Natural anticoagulant concentrates
A. Antithrombin concentrate (plasma-derived)
B. Protein C concentrate (plasma-derived)
C. Activated protein C concentrates (recombinant)
Direct antithrombins
A. Recombinant hirudin
B. Argantroban

Because the haemostatic system in infancy and throughout childhood is constantly maturing, the anticoagulant effects of un-fractionated heparin and warfarin are not predictable and therefore are deemed age-dependent (Table 10.4). Unfractionated heparins also need to be given frequently by the intravenous route; they usually take a long time to achieve the desired anticoagulant effect and also have the well-recognized side-effects of bleeding, osteoporosis and HIT/HITTS. On the other hand, low-molecular-weight heparins have a predictable anti-coagulant effect, can be administered sub-cutaneously, do not require regular monitor-ing, and have definite reduced incidences of HIT/HITTS and osteopenia. Until recently, their use in childhood was minimal, and although their true safety and efficacy have not been truly tested in a large randomized clinical trial, a number of pilot trials to date have shown them to be an important advance in both the treatment and prophylaxis of thromboembolic disease in children.

Warfarin on the other hand is less rarely used in the paediatric haematology clinic as the vast majority of patients on oral anticoag-ulation are children with complex congenital heart disease and cardiac heart valves. It should be remembered again that oral antico-agulation dosing in children is different from adults; namely, as the child grows, the amount of oral anticoagulation required will become less on a dose per kilogram basis with time. The ability of plasma from children to generate thrombin is lower than that seen in adult plasma. Because of this, it is most likely that the target prothrombin time and/or international normalized ratio (INR) level for an adult is inappropriate in children in the paediatric setting. Unfortunately, no trials have accessed this in any great detail, and therefore target INRs used in children are extrapolated from published adult data. See

Table 10.4 Profile of the commonly used anticoagulants			
	Warfarin	**Unfractionated heparin**	**LMWH**
Pharmacokinetics	Age-dependent	Age-dependent	Predictable
Monitoring	Frequent	Frequent	Minimal
Venous access	Essential	Essential	Not essential
Time to anticoagulation	Days	Hours–days	Immediate
Bleeding risk	Yes	Yes	Minimal
Osteoporosis risk	Increased	Increased	Decreased
HIT/HITTS	–	Increased	Decreased

HIT, heparin-induced thrombocytopenia; HITTS, heparin-induced thrombocytopenia thrombosis syndrome; LMWH, low-molecular-weight heparin.

Andrew et al (2000) for a full account of dosing (loading and maintenance). It should be remembered that there are numerous factors influencing the effect of warfarin, such as the concurrent dose of other drugs, change in diet, liver dysfunction, presence of a lupus anticoagulant and age (the older the child, the less oral anticoagulation will be required).

Natural anticoagulant concentrates are now available for protein C- and antithrombin-deficient states. These concentrates are being used more widely now, especially in the area of sepsis, where acquired protein C and antithrombin deficiency are regularly seen. Both plasma-derived and recombinant activated protein C concentrates are available. Plasma-derived protein C infusions have been used successfully (in terms of morbidity and mortality) in patients with purpura fulminans associated with meningococcal septicaemia. More recently, recombinant protein C in a phase III trial in adult sepsis was shown to have a favourable outcome at day 28 in terms of mortality. Antithrombin concentrates have been around for a lot longer and have been used effectively in patients with antithrombin deficiency requiring anticoagulation support, either to cover surgery or in the acute phase of a venous thrombosis. Their use in sepsis is less clearly defined.

Recombinant hirudin, which is a specific antithrombin, is increasingly used, especially in the case of HIT/HITTS. Most supporting data have come from studies in adults; however, there is increasing evidence showing its safety and efficacy in children.

CONCLUSION

The past quarter of a decade has seen advances in the treatment of life-threatening disease in children. One of the costs of achieving this has been more children developing thrombotic disease, the majority of which are related to indwelling vascular catheters. As a result, these children are commenced on anticoagulation therapy. Alongside these advances, there has been an explosion in knowledge of the understanding at the molecular level of blood coagulation, in particular how the natural anticoagulant pathways work. Stemming from these discoveries, new anticoagulant therapeutics have become available to the paediatrician, and over the next quarter of a century their true place in the treatment of childhood thrombotic disease will be established.

FURTHER READING

Andrew M, Monagle PT, Brooker L. (2000) *Thromboembolic Complications During Infancy and Childhood*. Hamilton, Ont.: BC Decker.

Seghatchian MJ, Samama MM, Hecker SP, eds. (1996) *Hypercoagulable States – Fundamental Aspects, Acquired Disorders and Congenital Thrombophilia*. Boca Raton, FL: CRC Press.

Lilleyman J, Hann I, Blanchette V, eds. (1999) *Pediatric Haematology*, 2nd edn. Edinburgh: Churchill Livingstone.

Bonduel M et al. (2000)Prothrombotic abnormalities in children with venous thromboembolism. *J Paediatr Haematol Oncol* **22** (1): 66–72.

Doupremepuich C ed. (1994) *Anticoagulation*. New York: Springer-Verlag.

11 Acute lymphoblastic leukaemia

Ian M Hann

INTRODUCTION

Acute lymphoblastic leukaemia (ALL) has been curable since the early 1970s, long before much success occurred with therapy for acute myeloid leukaemia (AML). It has been fortuitous that the earliest found anticancer drugs, including mercaptopurine, methotrexate, vincristine, corticosteroids, anthracyclines, epipodophyllotoxins and cytarabine, all have an effect on this disease. What is more, they can be used in a way that now produces minimal late toxicity in the majority of patients. In fact, ALL along with Hodgkin's disease are the best examples of a very fruitful approach whereby randomized trials have looked at toxicity and efficacy, hand in hand. Such studies continue today with large randomized trials that are investigating the best modes of treating the central nervous system (CNS), cranial irradiation having been already abandoned except in the highest-risk groups because of its adverse effects on intellectual and endocrine function. The other great advance of the last 15 years has been the introduction of intensification therapy, which has reduced the risk of relapse overall to a maximum of one-third. Therapy-related mortality with ALL was always low and has been further reduced by successful measles vaccine campaigns, which hopefully will continue, despite adverse publicity, and better antibacterial and antifungal agents (see Chapter 4). Currently, the diminishing role for allogeneic bone marrow transplantation (allo-BMT) is becoming confined to children with marrow relapse within three years of diagnosis. The 'Holy Grail' of therapy is to tailor the treatment to the individual patient, and current studies are investigating whether or not this is possible using molecular biological tests for minimal residual disease.

Thirty-five years ago, no children with ALL survived, with the median survival being about ten weeks. The great success story that led to more than two-thirds survival began in 1948, when Farber and colleagues induced remissions in terminally ill children with the folic acid antagonist aminopterin. In the early 1950s, more key drugs were developed, especially corticosteroids and mercaptopurine. Even more importantly, the drugs vincristine and asparaginase were developed in the 1960s, and the 1970s saw the introduction of cytarabine, epipodophyllotoxins and the anthracyclines. The ironic point is that there have been no new drugs since then, and because their introduction outstripped the contemporary knowledge we still have a lot to learn about the old ones. For instance, the very similar drugs thioguanine and mercaptopurine are being compared in the current Medical Research Council (MRC) ALL trial (ALL 97) and that trial also compares the steroids dexamethasone and prednisolone. There is still a debate over how best to use all of the other drugs in order to minimize toxicity and maximize efficacy. The best current example would be the controversy over various formulations of asparaginase, the frequency with which it should be used, the dosage and the number and mode of injections that should be given, and whether or not it should be attached to polyethyleneglycol.

In the early days, the concept of therapy was effectively palliative, although that may not have been accepted by everyone involved in the care of these children. Drugs were given singly and sequentially, until it was recognized that the effect was much greater and still tolerable if they were combined. The great breakthrough was in the late 1970s, pioneered in the USA by Don Pinkel, when he coined the phase 'total therapy', which is still a valid concept. He planned to induce remission as quickly as possible, by which time the child was fit to receive consolidation therapy in order to reduce the tumour burden to a level of minimal residual disease, finishing with a period of continuing therapy for several years. After some initial success was marred by CNS relapses in half of the patients, the concept of CNS-directed therapy was adopted. These phases of therapy remain unchanged to this day, and the major advances have been achieved by reducing toxicity, for example by largely abandoning cranial irradiation, increasing the dose and frequency of drug combinations (so-called dosage-intensity) and addressing the role of allo-BMT in the diminishing band of patients with very high-risk and/or recurrent disease.

AETIOLOGY, INHERITANCE AND EPIDEMIOLOGY

The incidence of ALL varies significantly throughout the world, with rates ranging from 9 per million to 47 per million for male children, and from 7 to 43 per million for females. Incidence rates are highest in the USA among whites and in Australia, Costa Rica and Germany. Intermediate rates occur in most of Europe, and the lowest quoted rates are in American blacks, India and Kuwait. There is a significant peak in incidence between 3 and 5 years of age, but this peak is noticeably absent in many developing countries, leading to theories that exposures, for example to infections associated with modern life styles, may lead to leukaemia. Boys are about 1.5 times more commonly affected than girls except in T-cell ALL, where the male-to-female ratio is 4:1, and in infant leukaemia, where there is a female preponderance.

The most striking genetic association is with Down's syndrome, in which there is a 12-fold increased risk of leukaemia. There is also an increased risk of ALL in neurofibromatosis*, Shwachman's* syndrome, Bloom's*

syndrome, ataxia telangiectasia*, Langerhans cell histiocytosis and Kleinfelter's syndrome. Those marked with an asterisk are also associated with an increased risk of AML.

Familial leukaemia cases have been described over many decades, and can cluster in families that experience a high risk of cancers, including brain tumours, colon and stomach cancer. This could suggest a genetic component to the aetiology but may also reflect a shared environmental exposure. Twin studies have shown a high degree of concordance among twins, particularly if they are monozygotic. The risk rises in infants, and approaches 100% for the unaffected twin sibling of a monozygotic twin diagnosed at less than one year of age, which is thought to be due to shared placental circulation.

Many environmental and demographic factors have been investigated for a potential role in the aetiology of ALL. A large case–control study of such factors has been completed within the UK, and the results should be available very soon. Currently, there is a suggestion that high birthweight may be associated, possibly due to the involvement of growth factors. Most studies have also shown an increased risk with a prior history of multiple fetal loss, indicating a genetic predisposition and/or chronic environmental exposure. The question of a predisposition to ALL related to paternal preconception exposure to radiation is controversial at present. In utero exposure to diagnostic radiation is an established risk factor, which, however, accounts for only a very few cases of ALL. The influence of other types of exposure to radiation and electromagnetic fields remains very controversial, and further results from epidemiological studies are keenly awaited. There is no good evidence for any other causative factors, but Greaves has proposed a hypothesis that early exposure to infection may be protective against the disease and delayed exposure (due to fewer siblings or delayed entry into day care) in susceptible individuals may predispose to ALL.

A variety of consistent structural chromosomal abnormalities have been described in ALL (Table 11.1). Besides being an aid to classification and diagnosis, the rearrangements almost certainly represent one of the genetic

Table 11.1 Commoner cytogenetic changes in ALL children: results from UK MRC trials, 1997

Chromosomal abnormalities	Approximate (%) positive
t(12;21)	30
t/del(9p)	8
t/del(12p)	7
del(6q)	6
t/del(11q)	6
t/del(11q) excl.	4
t(1;19)	4
t(4;11)	3
t(9;22)	2
Near-haploid (24–29)[a]	1
Hypodiploid (30–45)	9
Pseudodiploid (46)	29
Low hyperdiploid (47–49)	16
High hyperdiploid (50–59)	40
Near-triploid (69)	4
Near-tetraploid (96)	1

[a] Numbers in parentheses are numbers of chromosomes.

events that eventually result in leukaemia. Many of the genes involved are transcription factors and the altered function caused by the translocation leads to inappropriate expression of a normal gene or production of a fusion gene, leading to production of an abnormal chimaeric protein.

CLINICAL FEATURES (Table 11.2)

Differential diagnosis

Leukaemia is the great mimic of the modern era, and the differential diagnosis is potentially endless (Table 11.2). In fact, it is easy to make this problem much more difficult than it really is, because the diagnosis is clearly obvious when one is presented with a child who has hepatosplenomegaly, low platelets, low haemoglobin and neutropenia and who

is clinically infected along with obvious bruising and petechiae. Occasionally one can be caught out by subtler changes when, for instance, there is no organomegaly and an essentially normal blood count. There are two important points to be made here. First, a delay in diagnosis of acute leukaemia is very rarely of any clinical significance, because it is a blood-borne and disseminated disease from the outset. Thus, as long as the patient's general condition is good, there will be no adverse effect of the delays that frequently occur because of the non-specific symptoms and signs which may be present initially. Second, the gold standard diagnostic test remains simple morphological examination of a stained bone marrow aspirate. The cytogenic changes and immunophenotyping of white cell antigens are of additional diagnostic help in some circumstances, but are subject to over-interpretation.

Rather than run through all of the possible diagnoses, it is probably useful just to mention the major pitfalls. Failure to diagnose infections in patients who usually present with organomegaly and pancytopenia, or occasionally some blast cells in the blood, is a real risk. It must always be remembered that young children are capable of producing leukaemia-like reactions, with early B-cells, to the following infections: HIV, cytomegalovirus, Epstein–Barr virus, and *Leishmania*. This can also occur in the rare child with an autoimmune/vasculitic disorder. Over-reliance on immunophenotyping results is a particularly important mistake not to make. Ancillary tests such as these must never be taken in isolation from the morphology, and CD10$^+$ and TdT$^+$ cells (Table 11.3) can be found as a response to the infections above, as well as in other disorders such as Diamond–Blackfan anaemia and congenital neutropenias. Cytogenetic changes (Table 11.1) are often very helpful, but low-level clones, especially of monosomy 7, can disappear or fail to progress over long periods. Morphological changes are subjective and are merely part of an overall picture; for instance, all patients receiving cytotoxic chemotherapy display some degree of myelodysplasia. Children with neuroblastoma may have almost complete replacement of the marrow with

Table 11.2 Differential diagnosis of acute leukaemia	
(Hepato)splenomegaly	Infections:
	Tuberculosis and MAI
	Leishmaniasis
	SBE
	CMV
	Meningococcaemia
	Severe and overwhelming infections
	EBV
	HIV
	Hepatitis
	Storage diseases
	Metabolic diseases
	HLH
	Osteopetrosis
	Liver problems, e.g. hepatic fibrosis
	Malaria
	Chronic myeloid leukaemia
	Lymphomas
	Other myeloproliferative disorders and myelodysplasias, e.g. essential thrombocythaemia
Bone pain and bone changes	Autoimmune and rheumatoid diseases
	Tumours, e.g. neuroblastoma
	Osteomyelitis
Purpura/petechiae/bleeding	Coagulation disorders
	Protein C deficiency
	Meningococcaemia
	Non-accidental injury

MAI, *mycobacterium avium intracellulare*; SBE, subacute bacterial endocarditis; CMV, cytomegalovirus; EBV, Epstein–Barr virus; HLH, haemophagocytic lymphohistiocytosis.

malignant cells – which can and have been mistaken for leukaemia. Failures of classification continue to be made because of faulty methodology and aberrant expression of antigens. The best examples are the presence of CD13/33 (so-called 'myeloid' antigens) on approximately one-fifth of cases of common ALL, which are also of no prognostic significance. In a similar way, cytogenetic changes can easily be misinterpreted, for example, the 11q2,3 changes in ALL and AML. The prognosis is usually affected in the former and insignificantly in the latter. Major therapeutic decisions, for example the plan to go ahead with allo-BMT, are still made erroneously. Finally, it must not be forgotten that ALL can present like severe aplastic anaemia that unaccountably recovers rapidly and spontaneously, only to present as frank ALL a few weeks or months later. Also, children (especially with Down's syndrome) can produce leukaemoid reactions to infections or no obvious precipitating factor, and in babies a diagnosis of acute leukaemia must be made with great caution.

The morphological changes and the usual

Table 11.3 Immunological classification of leukaemias
B-lineage ALL Early pre-B ('null') $\quad$ CD19$^+$CD10$^-$TdT$^+$ 'Common' ALL $\quad$ CD19$^+$CD10$^-$TdT$^+$ Pre-B ALL $\quad$ CD19$^+$CD10$^-$TdT$^+$ cytoplasmic μ^+ Mature B ALL $\quad$ CD19$^+$CD22$^+$ surface membrane Ig$^+$ **T-lineage ALL** CD7$^+$ and/or CD2$^+$, TdT$^+$ **AML** FAB types M1−M5: CD13$^\pm$CD33$^+$, myeloperoxidase$^+$ FAB M6 (erythroid): glycophorin A$^+$ FAB M7 (megakaryoblastic): CD41$^\pm$CD61$^+$
μ, μ heavy chains; TdT, terminal deoxynucleotidyl transferase; Ig, immunoglobulin; FAB, French–American–British morphological classification.

Table 11.4 Morphological classification and relevance in ALL
L1 **Microlymphoblastic.** Usually more than 75% of cells are small with non-prominent nucleoli and high nucleo-cytoplasmic ratio and little nuclear folding. Tend to be Periodic Acid Schiff reagent (PAS)-positive. No clinical significance.
L2 **Macrolymphoblastic.** Usually more than 75% of cells are large, often with prominent nucleoli, nuclear folding, abundant cytoplasm and prominent nucleoli.
L3 Almost always associated with mature B-cell (surface membrane immunoglobulin-positive) ALL. Beware vacuolated L2 cases, which can look similar but have less basophilic cytoplasm (if the staining is adequate) and are surface membrane immunoglobulin-negative. Very important diagnosis, because these patients are at very high risk of urate nephropathy and often require dialysis. Also require different therapy – do very badly with straightforward ALL therapy and well with lymphoma-like regimens.

classification of ALL into L1, L2 and L3 subtypes are shown in Table 11.4. This was proposed by a French, American and British (FAB) collaborative group. In fact, the L3 subtype is almost always associated with the mature B-cell type of ALL. This is a very important subtype biologically, which used to carry an extremely poor prognosis. It does not respond well to the usual ALL-type therapy, but does do very well with a lymphoma-type high-dosage fractionated CHOP (cyclophosphamide, doxorubicin, vincristine, prednisolone) regimen. It is in fact a lymphomatous type of leukaemia that usually presents with bulky abdominal disease, related to Peyer's patches, pleural effusions and early CNS disease. A very high (usually >40%) proportion of the blast cells are in S phase of the cell cycle. Early management of the tumour lysis syndrome is essential in these cases, and most patients end up requiring dialysis owing to urate nephropathy with hyperkalaemia and hyperphosphataemia, despite therapy with allopurinol or uricozyme. Gut perforation is also common.

CLINICAL MANAGEMENT

There is a very real danger when splitting diseases like leukaemia into multiple subgroups and treating them differently when it is shown that they have different outcomes with standard therapy. Whereas this may sometimes be a justifiable approach, it must never be assumed that prognostication equates to a reliable response to altered therapy. A good example of a prejudice that was proven to be untrue was the vogue to reduce therapy for good-risk girls with ALL in the 1980s. It has subsequently been shown that all risk groups benefit from additional intensive blocks of chemotherapy following induction treatment. Having said that, information on prognosis does select out different biological types of leukaemia that may or may not respond differently to amended or different chemotherapy or more specific treatments such as gene therapy. In addition, the families of affected children find it helpful to be given a clearer idea of the eventual outcome.

Prognostic factors (Table 11.5)

It has already been said that not only does ALL of mature B-cells look different but it also responds differently to chemotherapy. Table 11.5 details the main bad- and good-risk groups have achieved international recognition. Although this is a long list of 13 features, for the great majority of patients it is age, gender and white blood cell count (WBC) at diagnosis that accounts for most of the variation in outcome. Within the infants less

---

Table 11.5 Important risk factors in ALL cases
Bad risk
MLL gene rearranged in infants
11q abnormalities
Philadelphia chromosome (maybe except high hyperdiploid)
Near-haploid chromosome number
Older age and less than 6 months
High white blood cell count
Male gender
Failure to remit within a month
9p chromosome abnormalities
Poor response at 7/14 days of treatment with >25% marrow blasts
Good risk
t(1;19)
High hyperdiploid
Age 2–5 years
Female gender
Low white blood cell count

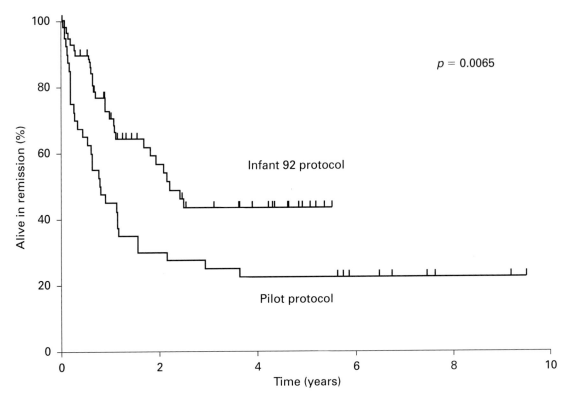

Figure 11.1

Disease-free survival of infants with ALL, showing the pilot study of the late 1980s and early 1990s in the UK, compared with the improved results of chemotherapy with hybrid (i.e. ALL- and AML-like) therapy since 1992.

than 2 years of age, there is a set of findings associated with a poor prognosis of less than 40% event-free survival at 5 years (see Fig. 11.1). This set of findings is age less than 6 months, rearrangement of the *MLL* gene (especially with high WBC and CNS disease at diagnosis) and possibly poor response to single-agent steroids. In older patients, to put it simply, the good features are low WBC, age between 2 and 5 years, and female gender. Boys with high WBC and older age do worse, as do patients who fail to show a rapid response over the first 7–14 days, and the rest are in the middle. Two or three out of every 100 patients do poorly, that is do not remit after the induction month of therapy. Other small poorly performing subgroups are those with the *BCR–ABL* translocation (the t(9;22)

Philadelphia chromosome), those with 11q cytogenetic abnormalities and those with a near-haploid chromosome number.

Remission induction (Table 11.6)

Prior to 1970 there were extremely few survivors, and up until the 1980s the cure rates ran between 40% and 50%. Since then, the real success (Fig. 11.2) has been the dramatic improvement in survival that has been achieved in the face of reduced toxicity – a medical form of 'double whammy'. Nowadays the results around the world show a two-thirds to three-quarters event-free survival at 5 years and overall survival rates with improved salvage therapy (chemotherapy and allo-BMT) in excess of 85% at 5 years in the

Table 11.6 Phases of therapy for ALL

Time	Phase[a]	Drugs used
0–4 weeks	Remission induction	Vincristine i.v. Asparaginase s.c. Prednisolone or dexamethasone p.o. Methotrexate i.t.
4–5+ weeks	Consolidation	Cytarabine Daunorubicin Etoposide — all i.v. Vincristine ± steroids
6–12 weeks	CNS-directed	Methotrexate i.t. or methotrexate high dose i.v. or cranial radiotherapy in high-risk cases
12–20+ weeks	Consolidation	As before
20 weeks until approx. 2 years for girls and 3 years for boys	Continuation	Usually — Mercaptopurine p.o. daily Methotrexate p.o. weekly Vincristine i.v. monthly Methotrexate i.t.

[a] The length and number of consolidation phases remains under investigation.
i.v., intravenous; s.c., subcutaneous; p.o., oral; i.t., intrathecal.

most recent international trials. To put it simply, the death rate from this disease has gone from close to 100% to about 15% in the space of less than 30 years. This is a great tribute to the success of a scientific approach with large randomized clinical trials and international collaboration, which is the best answer to the current anti-clinical-trials scientists who propose a reductionist (ad absurdum) approach to research. Long may the clinical trials approach last, because the last stretch in the home straight is going to be the most difficult because increasing success will leave a smaller number of difficult patients smaller, with more intransigent disease. Consequently, more not less international collaboration is required in order to recruit enough patients into trials. When reading Chapter 4, it is important to remem-

ber that an improvement in cure rates of the order of 10% can be attributed to lower rates of deaths due to infection.

The phases of therapy that are required to cure the disease are shown in Table 11.6 and are accepted internationally, although the details differ following the outcome of different trials. During the first four weeks, three-drug therapy with vincristine, L-asparaginase and steroids induces an apparent remission in about 98% of children. Failures may be due to presence of the *BCR–ABL* translocation or in some cases for no good reason. Such patients do very badly and therapeutic options include allo-BMT. This does emphasize the point that molecular methods are taking over from classical cytogenetic techniques and that the *BCR–ABL* translocation must be sought by the more sensitive molecular tests. One vari-

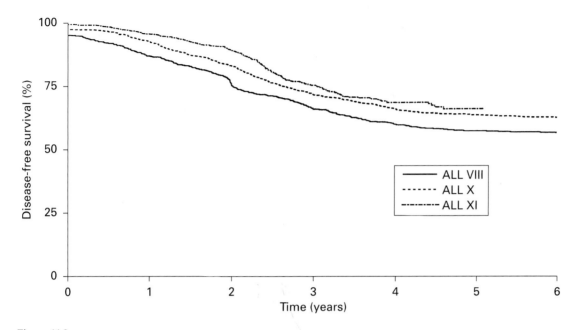

Figure 11.2

Disease-free survival in the last three UK Medical Research Council ALL trials (ALL VIII, X and XI), documenting gradual improvement consequent upon intensification of therapy and despite reduction in toxicity.

ation upon the induction regimen that is being adopted in some parts of the world is to use an initial few days of steroids and then to assess the proportion of blood and bone marrow blasts. Such steroid responsiveness may add more prognostic information, but it is as yet unclear as to whether this further subdivision of patients improves the ultimate outcome, or whether it negates the need for minimal residual disease testing or an approach (adopted in the UK and USA) of marrow assessment and subsequent therapy stratification following standard three-drug chemotherapy and bone marrow assessments.

There are two other controversial points at this stage. First, there is some evidence that dexamethasone may be more effective than prednisolone, at least in part because of its better ability to penetrate the CNS. This is now the subject of further large randomized studies because of the toxicity of dexamethasone, which is probably associated with more psychiatric disturbance, bone necrosis, myosi-

tis and gut bleeding. Second, the type, dose, route and frequency of asparaginase remains a difficult issue. It would appear at present that *Erwinia* asparaginase should be given every 48 hours in order to achieve maximal asparagine suppression and that perhaps 12 doses over 24 days during the first four weeks is the better approach.

Intensification therapy

Having finished the induction phase, 98% of patients will be in a state that is inaccurately called 'complete remission'. Testing for minimal residual disease using molecular biology techniques is now available for most cases, and now is the time to evaluate levels that are predictive of subsequent relapse and that can be investigated with regard to modification of therapy. Tests at about five months from diagnosis (possibly looking for 1 in a 1000 positive cells) appear to have the best predictive value at present, and we now have to learn how best to use this knowledge. At present, all we know is that the use of at least two intensive courses of chemotherapy has increased the event-free survival rate over the last 15 years by about 15%. The idea of such therapy is to hit the disease with new drugs at high dosage at a time when there is minimal residual disease that includes clones of cells that exhibit drug resistance. This resistance involves mechanisms such as P-glycoprotein, which encourages drug efflux from the cell. At present, there are no drugs that work in combating multidrug resistance, although cyclosporin A and verapamil have been tried. This is a potentially fruitful line of new drug development for the future.

The ideal approach to intensification therapy awaits the results of current trials and advances in molecular biological techniques. Various trials have shown that two intensive blocks produced better results than one and that one was better than none. Current trials have increased the intensity further for high-risk patients, including those not responding rapidly from the outset. Eventually, when minimal residual disease testing comes of age, we should be able to tailor treatment to the individual and give extra therapy when excessive levels are present, whilst stopping or modifying treatment when the level falls below that which the body can eradicate through programmed cell death (apoptosis) and other mechanisms.

Apart from the number of courses, we also do not know whether the intensification blocks should be short, sharp and of high dosage, or intensive and more extended in nature, that is lasting 6–8 weeks. Both are probably effective, but a combination of such approaches may be of added value.

Therapy directed at the CNS

Initial success in curing ALL depended upon eradication of the disease within the CNS, which cannot be achieved by the use of systemic chemotherapy. The initial success was achieved by using doses of about 24 Gy of irradiation to the brain, and the real success of recent years has been the realization that this can be achieved in the majority of cases without radiation therapy. Prognostic factors are not as reliable at predicting CNS relapse as they are at predicting marrow relapse, but the WBC (often taken at the level of $50 \times 10^9/l$) at diagnosis is the easiest test. Some centres also include patients with T-cell disease and those with the so-called leukaemia–lymphoma syndrome with large organomegaly, which may include a mediastinal mass, and relative preservation of marrow function with higher than usual haemoglobin and platelet levels.

The choice of the most effective and least toxic CNS-directed therapy has to remain under review and awaits the results of current trials. Various approaches have apparently proven successful, but nearly all trials have failed to produce a really helpful answer because of a failure to include prospective neuropsychometric assessments of toxicity. It is well known now that cranial irradiation can be damaging, and particularly so to the developing brain in very young children. This is often manifest in problems with concentration and short-term memory, which sadly have led to some children being labelled as lazy or badly behaved. There is now good evidence that intrathecal therapy given throughout the two years of treatment, with an initial burst of approximately 6 doses within the first 8 weeks of therapy, is effective in all risk groups other than those with overt CNS disease at diagnosis (CNS+). This treatment is also less toxic. There is also accumulating evidence that high-dose methotrexate with folinic acid (leucovorin) rescue, plus continuing intrathecal methotrexate, given in various types of schedule, is no more effective, with regard to overall survival, than intrathecal therapy. There is still uncertainty as to whether radiation therapy has any role other than in the CNS+ group. We should soon know whether the initial promise of an additional CNS anti-leukaemic effect from dexamethasone, over prednisolone, is realized.

Continuation therapy

ALL is an unusual malignancy in that all trials to date have shown that low-dose continuation therapy given over a long period remains an important part of therapy. In most other circumstances, this would be the worst way to treat cancer, and we must keep this approach under review because more effective intensive therapy may well reduce the need. The best example is allo-BMT given within 6 months of diagnosis in patients with very high-risk ALL, who have a low relapse rate without any subsequent continuation therapy.

The standard form of continuation therapy is daily oral mercaptopurine, weekly oral methotrexate and monthly pulses of intravenous vincristine and corticosteroid. This programme is usually continued for two or three years. The current theory is that such continued therapy encourages apoptosis.

The biggest problem with this phase of treatment is with doctor and patient compliance. For that reason, it is important that all patients have check blood counts at least fortnightly and neutrophil counts reliably suppressed to a level between 0.75 and $1.5 \times 10^9/l$. Intermittent testing of the thiopurine levels may also be of value. If more than 75% dosage on a surface area basis cannot be maintained, then the standard *Pneumocystis* pneumonia prophylaxis with co-trimoxazole (on two days per week, as widely separated from methotrexate dosage as possible) should be abandoned in order to optimize the anti-leukaemic effect. In this circumstance, it is probably adequate to have a very high level of diagnostic suspicion for the existence of *Pneumocystis* pneumonia. Early therapy with high-dose co-trimoxazole is usually successful, and when it is not, pentamidine, steroids and surfactant therapy can be used, with very rare failures nowadays.

Current trials are comparing the similar drugs thioguanine and mercaptopurine for safety and efficacy in continuation therapy.

Treatment after relapse (Fig. 11.3)

Major advances have been made with salvage procedures, such that at least one-third to a half of patients who relapse will ultimately survive. Patients who relapse after two years from diagnosis with isolated testicular relapse can be cured in over three-quarters of cases, with chemotherapy and 24 Gy radiotherapy to both testicles and inguinal canals and without the need for orchidectomy. Patients with an isolated CNS relapse can also be

cured without BMT, even if they relapse before the end of therapy. The level of knowledge about the best treatment after relapse for patients with differing previous CNS-directed therapies is limited at present. Those who have not been irradiated should receive cranial radiation and continuing intrathecal therapy, along with intensive chemotherapy to prevent marrow relapse. Patients who have been irradiated more than a year previously can be given radiation again, although it is damaging. However, the CNS relapse rates with modern therapy are low – for example, in the UK MRC ALL XI trial, the relapse rate is only 5% in the lower-WBC group, receiving intrathecal methotrexate only.

BMT is considered for all patients with marrow relapse at any time because the results are poor whenever the relapse occurs (Fig. 11.3 shows the results of the Great Ormond Street series), although they are exceedingly poor when relapse occurs within the first two years. The results with BMT in this latter very poor risk group are also very poor at the present time, and alternative BMT approaches such as inducing graft-versus-leukaemia (GVL) effects, along with new cytotoxic drugs, are needed. In the majority of patients (over 90% of cases at present), a donor can be found. Controversy rages over the best type of donor, there being evidence that the use of matched sibling donors (MSDs) leads to a lesser GVL effect than unrelated or mismatched (usually haplo-identical) relatives. It is, of course, known for sure that the highest relapse risk and lowest GVL effect occur with the most closely matched donors, that is syngeneic BMT. In practical terms, a donor will in the very near future be found for almost everyone, and the crucial question is when one should use it. The important fact to determine is the procedure-related mortality and late effects. Non-MSD BMT should now carry an approximately 5–10% mortality, and worse results within centres should be audited if they are dealing with the better-risk younger patients. A large and regular experience is required in order to achieve such results, and an expert team of BMT medical experts, nurses, trainee doctors, psychologists, scientific officers and psychosocial/nutritional/physiotherapy support staff must

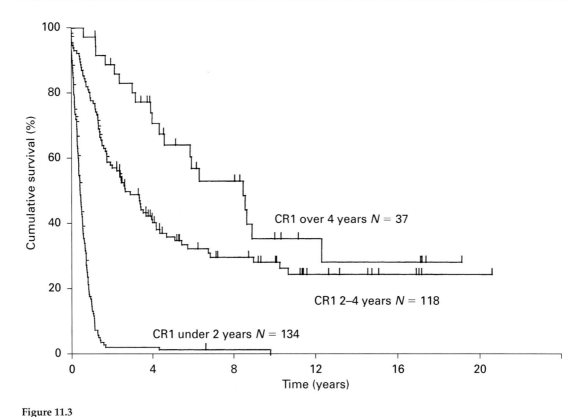

Figure 11.3

Survival in patients who have had a bone marrow or combined leukaemic relapse of ALL. This excludes mainly patients with isolated CNS or testicular relapse, who usually have a better prognosis.

be involved before embarking upon such procedures within a modern air-filtered environment.

The late effects of allo-BMT are considerable, and the problem is worse in the non-MSD area, where the incidence of debilitating and life-threatening chronic graft-versus-host disease (GVHD) approaches 20%. This causes auto-immune disorders, hepatitis, lung fibrosis, scleroderma and gut problems. In addition, all patients receiving total body irradiation, which with cyclophosphamide is the gold standard preparative regimen in this situation, will be infertile and require growth hormone, sex hormone and other hormone replacements. They are also at risk of cataracts and other organ damage such as cardiac failure, and all of the systems must be monitored carefully (see Chapter 17).

The headlong rush into BMT for most relapsed patients is on the one hand depressing because of all of the above problems. But, on the other hand, there are far fewer relapses nowadays and we can now salvage a lot of patients. The challenge is to do away with the need for BMT, by the use of more effective cytotoxic chemotherapy. There remains one very controversial area, which is the use of allo-BMT at first remission in very high-risk patients. Most experts would agree that, because of the lesser late effects and probably lower procedural mortality, this is mainly confined to MSD-BMT for the 2–4% worst-risk patients. This would include the rare patient with very resistant disease, those with a *BCR–ABL* translocation, patients with near-haploid disease and possibly those with 11q abnormalities.

Late effects of therapy (see Chapter 17)

This is becoming a branch of medicine in itself, and a Pandora's box of problems has been identified by its devotees. It is very important to keep these problems in context and always to work towards providing a cure at the least cost, and recognize that this is one area in which both have already been achieved to a large extent. A small and as yet undefined proportion of patients will develop cardiac failure over a period of decades. We have thus begun the process of reducing anthracycline doses to levels below the equivalent of $200 \, mg/m^2$ of daunorubicin and we must monitor all patients with accurate and hopefully reproducible echocardiography over a period of years. The extent of intellectual impairment in non-radiation schedules remains under active review and hopefully will be a small problem in the future. Early puberty and endocrine disturbances are rare but the patient must be monitored at regular intervals by clinical examination and anthropometry. Dental problems can occur and should be managed actively in the usual way and from the outset of treatment. Psychological disturbances can occur within families, not surprisingly in view of the potentially devastating effect of the disease, and expert assistance may be required to help with enuresis, nightmares and bad behaviour.

SUMMARY AND CONCLUSIONS

The overall survival of patients with ALL is creeping close to 90%. This great success has been accompanied by an overall reduction in serious toxicity. The treatment of ALL over the years has been marred by unjustified medical euphoria, which held back progress in the 1960s because intensification therapy and compliance with continuation therapy was not applied to all patients. We now run the risk again of deluding ourselves into thinking that ALL is an easy disease to cure with easily given therapy and little risk of early and late toxicity. Nothing could be much further from the truth, but the real as opposed to the illusory challenge is to cure all of the patients with less damaging therapy. There are exciting developments such as the availability of minimal residual disease testing and transplants for all, which we must properly evaluate and not abuse. The difficulty is that we currently have no new effective drugs, and management of this very difficult disease will continue to be a major challenge for the foreseeable future.

FURTHER READING

Hann IM, Lake BD, Lilleyman JS, Pritchard J. (1996) *Colour Atlas of Paediatric Haematology*, 3rd edn. Oxford: Oxford University Press.

Hann IM, Vora A, Richards S et al. (2000) Benefit of intensified treatment for all children with acute lymphoblastic leukaemia – MRC UKALL X and ALL 97. *Leukemia* **14**: 356–63.

Lampert F, Henze G. (1997) Acute lymphoblastic leukaemia. In: Pinkerton CR, Plowman PN, eds. *Paediatric Oncology*. London: Chapman & Hall: 258–78.

Lilleyman JS, Hann IM. (1995) Management of acute lymphoblastic leukaemia. In: Chessels JM, Hann IM, eds. *Leukaemia and Lymphoma, Baillière's Clinical Paediatrics*. Philadelphia: WB Saunders: 779–98.

Niemeyer CM, Sallan SE. (1998) Acute lymphoblastic leukaemia. In: Nathan DG, Orkin SH, eds. *Hematology of Infancy and Childhood*. Philadelphia: WB Saunders: 1245–85.

Schrappe M, Reiter A, Ludwig WD et al. (2000) Improved outcome in childhood acute lymphoblastic leukaemia – ALL-BFM 90. *Blood* **95**: 3310–22.

12 Acute myeloid leukaemia

Ian M Hann

INTRODUCTION

The management of acute myeloid leukaemia (AML) in young people has been one of the greatest cancer success stories. Prior to the early 1970s, there were very few survivors, and thereafter no more than one in ten survived until the advent of more intensive therapy and allogeneic bone marrow transplantation (allo-BMT) later in that decade. During the 1980s, some progress was made, but even in the childhood age group, wherein the cure rates had always been higher, only about a third were cured. Over the last ten years, survival rates have nudged over the 50% mark. A good-risk group of patients with t(8;21), t(15;17) translocations and inversion of chromosome 16 have survival rates equivalent to the better risk groups with acute lymphoblastic leukaemia (ALL), and the survival rates of young infants will ALL are significantly worse than those with AML. This progress has been achieved because supportive care, in the form of indwelling venous catheters, total parenteral nutrition, antibiotics, antifungals and intensive care, have allowed the use of extremely dosage-intensive regimens. There really is little evidence that so-called 'maintenance' or continuation therapy works in AML as opposed to ALL, and the UK Medical Research Council (MRC) studies have shown that cranial radiation has little role to play. The central nervous system (CNS) relapse rate is very low with the use of simple intrathecal chemotherapy, which has less long-term toxicity than cranial irradiation.

The value of autologous bone marrow rescue from high-dose therapy is probably very small. Marrow purging will probably not make a tangible difference. The real challenge for the future is to design even more successful chemotherapy regimens that preferably do not contain anthracyclines because of the looming problem of cardiotoxicity. In that vein, current evidence for one anthracycline being better than another is weak, and large randomized trials should be undertaken of cardio-protective agents or agents such as liposomal daunorubicin and doxorubicin that reduce the cardiotoxicity risk. There are already long survivors whose hearts are damaged enough to require heart transplant, and the aim must be for cure at least cost within the next decade. In that context, fludarabine- and cytokine-containing regimens and immunotherapy such as anti-CD33 must be explored in randomized clinical trials. High-dose cytarabine and asparaginase-containing regimens (so-called Capizzi schedules) are already in trials such as the MRC AML12.

Increased success has led to greater ability to predict outcome, based mainly upon good and poor (the latter being chromosomes 5, 7, 3q and complex changes) cytogenetic features. This certainly helps with planning therapy, but the temptation to tailor individual therapies must be resisted. However, significant numbers of patients can be cured without resort to BMT, and as chemotherapy improves, the hope is that it will mainly find use as a salvage therapy for patients with resistant disease and early relapse. Patients with poor-risk AML do badly with any type of therapy at present and less than one in five is cured, and thus it is essential to continue to search for better chemotherapeutic options.

The acute myeloid leukaemias are a heterogeneous group of haematological malignancies with similar morphological and biological factors in adults and children, although, as is often the case, the poorer-risk features become more prevalent with increasing age. Although a great deal of progress has been made and just over a half of affected children survive, a high proportion of patients still relapse and a large number of survivors will suffer late effects, in particular those related to cardiac dysfunction. Thus, a number of challenges remain and although the dismal results of 25 years ago have been rectified, this has been achieved at significant cost to health services and the patient. It is to be hoped that a better understanding of the biological and drug resistance mechanisms along with measures of minimal residual disease will allow a more scientific approach to therapy in the future.

AETIOLOGY AND EPIDEMIOLOGY

A number of predisposing factors have been associated with the development of childhood AML. Down's syndrome patients have an approximately 20-fold risk of developing leukaemia, which is usually of the megakaryoblastic M7 morphological subtype (see Table 12.1) when it occurs in the first three years of life. Neonates with Down's syndrome may also show a transient abnormality (transient abnormal myelopoiesis, TAM) that is indistinguishable from congenital leukaemia except that it is of M7 or erythroid type (M6, Table 12.1). However, this myeloproliferation resolves spontaneously within a few months, but subsequently up to a third of patients can develop true AML during the first three years of life. It should also be noted that patients with Fanconi anaemia, Bloom's syndrome, Kostmann's syndrome and possibly those exposed to benzene and nitrosoureas are at increased risk of developing AML. Treatment with alkylating agents is also associated with an increased incidence, and these leukaemias may present with a myelodysplastic (MDS) prodrome. Typically, these cases present within four to six years of initial therapy, with a much lower risk after 10 years, and commonly the associated cytogenetic abnormalities involve deletions of the long arms of chromosomes 5 and 7.

The development of AML after prolonged exposure to an epipodophyllotoxin is now well established, but the quantity of the risk is controversial. Within the MRC studies, the incidence in children treated primarily for ALL is 0.3% and has not increased overall since the introduction of two short intensive blocks of epipodophyllotoxin chemotherapy. Much higher incidences reported from the USA have been associated with different drug scheduling, usually given once or twice weekly for longer periods, and this information must not be allowed to cloud the real issue, which is that cure of leukaemia is paramount and the risk of secondary AML is very small if appropriate scheduling of epipodophyllotoxins is followed.

We are not a great deal closer to understanding the aetiology of AML, although we do now know the genes involved in many of the cases where chromosome abnormalities have been demonstrated. Examples include the transcription factors AML-1–ETO associated with t(8;21) and SMMHC–CBFβ associated with inv(16).

Homeobox proteins are involved with t(9;11) and 11q23 (various partners) translocations, and tyrosine kinases are involved in the t(9;22) translocation. The exciting development is that such findings mean that it will be possible to look into sensitive tests to detect when minimal residual disease exists and what it means and whether this can be manipulated with different treatment modalities such as allo-BMT. It also opens up the ability to produce specific therapeutic agents, for example those being developed that compete with tyrosine kinase binding sites.

CLINICAL FEATURES AND DIAGNOSIS

Children with AML usually present with weight loss, hepatosplenomegaly and various blood cytopenias. These may lead to the development of infection, bleeding and symptoms of anaemia. The differential diagnosis is in most cases obvious because this constellation of features is usually associated with the presence of obvious primitive myeloid blast forms in the blood. The crucial diagnostic test remains the morphological appearance of the bone marrow. The morphological sub-classification of AML is shown in Table 12.1 and will be discussed further below. There is a very wide differential diagnosis in patients who present with acute leukaemia, because the symptoms are potentially numerous and varied and the clinical signs of lymphadenopathy, hepatosplenomegaly, skin lesions, pallor, bruising and petechiae can signify many other diseases, including especially storage and metabolic and haemophagocytic disorders. Infections may also present in the same way, and a relatively common catch is to miss the travel history and sometimes subtle marrow changes of leishmaniasis. The main point to be made is that diagnosing leukaemia a few days earlier or later does not make a jot of difference to its curability, because it is always disseminated from the outset and delays only cause problems if the child's clinical condition deteriorates dramatically, which usually responds to appropriate supportive care.

Bone marrow appearances (Table 12.1)

A great deal has been made of the need to split up AML into various groups and there are in fact a few points relating to the morphological sub-classification that are of real importance. The promyelocytic or M3 type

---

Table 12.1 Morphological classification in AML and clinical relevance

M0	Undifferentiated, agranular or hypogranular blasts. Ensure not ALL by cytogenetics, cytochemistry and immunophenotype. If doubt still exists, treat as ALL and monitor response.
M1	Some myeloid differentiation with granulated blasts. Often Sudan Black and myeloperoxidase stain-positive.
M2	Differentiated myeloid with prominent granules and usually Auer rods. Sudan Black and myeloperoxidase-positive. Good-prognosis patients with t(8;21) usually have this variety.
M3	Promyelocytic leukaemia. Have abnormalities of the retinoic acid receptor gene due to t(15;17) and a good prognosis. But, they get DIC and should be treated from the outset with ATRA. **Beware:** high rises in WBC on ATRA leads to pulmonary and other problems, so start cytotoxics early.
M4	Myelomonocytic
M5	Monocytic and monoblastic

Tendency to high WBC and extramedullary disease, e.g. gums, skin, CNS.
Beware: problems of leukostasis, especially ARDS and ICH

M6	Erythroid leukaemia. Very rare in children. **Beware:** mixing up with dyserythropoietic anaemias. Juvenile myelomonocytic leukaemia may have a prominent erythroid element.
M7	Megakaryoblastic. Often associated with Down's syndrome. May present with osteosclerosis. Marrow often very difficult to aspirate due to myelofibrosis. Down's patients do very well without BMT.

DIC, disseminated intravascular coagulation; ICH, intracranial haemorrhage; ATRA, all-*trans*-retinoic acid; ARDS, acute respiratory distress syndrome.

was in the past associated with a poor outcome because of the early onset of disseminated intravascular coagulation (DIC). The pathogenesis of this process is still argued over but excess fibrinolysis and release of thromboplastins are probably involved. In fact, the M3 type and its variant form, wherein the blast granulation is much less prominent, responds well initially to treatment with all-*trans*-retinoic acid (ATRA), which is a differentiating agent. The disorder is probably always associated with the t(15;17) translocation, which involves the retinoic acid receptor. Nowadays, the outlook is extremely good, with more than two-thirds of patients being cured with intensive chemotherapy, and this is another instance whereby excellent supportive care has made a big difference. However, it is essential to start chemotherapy early, especially in patients with high white blood cell counts (WBC), because ATRA will cause a further rise and problems with leukostasis/ARDS etc., which can be fatal.

There is a clinical pattern of AML in young children that approaches the level of a syndrome and is one of the differences between children and adults. It consists of a high WBC, CNS disease at diagnosis, extramedullary subcutaneous lumps (which also commonly occur in the M2 type) and the M4 or M5 morphological type. These patients have a relatively poorer prognosis and are prone to bleeding, especially in the lungs and brain, wherein the large 'sticky' macrophages cause white cell 'plugging' and necrosis. These patients must not be transfused with red cells, unless they are in heart failure, and treatment should be started urgently and possibly combined with leukapheresis.

As already stated, the megakaryoblastic or M7 variant is much commoner in children with Down's syndrome and where marrow fibrosis (sometimes with bony sclerosis) is a prominent feature. This leads to problems with diagnosis because the bone marrow may be inaspirable. In that circumstance, immunohistochemistry of the bone marrow trephine using anti-factor VIII and platelet glycoprotein markers is sometimes helpful. Also, these patients essentially have marrow scarring and their blood counts take significantly longer to

recover after the first course of chemotherapy, during which the fibrosis gradually resolves. Thus, they are at risk of serious infections for longer than other patients.

Bone marrow cytochemistry (special stains) is of diminishing value now that cytogenetics and immunophenotyping are available, allowing accurate diagnosis and prognostication in most cases. In brief, the Sudan Black stain is positive in the M1, M2, M3 and M4 cases, and M6 cases are periodic acid Schiff (PAS)-reagent positive. M4 and M5 cases are positive with non-specific esterase and acid phosphatase.

Immunophenotyping (Fig. 12.1)

Looking for white cell antigens using monoclonal antibodies can be valuable, although it is of much less value in AML than in ALL. Probably the most useful test is that for myeloperoxidase, which is positive in AML and negative in ALL, and is of particular value in categorizing cases that would in the past have been labelled acute undifferentiated leukaemia. Very occasionally, it is also helpful in differentiating AML or ALL from infiltrating tumours such as neuroblastoma. In addition, the platelet glycoprotein markers CD41, CD42 and CD61 are very helpful in the M7 megakaryoblastic cases, with glycophorin being present in the rare M6 erythroleukaemias. CD14 and CD11 positivity may indicate a monocytic variant (M4/5). CD13 and CD33 positivity are difficult to interpret because up to a quarter of B-cell lineage cases may be positive. However, in the absence of CD19 (early pre-B cell marker), strong CD13 and CD33 positivity is very suggestive of a myeloid subtype.

Cytogenetics (Tables 12.2 and 12.3)

Looking for chromosome changes, usually with molecular biological techniques, has at last come of age in the management of AML. Table 12.2 details the changes that occur and the proportion of cases that display these changes, and Table 12.3 categorizes patients into bad- and good-risk groups based mainly on the cytogenetic features. Thus, the use of these techniques aids specific

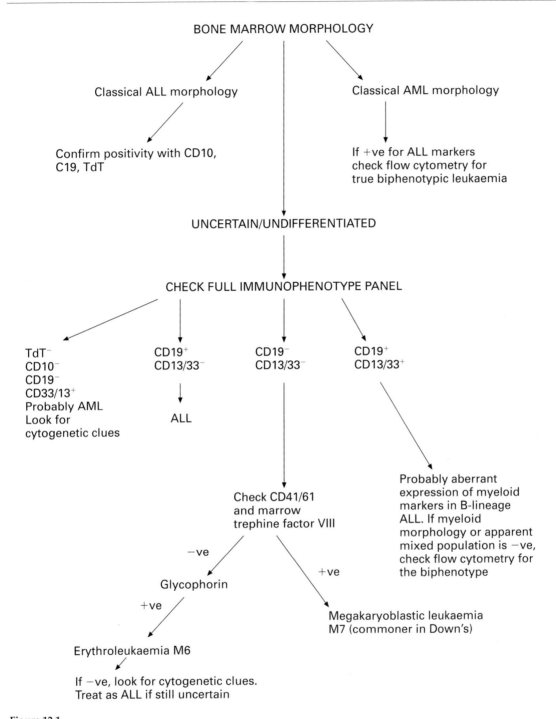

Figure 12.1

Algorithm for confirmation of leukaemia type

Table 12.2 Commoner cytogenetic changes in AML in children	
Chromosomal abnormalities	**Approximate % positive**
+8	14
t(8;21)	12
t(15;17)	9
11q2,3	8
+21	7
inv(16)	5
−7	4
del(9q)	4
abn(3q)	2
del(7q)	2
del(5q)	1
−5	1
+22	1

Table 12.3 Important risk factors in AML cases

Bad risk
−5
del(5q)
−7
abn(3q)
Failure to remit after first chemotherapy course
Complex cytogenetic changes (a clone with at least 5 unrelated cytogenetic changes)
Secondary AML

Good risk
t(8;21)
t(15;17)
inv(16)
Down's megakaryoblastic leukaemia (M7)

diagnosis and planning of therapy. The only useful additional information is the finding of a Down's syndrome-associated M7 AML, which carries a very good prognosis with survival rates approaching 90% without the need to resort to BMT or high anthracycline doses. It can be seen from Table 12.3 that failure to remit after the first chemotherapy course is an additional adverse risk factor, but this eventuality rarely occurs outside of the poor-risk cytogenic group and thus adds little to the power of prognostication. It should also be noted that the adverse cytogenetic features only represent 10% of the total, that is 6–7 cases per year in the whole UK, and that this proportion is higher in older age groups, accounting for some of the worse outcome with increasing age. Additionally, the incidence of secondary leukaemia also increases with age and accounts for less than 1% of the total in children. The good-risk group includes about a quarter of the children, and the rest (about 57%) fall into an intermediate- or standard-risk group.

CLINICAL MANAGEMENT

As stated in Chapter 4, the key to curing AML is dosage-intensive chemotherapy allied to excellent supportive care, along with allo-BMT in selected cases. The role of autologous bone marrow rescue from high-dosage therapy (ABMT) is controversial and will be discussed further below. In the preceding paragraphs it should have become obvious to the reader that dramatic improvements in therapy have allowed selection of groups who do badly with current chemotherapy for more innovative therapies, which will also be discussed below. Between a quarter and a third of patients fall into the good-risk category, having t(8;21) t(15;17) translocations, inv(16) or Down's M7 AML, and can be spared from having a BMT in most cases. One in ten have chromosome 3q, 7 or 5 abnormalities, and the rest (57% of the total) fall into a standard-risk group. Thus, discussion of therapeutic approaches now depends on these groupings, which are widely accepted throughout the world.

Autologous bone marrow rescue from high-dosage therapy (ABMT)

The MRC AML10 trial (see Fig. 12.2) demonstrated that the ABMT procedure with cyclophosphamide and total body irradiation (Cy-TBI), or busulphan–cyclophosphamide (BuCy) in the youngest patients, reduced the risk of relapse by about 10% over no further therapy, after four intensive initial courses in both instances. This is a very problematic approach in children because of the severe late effects on the heart, growth, fertility and endocrine function. The belief is that it is possible, and indeed essential, to find a less toxic alternative chemotherapy regimen (because that is all that ABMT is) that can achieve the same antileukaemic effect, and that is precisely what the current series of trials is attempting to do (MRC AML12 in particular), often using high-dose cytarabine/asparaginase regimens.

A debate rages over whether purging the marrow that is subsequently infused into the recipient will further reduce the relapse rate. In the absence of leukaemia-specific antigens, various approaches have been considered, and in particular the use of the cytotoxic drug mafosfamide. There is no convincing

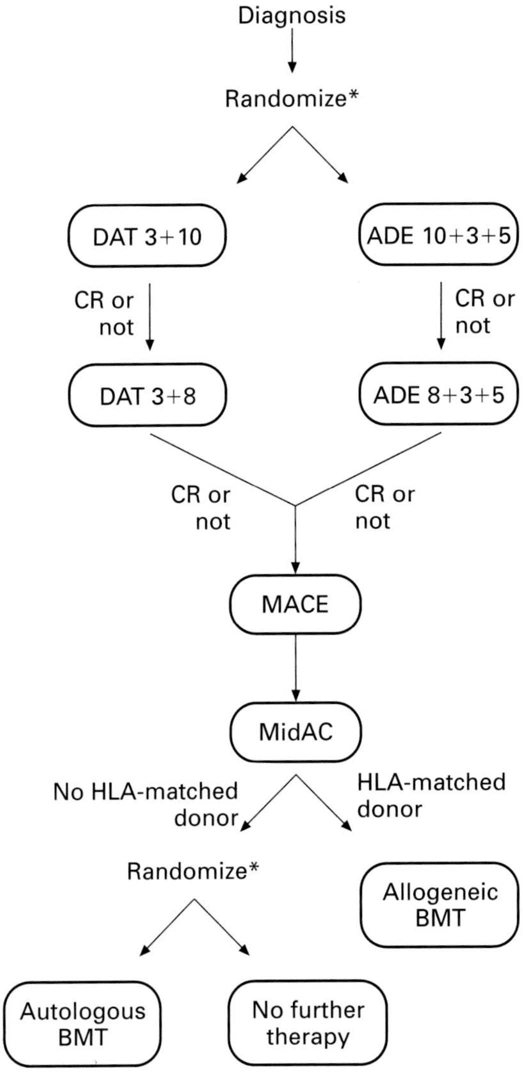

Figure 12.2

AML10 protocol flow chart.

*Randomization actually occurred before course 4.

DAT 3 + 10	Daunorubicin 50 mg/m^2 slow i.v. push days 1, 3, 5
	Cytarabine 100 mg/m^2 12-hourly i.v. push days 1–10
	6-Thioguanine 100 mg/m^2 12-hourly orally days 1–10
ADE 10 + 3 + 5	Daunorubicin 50 mg/m^2 slow i.v. push days 1, 3, 5
	Cytarabine 100 mg/m^2 12-hourly i.v. push days 1–10
	Etoposide (VP-16) 100 mg/m^2 i.v. (1-hour infusion) days 1–5
DAT 3 + 8	As DAT 3 + 10 but cytarabine and 6-thioguanine days 1–8 only
ADE 8 + 3 + 5	As ADE 10 + 3 + 5 but cytarabine days 1–8 only
MACE	Amsacrine (m-amsa) 100 mg/m^2 i.v. (1-hour infusion) days 1–5
	Cytarabine 200 mg/m^2/day i.v. (continuous infusion) days 1–5
	Etoposide 100 mg/m^2 i.v. (1-hour infusion) days 1–5
MidAC	Mitoxantrone 10 mg/m^2 i.v. (short infusion) days 1–5
	Cytarabine 1.0 g/m^2 12-hourly i.v. (2-hour infusion) days 1–3

Note: All doses were reduced by 25% for children less than 1 year old.

evidence that this approach is going to make a major contribution in eradicating the disease from the rest of the body, and the issues of severe late effects remain (see Chapter 17).

Allogeneic bone marrow transplantation (allo-BMT)

There are essentially two main types of allo-BMT: from matched sibling donors (MSDs) and from others, usually including unrelated donors (of which cord blood donations is one modality) and haplo-identical family donors. Although this is currently not universally accepted, it is very likely that the procedure-related mortality rates of MSDs will continue to be less than that with alternative donors, and this has a major impact upon therapeutic plans. The disparity could be as great as a 5% mortality for MSDs and 20% for less closely matched non-MSD donors. It also seems very likely that late effects will be greater in the non-MSD group because of a higher incidence of graft-versus-host disease (GVHD), veno-occlusive disease and severe infections, such as those due to non-herpes group viruses, because of the persisting severe immune suppression. Thus, it would seem reasonable to have the following current approach, which has some international acceptance. Patients in the good risk group are transplanted with an MSD allo-BMT only if they relapse. If a patient relapses within a year of diagnosis, a non-MSD should be sought if an MSD cannot be found, because any patient relapsing early has a very poor prognosis. However, within this group it is justified to try intensive chemotherapy again if relapse occurs after a year and no MSD is available, although there is a high relapse rate and some units would now transplant from alternative donor sources.

At present, MSD allo-BMT is recommended for and high-risk patients during first remission and after 3–5 courses of chemotherapy. Management of standard-risk patients who have a matched sibling donor is controversial, with a drift towards reserving BMT for patients who relapse. If an MSD is not available, first-remission non-MSD BMT is usually only considered for patients within the poor-

risk group and then only when they fail to remit after one course of chemotherapy. Within the standard- and poor-risk groups, allo-BMT from an unrelated donor is also the recommended option if they relapse after chemotherapy, a MSD not having been available. The evidence that multiple BMTs of different types is of value is lacking. In this circumstance, the infusion of donor lymphocytes to a recipient who previously had a marrow graft is being investigated, but shows little promise at present.

Therapy directed at the CNS

Within the MRC AML10 protocol, the patients received five doses of intrathecal methotrexate, cytarabine and hydrocortisone. Overall, only 4% of relapses involved the CNS and there was only one isolated CNS relapse out of 341 children treated. Thus, the previous vogue for cranial irradiation should be abandoned and should only be used in the rare instances (24 of 341, or 7%) where CNS disease occurs at diagnosis. Most of these cases occur in the children with monocytic (M4 or M5) variants, and the option for these patients is an allo-BMT if an MSD is available, or cranial irradiation at the end of therapy. Sadly, these children tend to be very young and the CNS damage, therefore, is significant, and it is to be hoped that we can eventually abandon cranial irradiation altogether when effective chemotherapy is available.

Chemotherapy schedules (Table 12.4)

The results of the most recent large trials of AML in childhood are shown in Table 12.4. In summary, it should now be the aim of every person who treats AML to achieve a greater than 90% complete remission rate and greater than 50% overall survival. It must be remembered that survival no longer just involves first-line therapy and that it is possible to rescue about a quarter of patients who relapse. The vast majority of currently salvageable patients are those who relapse after a year from first diagnosis. The other challenge (see Chapter 4) is to reduce the toxic mortality rate. This was in fact achieved in the MRC AML10 trial, wherein the mortality rate fell by

Table 12.4 Treatment results of five recent multicentre childhood AML trials					
	CCG-2891[a]	POG-8821[b]	MRC-10[c]	BFM87[d]	NOPHo93[e]
Trial period	1989–1994	1988–1993	1988–1995	1987–1992	1993–1998
No. of patients	558	649	341	307	148
Early death	42 (7.5%)	26 (4%)	15 (4.5%)	28 (9.1%)	4 (2.7%)
Resistant disease	109 (19.5%)	71 (11%)	12 (3.5%)	49 (16%)	8 (5.4%)
Complete remission	407 (73%)	552 (85%)	314 (92%)	230 (75%)	136 (92%)
No. of allogeneic BMT	105	89	63	17 (5.5%)	n.a.
No. of autologous BMT	107	115	60	6 (1.9%)	0
Death in CR	n.a.	19	30	8 (2.6%)	9 (6%)
Estimated probability of event-free survival at 5 years	43 ± 6%	n.a.	48 ± 2%	43 ± 3%	57 ± 1%
Estimated probability of disease-free survival at 5 years	46 ± 6%	37 ± 6%	54 ± 2%	55 ± 3%	50 ± 3%
Overall survival	n.a.	42% (3 yrs)	58% (5 yrs)	49 ± 3%	n.a.
Comments	*	**	**	**	

[a] Woods 1996.
[b] Ravindranath 1996.
[c] Stevens 1998.
[d] Creutzig 1997 (updated February 1998).
[e] Lie 2001.
* A short interval between the first two induction cycles improved the end result in all branches.
** No difference in the end results of the different branches.
n.a., not available.

a half in the latter few years of the trial. However, mortality rates greater than 5% persist and are related mainly to *Aspergillus* infections and some other difficult problems such as bleeding and leukostasis in high-WBC patients with M4 and M5 subtypes. The toxic mortality rate will also undoubtedly fall now that a much smaller proportion of patients (probably less than 20%) receive a first-remission BMT.

The common feature of all successful modern trials has been the use of dosage-intensive chemotherapy protocols that contain high-dose cytarabine and some anthracycline. There is no really convincing evidence that one anthracycline is better than another, and attention must now be turned to reducing the amount that is given and to large randomized trials of cardioprotective agents such as cardioxane and cardiac sparing liposomal anthracyclines. There are already a number of patients treated on modern protocols who require cardiac transplant, and considerable energy must be directed at reducing this problem.

Table 12.4 also demonstrates another problem, which is with patients who have resistant disease. It is now possible to predict this problem in most cases, because it usually occurs only within the poor-risk cytogenetic group. Although there are only very few patients, new therapeutic modalities must be tried in these children, in order to give them any real chance of success. This is of course particularly true in the worst group of all, who have a high percentage of residual marrow disease after one course of chemotherapy. These are the patients for whom new drugs such as fludarabine, multidrug resistance modifiers when they become available, immunotherapy such as anti-CD33, and altered old regimens such as high-dose cytarabine and asparaginase are being investigated. This is also the group within which allo-BMT may add a little anti-leukaemic effect that may benefit some patients.

NEW DEVELOPMENTS

The situation has now been reached where it is at last possible to cure the majority of children with AML, but at great cost to them and the health services. However, at least a third of patients still die and a significant proportion of survivors are severely damaged. What needs to be done now is to assess the addition of new non-anthracycline regimes such as CLASP (high-dose cytarabine and timed sequential asparaginase), which is the subject of the MRC AML12 protocol, and fludarabine with or without granulocyte colony stimulating factor

(G-CSF) which is the subject of early randomized trials in relapsed patients. Certain agents such as anti-CD33 and liposomal daunorubicin (DaunoXome) are in relatively early-phase protocols and it is to be hoped that the dearth of other newer drugs will soon be rectified and they can also be tried out in earlier phase studies. Finally, minimal residual disease (MRD) testing is beginning to come of age and may eventually lead to more specific individual tailoring of treatment, but it is important not to fall into the trap of believing that it is known what levels of MRD matter and when, before proof is at hand. Even more importantly, there must be no delusion that modalities of therapy are available that will definitely alter the outcome in patients with MRD. This must first be the subject of randomized trials.

CONCLUDING COMMENT

This is an exciting era in AML therapy following much success already achieved (Fig. 12.3). The challenge is to build on this success of the

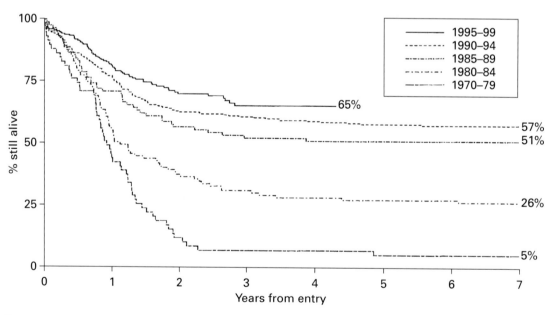

Figure 12.3

MRC AML trials: survival at ages 0–14. Over a 30-year period, AML has been transformed from a disease that was nearly always fatal into one where two-thirds of children are cured. Figure reproduced with many thanks to Dr Keith Wheatley and the Clinical Trials Service Unit, Oxford, UK.

last 30 years and not to 'throw the baby out with the bathwater' through medical prejudice. Therapies such as multidrug resistance modification, MRD modification, new drug therapies, cardioprotection and allo-BMT must be studied vigorously and in a proper scientific fashion if effective cure at least cost is to be achieved.

FURTHER READING

Craze JL, Harrison G, Wheatley K, Hann I. (1999) Improved outcome of acute myeloid leukaemia in Down's syndrome. *Arch Dis Child* **81:** 32–7.

Creutzig, U. (1996) Diagnosis and treatment of acute myelogenous leukaemia in childhood. *Crit Rev Oncol Haematol* **22:** 183–96.

Hann IM, Stevens RF, Goldstone AH et al. (1998) Marked improvements in outcome with chemotherapy alone in paediatric acute myeloid leukaemia. *Br J Haematol* **101:** 130–40.

Stevens RF, Hann IM, Wheatley K et al. (1998) Marked improvements in outcome with chemotherapy alone in paediatric acute myeloid leukaemia. *Br J Haematol* **101:** 130–40.

Wheatley K, Burnett AK, Goldstone AH et al. (1999) A simple robust, validated and highly predictive index for determining directed therapy in AML. *Br J Haematol* **107:** 69–79.

Woods WG, Kobrinsky N, Buckley JD et al. (1998) Timed-sequential induction therapy improves postremission outcome in acute myeloid leukaemia; a report from the Children's Cancer Group. *Blood* **87:** 4979–89.

13 Myelodysplastic and myeloproliferative disorders

Ian M Hann

INTRODUCTION

Myelodysplastic syndrome (MDS) and myeloproliferative (MP) disorders have been the poor relations among malignancies in childhood, attracting little research prior to 1990. There has also been a major problem because the various classifications used in adults have been of extremely limited value in children. These disorders are very much commoner in adults, in whom they have a different natural history, relative prevalence and response to treatment. Over the last decade, efforts to sort out the classification and management of these rare and difficult diseases in children has been allied with a greatly increased interest in scientific research. The understanding of these disorders is still at a primitive stage, and it is very important that they are not split up into artificial classifications that have no biological meaning or clinical relevance. There is a move to more discipline in diagnosis, and the national registries are producing interesting epidemiological data. Relatively simple prognostic criteria are now available, for instance showing that a high haemoglobin F (HbF) level, low platelet count and cytogenetic complexity are poor-risk features in juvenile myelomonocytic leukaemia (JMML). It is now known that chromosome 7 abnormalities are the commonest in children, and candidate genes on this chromosome are currently being mapped. In addition, some new problems have arisen, mainly related to the improved survival in certain disorders such as Shwachman–Diamond syndrome (see Chapter 7), where MDS is being recognized often at a late stage. Modern chemotherapy is also throwing up cases of secondary myelodysplasia, and this problem must be

monitored carefully, so that the types of drug schedules that cause problems can be omitted, without seriously compromising the cytotoxic effect.

Far too much time has been wasted on nosological arguments and far too little spent on clinical management issues in the rare and difficult myelodysplastic and myeloproliferative disorders of children. Haematologists mainly engaged in the adult field worry about whether a disease is MDS or an MP disorder, but the difference is a semantic one and the biological and clinical processes are the same or similar. MDS has been loosely used to cover those disorders that would previously have been called 'pre-leukaemia' or 'sub-leukaemia' or 'grumbling leukaemia', all of which are meaningless terms that have now been abandoned, and rightly so. This group of patients usually presents with organomegaly, pancytopenia, and a normo- or hypercellular marrow that shows dysplasia and a varying percentage of blast cells, from 0 to 25% (at which stage it is very arbitrarily deemed to deserve the cachet of 'leukaemia'). The term 'MP disorders' has usually been reserved for the abnormal proliferation of various single elements, that is essential thrombocythaemia, polycythaemia, eosinophilia and sometimes myelomonocytic proliferations (which have now been called juvenile myelomonocytic leukaemia, JMML). In order to prevent further confusion and turning of attention away from real differences, most paediatric haematologists have agreed that MDS and MP disorders should be considered together until the molecular mechanisms involved are understood. The term 'MDS' will be the only one used for the rest of this chapter.

MDS accounts for only 5% of malignant

blood disorders of childhood. In other words, in areas where there are about five million people, one would expect to see one or two cases a year on average. Although there is some degree of under-diagnosis, due to the difficulty in accurately distinguishing myelo-proliferations such as eosinophilia from benign causes such as infection and allergy and the lack of a specific test as in refractory anaemia, these are of course very rare diseases. However, they are difficult to diagnose and manage and carry a high mortality. Should further justification be required for this separate chapter on the topic, then one may add that investigation of these nasty proliferations may well lead to a better understanding of how blood is regulated and what goes wrong in leukaemias and MDS. The aim of this chapter is to clarify the diagnostic difficulties and classification and to begin the process of more rational management of these difficult diseases.

It was recognized very early on that chronic lymphocytic leukaemia (CLL), whilst being a common disease of the elderly, rarely if ever occurred in children and that lymphocytic reactions were common responses to infections such as pertussis, cytomegalovirus (CMV) and Epstein–Barr virus (EBV). In 1950, Dameshek coined the term 'myeloproliferative disorder', and it was not until considerably later that it was shown that myeloproliferative and myelodysplastic disorders both arose from an abnormal clone of cells and carried a risk of progression to acute leukaemia, sometimes at a slow pace. In 1964, Hardisty et al distinguished two types of chronic granulocytic leukaemia (CGL) in children – the adult type of CGL with the *BCR–ABL* oncogene and Philadelphia chromosome behaves exactly as it does in adults. The other type was initially called juvenile chronic myeloid leukaemia (JCML) and was shown to be associated with wasting infections, suppurative skin rashes, low platelets, huge liver and spleen, high HbF and a reversion to fetal red cell characteristics. Subsequently, other workers described what was initially called the infantile monosomy 7 syndrome, which had similar blood features, including a myelomonocytic proliferation. Only recently has the situation been rational-ized with the adoption of the term juvenile myelomonocytic leukaemia (JMML), within which group various prognostic factors have been identified.

AETIOLOGY, INHERITANCE AND EPIDEMIOLOGY

Recent research has confirmed that MDS is a clonal disorder, which in some cases has been shown to arise in progenitor cells restricted to myelopoiesis and erythropoiesis, whilst in others the lymphoid series is also involved. In the latter cases, a primitive haemopoietic cell has presumably undergone transformation, but the initiating events are currently unknown. Many of the chromosome abnormalities in MDS involve 5q and 7q, regions that are rich in genes with a role in haemopoiesis, and the current theory is that loss of suppressor gene activity leads to an abnormal myeloproliferation. It should also be remembered that monosomy of chromosome 7 frequently occurs in many conditions with a predisposition to leukaemia, including the congenital bone marrow disorders, for example Shwachman–Diamond syndrome. It seems most likely that genes located there contribute to leukaemogenesis as part of a final common pathway following a number of genetic events, including possibly *p53* and *ras* mutations.

There has been a lot of interest in the ineffective haemopoiesis in these disorders, which leads to the paradoxical presence of cytopenias, despite the apparent hypercellularity of the marrow that is often seen. Recent studies have shown that there is in fact a high rate of cell proliferation, but that these cells rapidly undergo premature programmed cell death (apoptosis) and never enter the circulation. Proliferation and apoptosis are influenced by haemopoietic cytokines, and recent studies have clearly demonstrated elevated tumour necrosis factor α (TNF-α), transforming growth factor β (TGF-β) and interleukin-1β (IL-1β).

The true incidence of MDS in children is not yet clearly known, but a population-based study in Denmark has estimated the incidence to be 4.0 cases per million children per year, whilst in the northern region of England a figure of 0.5 per million was found, underlining the problems of definition and case acquisition. National registries with independent data and morphological review are now in progress within the UK and elsewhere, and over the last decade the UK national database has revealed an incidence of 2 per million. The median age of registered patients was 31 months (17 months for JMML).

Childhood MDS is frequently associated with other clinical abnormalities, occurring in between a fifth (in the UK series) and a half of all cases. Some are non-specific, such as mental impairment and short stature. Other cases have recognized genetic conditions; for example, Down's syndrome children have an increased risk of developing megakaryoblastic leukaemia, which often has a preceding phase of MDS that may last some weeks or months. This evolving myeloid leukaemia must be carefully differentiated from transient abnormal myelopoiesis (TAM) seen in newborn Down's babies and occasionally in normal neonates, which resolves in about two-thirds of cases without specific treatment.

Constitutional trisomy 8 presents with facial dysmorphism, skeletal abnormalities and mild to moderate mental impairment. Trisomy 8 is commonly found as a nonsomatic change in blood malignancies, but MDS can also occur with the somatic changes. Neurofibromatosis carries an increased risk of JMML. Severe congenital neutropenia (Kostmann's disease, see Chapter 7) is treated with granulocyte colony stimulating factor (G-CSF) and can then develop MDS with monosomy 7. The Shwachman–Diamond syndrome of pancreatic exocrine insufficiency and neutropenia is associated with an increased risk of acute myeloid and lymphoblastic leukaemias (AML and ALL) and MDS. Fanconi anaemia patients are at significant risk of AML and MDS. Familial cases of MDS with no apparent precipitating factor have been described, and there is a link in some cases with familial platelet storage pool disorders.

So-called 'secondary' MDS was first described in patients with Hodgkin's disease, multiple myeloma and ovarian cancer, and more recently after high-dose chemoradiotherapy and infusion of autologous bone marrow and intensive immunosuppressive therapy for aplastic anaemia. By contrast, secondary acute leukaemia in patients who have been treated with topoisomerase II inhibitors usually occurs without any dysplastic prodrome, and appears earlier than those due to alkylating agents, which present after 4–5 years. Alkylating agents (e.g. nitrosoureas, cyclophosphamide) induce MDS that has a poor prognosis, and the majority of cases exhibit clonal abnormalities involving chromosomes 5 and 7. Much recent interest has been generated by reports of secondary AML following intensive treatment of ALL with regimens containing high dosages of epipodophyllotoxins which are topoisomerase II inhibitors. The AML is often of M4 subtype and usually the cytogenetic change involves the 11q2,3 region (t(9;11) or t(11;19)). An incidence of secondary AML of 12% was described in regimens using an epipodophyllotoxin weekly or twice-weekly. This emphasizes the importance of total dose as well as scheduling, because within the MRC (UK) ALL trials the incidence remains unchanged and below 1% despite the introduction of two blocks of 5-day intensive epipodophyllotoxin therapy.

CLINICAL FEATURES AND DIFFERENTIAL DIAGNOSIS

The differential diagnosis of MDS is very similar to that of the leukaemias (see Chapters 11 and 12). The crucial test that differentiates this disease from aplastic anaemia and other causes of pancytopenia is the bone marrow with a trephine and marrow iron stain and a blood count with HbF level. Whereas the bone marrow can sometimes appear hypocellular in MDS, in the great majority of cases it is normocellular and mainly hypercellular, sometimes grossly so. If there is associated gross dysplasia then the diagnosis is easy, but there is a great risk in diagnosing myelodysplasia in the face of mild or moderate dysplasia in a very active marrow in a child. This degree of dysplasia

Table 13.1 Comparison of paediatric with adult myelodysplasia

French–American–British (FAB) classification	Children[a] (%)	Adults[b] (%)
RA: refractory anaemia	22	28
RARS: refractory anaemia with ring sideroblasts	(1)	24
RAEB: refractory anaemia with excess blasts	13	23
RAEB-t: refractory anaemia with excess blasts in transformation	12	9
CMML: chronic myelomonocytic leukaemia	50	16
Eosinophilia	(2)	–

[a] Children's data is from the UK National Paediatric Myelodysplasia Registry 1990–99 (10.4 cases per annum) with thanks to the United Kingdom Children's Cancer Study Group and Children's Cancer Research Group, Oxford.
[b] Adult data based on the Third MIC Workshop (*Cancer Genet Cytogenet* **32**: 1–10) and Fenaux P et al. (1996) *Semin Haematol* **33**: 127–38.

frequently occurs in response to a stimulus such as infection, when the marrow is 'driven' to produce abnormal-looking cells. In fact, the differentiation between aplastic anaemia and MDS can be very tricky because aplastic anaemia bone marrows can be really quite dysplastic at times. In that situation, the management of the case can be very difficult if a clonal cytogenetic change is not found to bolster the diagnosis of MDS. In such cases, it may be wise to wait and repeat the tests if the clinical condition permits, prior to the institution of immunosuppressive therapy for aplastic anaemia.

In cases of essential thrombocythaemia and polycythaemia, it is essential to rule out a temporary excess, for instance following bleeding or infection, by careful follow-up. In polycythaemics, haemoglobin affinity disorders must also be ruled out along with cardiac abnormalities and erythropoietin-producing tumours.

Table 13.1 shows the classification of cases that have resulted from the UK national MDS registry, and Table 13.2 shows the commoner cytogenetic changes. It is clearly seen that over a third of children will have a chromosome 7 abnormality and that only about one in seven children will be devoid of a detectable abnormality using classical cytogenetic tests and fluorescence in situ hybridiza-

tion (FISH). Unfortunately, in some cases one is left with a child who has a moderately dysplastic marrow, minimal or no organomegaly and variable cytopenias with no cytogenetic change detected. Such cases fall into the refractory anaemia (RA) subtype according to the French–American–British (FAB) classification, which carries a relatively good prognosis (Fig. 13.1). Some of these cases progress to AML, but others improve or remain unchanged for many years and it remains to be seen what their ultimate fate will be.

Table 13.2 UK National and Great Ormond Street MDS Registry: cytogenetic data

Cytogenetic change	Patients (%)
Normal	14
Non-clonal abnormality	32
Monosomy 7	32
Abnormal structural 7	4
Trisomy 8	8
Other abnormalities[a]	10

[a] In eosinophilia, usually involves chromosome 5 in regions that may involve interleukin-5 (IL-5; eosinopoietin).

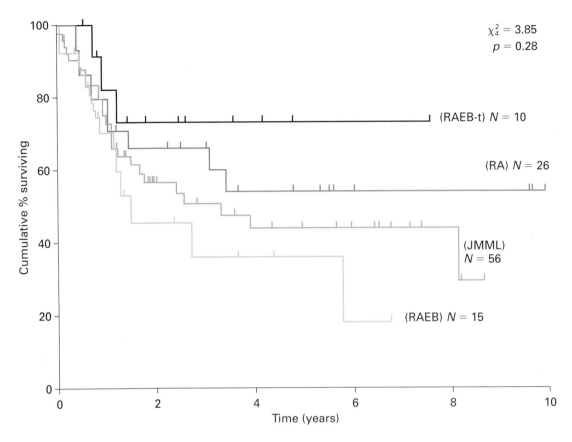

Figure 13.1

Results from United Kingdom Children's Cancer Study Group Database 1990–99 broken down by subtype: RA, refractory anaemia; RAEB, refractory anaemia with excess blasts; RAEB-t, refractory anaemia with excess blasts in transformation; JMML, juvenile myelomonocytic leukaemia.

Several points need to be made about Table 13.1. Not surprisingly, for those of us who believe that children are not just small adults, the disease is different. Nearly a quarter of adults have refractory anaemia with ring sideroblasts (RARS), whereas <1% of children have this disorder. In morphological terms, RARS is like refractory anaemia, that is with ill-defined moderate dysplasia, but with the presence of ring sideroblasts with the iron stain. In childhood, it is vitally important to recognize that most cases presenting like this have in fact a mitochondrial cytopathy, or Pearson's syndrome. An additional clue may

be the variable presence of vaculation of the cytoplasm of cells within the bone marrow. These children usually present with a transfusion-dependent anaemia and then go on to develop various serious metabolic disorders, including diabetes mellitus. Congenital sideroblastic anaemia, due to abnormalities of haem synthesis, is usually associated with a dimorphic blood film and normal white cells and megakaryocytes.

The blood film is a crucially important piece in the jigsaw that goes into making the diagnosis of MDS. The degree of blood dysplasia is often much clearer than that which is seen in the marrow, and one can particularly see hypogranulation of the neutrophils, with abnormally large forms and distorted nuclei. In JMML, there is a marked blood monocytosis with unusual nuclear forms; and in cases of refractory anaemia with excess blasts (RAEB), and the same in transformation (RAEB-t), there may be some blast cells, which may also be present in JMML. A HbF level of greater than 10% clinches the diagnosis of JMML and has prognostic importance (see below and Fig. 13.2). The UK national registry data shows that the so-called FPC score (score 1 for each of

the following: platelets $<40 \times 10^9/l$, HbF >10%, more than two cytogenetic abnormalities) predicts for the outcome in JMML.

The bone marrow trephine histology can give useful confirmatory information. Many cases of MDS show myelofibrosis, and in very rare cases this may be associated with acute myelofibrosis as seen in adults, along with teardrop poikilocyte red cells on the blood film. Of more value is the presence of blast cells towards the centre of the marrow cavity, away from their usual paratrabecular location – so-called abnormal localization of immature

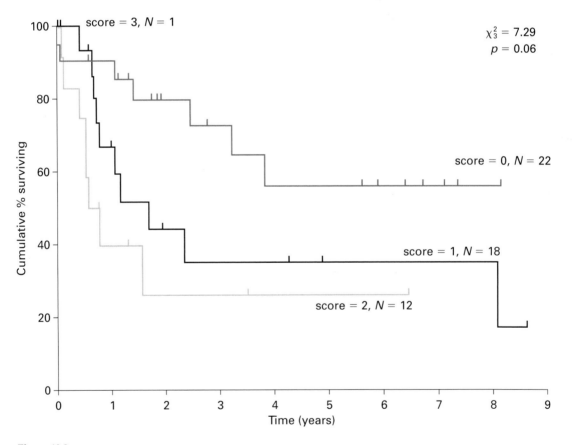

Figure 13.2

The actuarial survival of JMML in the United Kingdom Children's Cancer Study Group 1990–99 Series by FPC; (HbF, platelets, cytogenetic complexity) score, where each feature (HbF > 10%, cytogenetic complexity, platelets $<40 \times 10^9/l$) scores one point. Higher scores do worse. With many thanks to Dr Jane Passmore, Dr Gerald Draper and Dr Charles Stiller at the Children's Cancer Research Group, Oxford, UK.

progenitors (ALIP). In myeloproliferative disorders, such as essential thrombocythaemia, polycythaemia rubra vera and eosinophilia, the trephine demonstrates a gross excess of the relevant precursors.

To cut a long story short, the classification in Table 13.1 requires the presence of an excess of blood or marrow monocytes in order to make the diagnosis of JMML. Unlike adults, this is the commonest form of MDS, occurring in up to half of cases. The other diagnostic group is of RA, RAEB and RAEB-t. There is no real logic in the differentiation of RAEB from RAEB-t or AML, because they are essentially just stages along the route to AML in childhood that have been artificially separated at arbitrary blast percentages. It would be much better to accept that RA is dysplasia without excess of blasts and that RAEB → AML have an excess of blasts.

CLINICAL MANAGEMENT

Prognosis and natural history

The biggest problem with managing children with MDS has been in trying to predict what will happen to them over the ensuing months. Some deteriorated and died rapidly, usually with bone marrow failure, and others proved to have very indolent disease, thus making clinicians very nervous about starting very intensive therapy at an early stage. There is now better, although not perfect, prognostic information and a better 'handle' on the natural history in some cases.

Transformation to AML is confined to patients with RA, RAEB and RAEB-t. However, deterioration in JMML is associated with progressive marrow failure, increasing the need for blood product and antimicrobial support, and general deterioration in physical condition, rather than the development of a frank new leukaemia. Analysis of prognostic factors in the UK national MDS and other surveys has shown that gender is of no importance and that age is only of marginal importance (and then only in JMML, for which younger children had a better prognosis). The most important adverse factors are shown in Table 13.3. The most important pre-

Table 13.3 Adverse prognostic factors in MDS
• Age >2 years in JMML
• HbF > 10% in JMML
• Platelets <40 × 10^9/l in JMML
• Complex cytogenetic abnormalities (two or more)
• Monosomy 7 in RAEB/RAEB-t

HbF, haemoglobin F blood level. Data taken from UK National MDS Registry.

dictors for a poor outcome in JMML are low platelets, high level of HbF and complex cytogenetic change. Similar to AML, monosomy 7 is associated with a poor prognosis is RAEB/RAEB-t. There is some controversy as to whether the percentage of bone marrow blasts adds to this prognostic scoring.

Various other attempts to predict outcome have been made and remain under investigation. The only one to help so far is the presence of autonomous granulocyte–macrophage colony growth in vitro in a proportion of patients with JMML who appear to do worse than those who do not display this abnormality on cell culture.

Treatment: cytotoxics and other drugs

Various haemopoietic growth factors have been used with a view to improving the various cytopenias that occur with MDS. Granulocyte colony stimulating factor (G-CSF) and its granulocyte–macrophage equivalent (GM-CSF) have largely been abandoned because the blasts may express cytokine receptors and increased numbers of blast cells in vivo have been induced. It is likely that platelet growth factors such as thrombopoietin and stem cell growth factors will be evaluated in the same way, and in some cases where more active therapy is not possible combinations of such agents may prove useful in the short term. There is also some interest in the use of differentiating agents such as cis-retinoic acid, particularly for JMML, but there is no real evidence that anything other than a palliative effect in some cases is achieved. In the same way, drugs such as mercaptopurine and hydroxyurea can damp down an excess of monocytes and macrophages in JMML and eosinophils in clonal proliferations. This may be of palliative value and in the run-up to allogeneic bone marrow transplantation (allo-BMT). The main treatment for essential thrombocythaemia is aspirin to prevent thrombosis, although ana-grelide is now entering paediatric usage, and in polycythaemia rubra vera it is venesection.

The biggest problem with MDS is knowing which patients to treat with cytotoxic therapy. In patients with RA, cytotoxic chemotherapy is not usually considered because progression may be very slow or non-existent. The usual progression is to develop an excess of blasts, and at that stage most clinicians would choose to treat with chemotherapy. Rarely, the patient can become dependent on blood products without developing leukaemia, and in that situation the clinical picture is very similar to thalassaemia, with markedly inef-fective erythropoiesis and the need for regular blood transfusion and iron chelation. This situation is not tolerable in the long term, and allo-BMT should be strongly considered even if a matched sibling donor is not avail-able.

There is little reliable information on the use of chemotherapy for RAEB and RAEB-t, but in the UK outcomes are similar to those for AML. Since RAEB/RAEB-t is a stem cell disorder, or at least a disease affecting early haemopoietic cells, usually of several lin-eages, it is not surprising that these patients are at greater risk than AML patients of severe toxicity related to prolonged and pro-found marrow hypoplasia. Factors that may predict a good response are the presence of Auer rods, normal karyotype or possibly monosomy 7 when it is associated with a JMML morphological picture and the classifi-cation of RAEB and RAEB-t. Other patients with JMML do not respond well to chemotherapy, and it is rarely curative. It must also be remembered that younger chil-dren with low levels of HbF, relatively pre-served platelet counts and the absence of autonomous in vitro colony growth can run a

very indolent course, which can be managed sometimes by splenectomy with or without intermittent hydroxyurea.

The available information suggests that chemotherapy-induced complete remission rates may be as low as one-third, with very resistant disease being present in as many as a third of cases. However, the reported series have clouded the picture by including JMML, and the actual response rates may be at least double these depressing figures. There is no doubt that procedure-related mortality was very high in the past and these patients above all others need to be managed with excellent supportive care. Newer agents have been tried, but so far the only one with real promise is topotecan, which is a topoisomerase I inhibitor.

It must again be stressed that the decision to give active chemotherapy to patients with MDS depends on making as firm a diagnosis as possible and ruling out all other possible causes, because these are at least in part diag-noses of exclusion. At Great Ormond Street over the last two decades, we have seen apparent JMML turn out to be due to infec-tion with CMV, EBV, *Leishmania* and par-vovirus. We have seen cases mimicking idiopathic myelofibrosis of adults, which turned out to be due to toxoplasmosis and auto-immune disorders. We have seen chil-dren with apparent RAEB who turned out to have a retroviral infection, and have recog-nized a number of times that the distinction between immune deficiency and MDS can be a fine one. A number of patients have features of both, and the genetic defect presumably can involve a myeloproliferative and immuno-regulatory defect, with one or the other being more prominent. In this situation, auto-immune phenomena such as Coombs-positive haemolytic anaemias can occur.

Bone marrow transplantation

To put it simply, the only cure for MDS in most cases is an allo-BMT of some kind, because the disease affects early progenitor cells and cytotoxic chemotherapy does not work in most instances. (However, children with RAEB/RAEB-t may be treated with standard regimens for AML.) As stated above, the exceptions are RA, essential thrombocythaemia and polycythaemia rubra vera, eosinophilia and some good-risk cases of JMML. It must also be remembered that in those cases where there are other disorders, a BMT may not be relevant or may not cure all of the problems, even if a new functional marrow results from the procedure. For instance, BMT will not cure neurofibromatosis and will not correct the exocrine pancreatic problems of Shwachman–Diamond syndrome. In Pearson's syndrome, the MDS may be the minor element and the various metabolic and cerebral disturbances preclude a BMT.

It must also be remembered that the late effects of allo-BMT in this generally very young group of patients may be very severe, because of the preparative regimens used and the pre-existing organ dysfunction, which, for instance, can lead to a higher incidence of veno-occlusive disease (VOD) of the liver. Also, BMT is usually performed in other groups of patients when they have reached a state of minimal residual disease, but, in JMML in particular, this may well not be the case. Thus, the problems of disease eradication make the choice of preparative regimen doubly difficult, because of the need to enhance the 'antitumour' effect.

Early attempts to eradicate the disease in JMML included the use of total body irradiation in very young children, with consequent severe late effects on growth, endocrine, intellectual, cardiac, optic and fertility function. More recent transplant programmes have thankfully shown that this is a set of diseases where chemotherapy-only preparative regimens may be more effective and are most likely to be associated with very significant but less severe late toxicity. Various regimens have been tried, although the protocol of high-dose cyclophosphamide and busulphan (Bu/Cy) is that with which others should be compared. The addition of melphalan or less likely an epipodophyllotoxin may enhance the antileukaemic effect with tolerable early toxicity.

The development that has made all the difference in MDS is the availability of a donor in more than 80% of cases, compared with only 33% a few years ago. It seems likely that within a short space of time all patients will have a reasonably matched donor, using molecular matching techniques for unrelated and related haplo-identical donors. The technique that has made the difference was pioneered by Prentice in London and others, whereby T cells are removed from the marrow and anti-T-cell monoclonal antibodies given to the recipient. The problem has been working out precisely how many T cells and which variety need to be present in the donated marrow in order to preserve their graft-versus-leukaemia (GVL) effect whilst minimizing their graft-versus-host disease (GVHD) effect (hepatitis, gastroenteritis, pneumonitis, dermatitis). This has to be delicately balanced against the need to prevent T cells of the recipient from rejecting the graft, by the use of adequate immunosuppression (antibodies, cyclophosphamide, etc.) within the preparative regimen. Such techniques are still developing, and at present it requires a great deal of skill and expertise to achieve the correct balance, depending on the underlying disease, closeness of tissue match, etc.

The best tests of a good BMT programme are the levels of procedural mortality and the incidence of disease relapse, rejection rate, VOD, GVHD and late effects. BMT centres should always have a good throughput of patients and a dedicated team of nurses, doctors and ancillary staff and a filtered-air facility. The procedural mortality that should currently be aimed for is 5–10% for allo-BMT from a matched sibling donor and 10–15% for allo-BMT otherwise, depending on the age of patients and underlying diseases. In order to achieve this, first-rate supportive care is required. This is a group of patients wherein there is a large amount of scope for randomized trials of supportive care, and interesting new therapies for trial include antithrombin and protein C therapy of VOD, itraconazole and echinocand, prevention of fungal infection, and various agents purported to reduce the incidence and severity of GVHD. There is a great tendency in this area, which must be resisted, to adopt expensive and potentially toxic and ineffective therapies with largely unknown toxicity profiles based on a few anecdotal stories of success. There is no substitute for scientific rigour in this or any other area of haematology. This statement also applies to the use of donor leukocyte infusions in order to attempt to achieve a greater GVL effect in patients whose disease relapses after BMT. There is no evidence of efficacy in MDS in children at this time, but this approach would be suitable for randomized study.

CONCLUSIONS AND SUMMARY

Diagnosis and management of childhood MDS is completely different from the biologically diverse disease seen in the elderly. There is a dearth of RARS cases and a preponderance of JMML. It is now possible to produce a prognostic scoring that identifies a poorer-risk group of patients with older age, high HbF, low platelets and complex cytogenetic changes. We have begun to feel our way towards more rational management of these rare and difficult diseases, partly because of good international collaboration, which will hopefully continue. At the same time, greater scientific interest is at long last producing exciting insights into the pathogenesis of these diseases and into the control of haemopoiesis. Chemotherapy has a small rôle to play in the cure of these diseases, and at present it is necessary to rely on the vastly improved area of BMT, albeit at great cost in late toxicity to patients. Much needs to be learnt about preventing toxicity and enhancing the antileukaemic effect of this type of treatment and we are on the verge of having a donor for everyone. It is to be hoped that in the future safer treatments will be developed that may obviate the use of donors.

FURTHER READING

Chan GC, Wang WC, Raimondi SC et al. (1997) Myelodysplastic syndrome in children: differentiation from acute myeloid leukaemia with a low blast count. *Leukaemia* **11:** 206–11.

Chessels JM. (1991) Myelodysplasia. *Baillière's Clin Haematol* **4:** 459–82.

Chessels JM. (1999) Myelodysplastic syndromes. In: Lilleyman JS, Hann I, Blanchette V, eds. *Paediatric Haematology*. Edinburgh: Churchill Livingstone: 83–104.

Haas OA, Gadner H. (1996) Pathogenesis, biology and management of myelodysplastic syndromes in children. *Semin Haematol* **33:** 225–35.

Passmore SJ, Hann IM, Stiller CA et al. (1995) Paediatric myelodysplasia: a study of 68 children and a new prognostic scoring system. *Blood* **85:** 1742–50.

Webb DKH, Passmore SJ, Harrison G, Wheatley K, Hann IM, Chessels JM. (2002) Outcome for children with refractory anaemia with excess blasts (RAEB) and in transition (RAEBt) in Britain. *Br J Haematol* (in press).

Zipursky A, Thorner P, De Harven E et al. (1994) Myelodysplasia and acute megakaryoblastic leukaemia in Down's syndrome. *Leukemia Res* **18:** 163–77.

14 Non-Hodgkin's lymphoma

Ian M Hann

INTRODUCTION

The great majority of cases of childhood non-Hodgkin's lymphoma (NHL) occur in the mediastinum, where it is nearly always T-cell high-grade lymphoblastic in nature, and in the abdomen, where it is almost always high-grade lymphoblastic of mature B cells. All other types are much less common, but it has recently been recognized that another group of high-grade lymphomas exist, called the anaplastic large cell (ALC) group, which may be positive for the Ki-1 (CD30) antibody with ALK protein expression and was previously called malignant histiocytosis, as well as some cases of peripheral T-cell NHL. The ALC group tends to present with nodal involvement, and there is often skin disease and sometimes lung involvement, along with prominent systemic features including fever and weight loss, which tends to mimic other causes of fever of unknown origin. In addition to these presentations, some ALC patients can present with head and neck tumours, generally involving Waldeyer's ring or maxillary and/or mandibular bones or lymph nodes. The remaining uncommon primary sites of NHL are bone (when it is often like a solid lump of early pre-B acute lymphoblastic leukaemia, ALL), kidney, thyroid, orbit, eyelid, skin and epidural. No particular histology is associated with these sites. Treatment results dramatically improved in the early 1980s, before which most children with NHL died. Now the great majority are cured with chemotherapy alone. Resort to bone marrow transplantation (BMT) is only necessary in less than one in ten with primarily resistant disease and the approximately one-fifth whose disease relapses and a good stable remission is obtained. Initially cardiotoxicity and infertility were very problematic late effects of the anthracyclines and cyclophosphamide used in the therapy of these disorders. In addition, second cancers followed some of the early regimens that contained nitrosoureas and cyclophosphamide. It would appear so far that these problems will be much less common with modern cytotoxic regimens (see Chapter 17).

The NHL's of childhood were a depressing set of diseases to treat 20 years ago, with the majority of patients dying – often very rapidly with resistant disease or, in the case of advanced-stage B-NHL and B-ALL of mature B cells, with early and extensive central nervous system (CNS) disease. The only advantage that the paediatric haematologist/oncologist had over his or her adult-treating counterpart was the lack of a need to split the disease into multitudinous histological subtypes of dubious clinical and biological relevance. Everything has now changed radically. Not only are more than three-quarters of the patients curable without the need to resort to BMT, but the last decade has been spent in refining the schedules such that the late toxicities, in particular infertility and cardiotoxicity, have been minimized. During this time, a new disease entity has been recognized that is not yet another histological 'splitting' exercise, namely anaplastic large cell lymphoma (ALCL), which has a good biological basis. Previously, this was called malignant histiocytosis (an extremely misleading term) and peripheral T-cell lymphoma, although the latter classification still lives on in rare cases. ALCL patients can be very difficult to diagnose because the primary can be very small (e.g. a small lung focus or small lymph node or tiny skin lesion) yet the systemic symptoms of hectic fevers, weight loss and being generally unwell are dramatic and can be confused with diseases such as vasculitis (e.g. in systemic lupus erythematosus, SLE), tuberculosis and familial Mediterranean fever.

Immunophenotyping has helped to make the diagnosis secure in some cases, but setting aside the rarities such as ALCL, peripheral T-cell lymphoma etc., there are mainly three types of presentation: mediastinal T-cell disease; abdominal B-cell disease; and head and neck localized disease of the facial bones and lymph nodes of both immunophenotypes. Almost all cases in childhood are diffuse and lymphoblastic, and low-grade lymphomas are so rare as to warrant only a very brief mention. In fact, before accepting the diagnosis of low- and intermediate-grade B-follicular lymphomas in children, it must always be remembered that lymphadenopathy with florid reactive change is very common in children and follicular lymphoma excessively rare, accounting for less than 1% of all NHL of childhood. Disease is usually localized to nodes and/or tonsils, systemic symptoms are rare, and mixed follicular and diffuse forms are more common than the pure follicular form. Clinical management of these low-grade cases is difficult because of the relative inefficacy of chemotherapy.

AETIOLOGY AND EPIDEMIOLOGY

There are remarkable international differences in the incidence of NHL. In Africa, there is a three times higher incidence of NHL than average because of endemic Burkitt's lymphoma. Brazil, Israel and Cuba also have high rates, and intermediate rates occur in Australia and Costa Rica. The lowest rates are in Hungary, American blacks and Norway. There is a male preponderance throughout the world, and in most developed countries there is an increased incidence with older age in childhood. Of interest is the incidence in America, where whites have 9.0 cases per million population and blacks only 5.4 per million.

It has been known for a long time that there is a higher risk of NHL in immunocompromised patients, both congenital and following HIV infection. Patients who have undergone organ transplantation are at considerable risk of lymphoproliferative disease (LPD), which is usually an Epstein–Barr virus (EBV)-driven lymphomatous disease that may or may not respond to reduced immunosuppression. The incidence of LPD cases is rising with the rising number of transplant procedures, and the UK Children's Cancer Study Group (UKCCSG) national register is picking up approximately one new case per month.

Burkitt's lymphomas are characterized by one of three cytogenetic translocations, t(8;14), t(8;22) and t(2;8), in each of which the c-*myc* gene is juxtaposed to an immunoglobulin chain gene, leading to abnormal proliferation of mature immunoglobulin-producing B cells. There is ongoing speculation as to the role of EBV in the pathogenesis of Burkitt's lymphoma and speculation about a predisposition to NHL following exposure to hair dyes and pesticides, but no real proof of anything at present and the results of national case-controlled epidemiological studies in this area as well as all other childhood malignancies are awaited.

Most of the rest of the research into the aetiology of NHL is at an early stage, and that related to T-NHL is obviously relevant to ALL, because the difference between T-NHL and T-ALL is largely semantic. Work continues to distinguish endemic Burkitt's lymphoma from non-endemic Burkitt-like NHL (i.e. they look histologically alike), and this work has concentrated on molecular studies. The endemic type shows consistent rearrangements of c-*myc*, bcl-2 and bcl-1, whereas the non-endemic cases show a much lower proportion of bcl-2 rearrangements and no rearrangements of c-*myc* or bcl-1, suggesting that apoptotic mechanisms and cell proliferation are involved in pathogenesis.

Cytogenetic changes also occur in the ALCL cases and may be of great diagnostic help in the relatively common cases where diagnosis may be difficult. The translocation t(2;5)(p23;q35) was described in 1986 and may involve the fusion of the nucleolar phosphoprotein gene NPM on chromosome 5 and a protein kinase gene ALK on chromosome 2, producing a hybrid protein with tyrosine kinase activity.

DIAGNOSIS (Table 14.1)

As stated above, there are four main patterns of presentation and in most cases the diagnosis is fairly obvious. The necessary tests are shown in Table 14.1. Thus, there is a mediastinal mass form, an abdominal mass form, the ALC presentation and patients with localized disease, usually of the head and neck. Whatever the presentation, it is always necessary to get a piece of tissue for histological diagnosis, and Table 14.2 shows the immunohistochemical techniques that are now being used to confirm the morphological diagnosis and help categorize the patients into the classification shown in Table 14.3. It is, however, necessary to sound a strong word of caution here, which is that antibody testing does not always work perfectly, due to aberrant expression of antigens or problems with tech-niques. The gold standard of diagnosis remains the standard histological stained slides, and whenever the diagnosis does not make sense, for example a B-cell immunophenotype on a standard mediastinal lymphoblastic lymphoma, then the tests should be repeated and interpreted with caution.

In future, it is likely that interventional radiology and fine-needle aspiration will greatly simplify the diagnosis of NHL and other solid tumours of childhood, but this must await proper evaluation and probably the development of incontrovertible tests such as molecular translocations like t(2;5) in ALCL.

The great majority of anterior mediastinal masses in children are T-NHL, with a small number of cases of Hodgkin's disease, usually in older children, and the rarities such as sclerosing B-cell mediastinal NHL and ter-atomas. Chronic granulomatous disease can also present in this way, due to *Aspergillus* infection and granulomatous reaction. Thus, getting a histological diagnosis is very important, but may not always be clinically possible. Patients with mediastinal T-NHL frequently present as a medical emergency with superior mediastinal syndrome and compromise of the airways, which can make anaesthesia very hazardous. In this circumstance, it is essential to check whether or not the patient has hepatosplenomegaly or an abnormal blood count, because if that is the case then it is much more likely that this is T-ALL, and the diagnosis could be made from a bone marrow performed under local anaesthesia, or by examination of the blood film and immunophenotyping if there are circulating blast cells. If this is not the case (and often it is not) then a mediastinal biopsy should be carried out when the patient is fit. If superior vena cava (SVC) obstruction exists then a couple of days of steroid and vincristine will usually dramatically improve the problem. There is then a risk of getting non-diagnostic material, because T-NHL responds dramatically to therapy – but one cannot always have it all ways! The fact is that the other tumour types would very rarely respond so rapidly anyway, and thus a dramatic response is in itself of great diagnostic importance.

Table 14.1 Investigation of NHL in childhood
Mandatory Physical examination and history Chest x-ray Abdominal ultrasonography Bone marrow aspirate Cerebrospinal fluid cytospin examination Full blood count and film Electrolytes, proteins, liver function tests Urate, creatinine Biopsy of lesion
Required in certain circumstances Scans of affected areas, e.g. nasopharynx, abdomen Marrow trephine if aspirate difficult Glomerular filtration rate: B-cell high-stage protocols Echocardiogram: anthracycline-containing protocols Investigation of immune status and for ataxia telangiectasia in very young patients and those with infectious history

Table 14.2 Antibodies commonly used in the tissue diagnosis of lymphoblastic leukaemia and lymphomas

CD designation[a]	Role of cell surface antigen	Distribution	Comments
CD1a	Part of a family of 5 genes: structure similar to MHC class I molecules	Cortical thymocytes, dendritic cells	Expression is minorly related with TCR and MHC class I expression
CD2	Interacts with CD58, through which signal transduction may occur	All mature T cells, NK cells and thymocytes	
CD3	Actually a complex of 5 peptides (γ, δ, ϵ, ν and ξ) associated with the TCR, and involved with signal transduction	Increasing expression with T-cell maturation	Paraffin antibody available
CD4	Co-receptor with TCR for binding antigen in association with MHC class II	Most thymocytes (also CD8$^+$) and T-helper cells (CD8$^-$): monocytes and macrophages	HIV-binding receptor
CD5	T-cell activation and proliferation: CD5$^+$ B cells produce polyreactive antibodies	Most thymocytes, all mature T cells and a subset of mature B-cells	Binds to CD72
CD7	A glycoprotein involved in signal transduction	Primitive haemopoietic cells, thymocytes, many mature T cells	
CD8	Co-receptor with TCR for binding antigen in association with MHC class I	Most thymocytes (also CD4$^+$) and CD4$^-$ mature T cells	
CD10	CALLA (common acute lymphoblastic leukaemia antigen). Neutral endopeptidase that clears various peptides including enkephalins and angiotensin	Wide: early B and T cells, some myeloid cells, bone marrow stromal cells, some epithelia, some soft tissues and glia	
CD13	Aminopeptidase, possibly involved in peptide-mediated signalling	Myeloid precursors and mature myeloid cells, including monocytes: also some epithelia and soft tissues	
CD15	Involved in cell adhesion and phagocytosis by myeloid cells	Mature myeloid cells, including monocytes, adenocarcinomas and Reed–Sternberg and Hodgkin cells	Binds to CD62 and ELAM-1: paraffin antibody available
CD19	Regulation of B-cell proliferation	Early B-cell precursors and mature B cells (not plasma cells); follicular dendritic cells	Paraffin antibody available
CD20	Regulation of B-cell activation and proliferation	B-cell precursors and mature B cells (not plasma cells)	
CD21	Regulation of B-cell activation and proliferation	Mature B cells: follicular dendritic cells; some thymocytes: some epithelia	EBV receptor
CD22	Cell adhesion to monocytes, T cells, B cells and erythrocytes	B-cell precursor and some mature B cells: hairy cell leukaemia	

CD25	Interleukin-2 (IL-2) receptor comprises α and β subunits; binding with IL-2 reduces activation and proliferation	Activated T cells, B cells and monocytes	
CD30	Member of nerve growth factor receptor family: involved in transduction of a cell death signal	Activated T cells, B cells. Hodgkin and Reed–Sternberg cells: some cases of embryonal carcinoma	Paraffin antibody available
CD33	Function unknown	Myeloid precursors, monocytes	
CD34	Function unknown; possible role in cell adhesion	Primitive haemopoietic precursors: endothelium	
CD45	Four isoforms are relevant (CD45RA, RB, RC and RO): formed by alternative splicing; function appears to be signal transduction	All haemopoietic cells (except erythroid cells)	Paraffin antibody available (detects all isoforms)
CD45RO	Splice variant of CD45	Memory T-helper cells (not naive T cells)	Specific paraffin antibody available
CD68	Lysosomal glycoprotein of uncertain function	Monocytic cells, basophils, neutrophils and large lymphocytes: hepatocytes and renal epithelium	Paraffin antibody available
EMA	Found on secretor epithelia	Many epithelia, some soft tissues, large cell anaplastic lymphoma	Paraffin antibody available
TdT	Terminal deoxynucleotidyl transferase: inserts nucleotides randomly at junctions during antigen receptor gene rearrangement	Early B-cell and T-cell precursors	

^{a} The CD designation refers to 'cluster of differentiation', which is a statistically derived group of antibodies reacting with epitopes on the same antigen. This has proved invaluable in clarifying the confusion in antibody terminology and in facilitating research into the characterization of cell surface antigens. MHC, major histocompatibility complex; TCR, T-cell receptor.

Table 14.3 Revised European–American classification of lymphoid neoplasms

B-cell neoplasms

I   Precursor B-cell neoplasms: precursor B-lymphoblastic leukaemia/lymphoma

II Peripheral B-cell neoplasms
   1 B-cell chronic lymphocytic leukaemia/prolymphocytic leukaemia/small lymphocytic lymphoma
   2 Lymphoplasmacytoid lymphoma/immunocytoma
   3 Mantle cell lymphoma
   4 Follicle centre lymphoma, follicular
      Provisional cytologic grades I (small cell), II (mixed small and large cell), III (large cell)
      Provisional subtype: diffuse, predominantly small cell type
   5 Marginal zone B-cell lymphoma. Extranodal (MALT type ± monocytoid B cells)
      Provisional subtype: Nodal (± monocytoid B cells)
   6 Provisional entity: splenic marginal zone lymphoma (± villous lymphocytes)
   7 Hairy cell leukaemia
   8 Plasmacytoma/plasma cell myeloma
   9 Diffuse large cell B-cell lymphoma
         Subtype: primary mediastinal (thymic) B-cell lymphoma
   10 Burkitt's lymphoma
   11 Provisional entity: high-grade B-cell lymphoma Burkitt-like[a]

T-cell and putative NK-cell neoplasms

I   Precursor T-cell neoplasm: Precursor T-lymphoblastic lymphoma/leukaemia

II Peripheral T-cell and NK-cell neoplasms
   1 T-cell chronic lymphocytic leukaemia/prolymphocytic leukaemia
   2 Large cell granular lymphocytic leukaemia (LGL)
         T-cell type
         NK-cell type
   3 Mycosis fungoides/Sezary's syndrome
   4 Peripheral T-cell lymphomas unspecified
      Provisional cytologic categories: medium sized cell, mixed medium and large cell, large cell, lymphoepithelioid cell
      Provisional subtype: hepatosplenic γδ T-cell lymphoma
      Provisional subtype: subcutaneous T-cell lymphoma
   5 Angioimmunoblastic T-cell lymphoma (AILD)
   6 Angiocentric lymphoma
   7 Intestinal T-cell lymphoma (± enteropathy-associated)
   8 Adult T-cell lymphoma/leukaemia (ATLL)
   9 Anaplastic large cell lymphoma (ALCL), CD30[+], T- and null-cell types
   10 Provisional entity: anaplastic large cell lymphoma, Hodgkin's-like

[a] This catagory is thought likely to include more than one disease entity.
Adapted from Harris NL, Jaffe ES, Stein H et al. A revised European–American classification of lymphiod neoplasms: a proposal from the International Lymphoma Study Group. *Blood* 1994; **84:** 1361–92. Copyright American Society of Hematology, used by permission.

In the past, surgeons have sadly carried out heroic operations in an attempt to diagnose and 'treat' abdominal B-NHL. This is obviously unnecessary, dangerous and ineffective. Surgical removal should be limited to rare cases where simple resection of intussuscepted bowel is required. Abdominal B-NHL classically presents with multiple masses arising from the gut or mesentery, often involving other intra-abdominal or retroperitoneal structures and sometimes associated with ascites, pleural effusions, wasting and fever. Diagnosis can sometime be made by the presence within pleural (and maybe ascitic) fluid of sheets of L3-type mature B-cell lymphoblasts. In some cases, the blood count is abnormal, and here a bone marrow aspirate may give the diagnosis of L3-type mature B-cell ALL. The blood film may give the diagnosis away and in such cases the diagnostic test is a bone marrow aspirate, and this again underlines the mainly semantic differences between ALL and NHL in childhood. They appear to be liquid and solid forms of the same disease. In most cases, a biopsy is required and hopefully this can be via interventional radiology in future, without the need for laparotomy.

NHL in isolated sites such as bone, thyroid, kidney, skin, eyelid, epidural, Waldeyer's ring and lymph nodes should obviously be biopsied. At present, the tissue architecture is necessary for diagnosis, but hopefully in the very near future, fine-needle aspirates may take over. This will ease the biggest problem, which is the child with glands in the neck referred with a possibility of a malignancy. To put this in context, a paediatric haematologist/oncologist working within a children's cancer centre can expect to see at least 10–15 such cases per year, and in more than 20 years the present author has personally only picked up one case of Hodgkin's disease and one of NHL from such referrals. General practitioners and district general hospital paediatricians see such cases very frequently. The likelihood of missing a serious disease that needs to be picked up early is extremely small if the child is generally well with no hepatosplenomegaly and no signs of bruising/bleeding/petechiae or signs or symptoms of anaemia. If the nodes are relatively small and smooth and not fixed and do not increase in size over several weeks then there is almost certainly no need to do more than keep an eye on the situation, especially if there is a reason for lymphadenopathy, for example recurrent upper respiratory infections.

As previously stated, the main differential diagnosis of T-NHL is other tumours occurring in the relevant areas, and infections. Agents such as *Toxoplasma, Yersinia, Toxocara*, cat-scratch, cytomegalovirus (CMV), EBV and adenovirus can mimic NHL, as can the autoimmune lymphoproliferative syndrome (ALPS) due to Fas deficiency.

CLINICAL MANAGEMENT (Tables 14.4 and 14.5)

Table 14.4 details the generally accepted staging system for NHL.

T-cell lymphoblastic lymphoma

This disease behaves very much like T-ALL, and thus many of the details of therapy are covered in Chapter 11. The specific issues with regard to T-NHL will be dealt with here. As previously stated, the most difficult challenge is to make a precise histological diagnosis, and sometimes one has to accept that it really could be nothing else and continue therapy on the protocol. It should be noted that only about one in five to one in ten cases has morphologically defined bone marrow disease at diagnosis and that there is no convincing evidence that these patients do worse. The overall survival rate is about 80%, similar to ALL, and the division between stage IV T-NHL and T-ALL at a marrow blast percentage of 25% is arbitrary.

Patients with T-NHL at diagnosis are at high risk of both SVC obstruction and urate nephropathy, due to rapid breakdown of the large tumour mass. Thus, the initial approach is to use excellent supportive care along with vincristine and steroid anti-NHL therapy. The patient is treated with the xanthine oxidase inhibitor allopurinol or uricozyme to counteract hyperuricaemia, and 3 litres/m^2 (body surface area) of fluid, taking care to prevent

Table 14.4 Staging classification of childhood NHL

Stage	Criteria for extent of disease
I	A single tumour (extranodal) or single anatomic area (nodal), with the exclusion of mediastinum or abdomen
II	A single tumour (extranodal) with regional node involvement Two or more nodal areas on the same side of the diaphragm Two single (extranodal) tumours with or without regional node involvement on the same side of the diaphragm A primary gastrointestinal tumour, usually in the ileocaecal area, with or without involvement of associated mesteric nodes only, grossly completely resected
III	Two single tumours (extranodal) on opposite sides of the diaphragm Two or more nodal areas above and below the diaphragm All primary intrathoracic tumours (mediastinal pleural, thymic) All extensive primary intra-abdominal disease All paraspinal or epidural tumours, regardless of other tumour site(s)
IV	Any of the above with initial central nervous system and/or bone marrow involvement

Table 14.5 General scheme of B-NHL protocols

Induction	Low-dose vincristine, cyclophosphamide, and prednisolone (COP). Induce a good tumour reduction and allow time to deal with urate nephropathy, infection and occasional gut perforations
Two further induction courses	Based on fractionated high-dose cyclophosphamide and high-dose methotrexate along with prednisolone, doxorubicin and vincristine (COPAD-M)
Two consolidation courses	Based on cytarabine by continuous infusion
Continuation	Monthly courses using the same drugs as above but at lower dose
CNS-directed therapy	Based on high-dose methotrexate ($3 \, g/m^2$) by 3-hour infusion, and intrathecal methotrexate started early and continued during treatment

fluid overload with diuretics, if required. Alkalinization of the urine probably also helps, and it is mandatory to monitor regularly and carefully for the often consequent hyperphosphataemia, hyperkalaemia, azotaemia and hypocalcaemia, which are life-threatening. The key to preventing fatalities is the early introduction of dialysis (usually haemodialysis via a vas-cath) at the first sign of an escalation in the level of phosphate and potassium. The help of expert nephrologists is vital, and their involvement at a very early stage usually prevents the need for pyelostomy and most fatalities. During this period (which lasts up to a week usually), the patient is at high risk of infection, and the other vital element of supportive care is antimicrobial therapy (Chapter 4). The additional problem is SVC obstruction, and a high proportion of patients require mechanical ventilatory support, which is usually a short-lived requirement if the expected rapid response to therapy occurs. Very occasionally, a delayed or inadequate response occurs, and this should make one search for an alternative diagnosis because this would be relatively commoner in Hodgkin's disease, for instance. The addition of anthracyclines, asparaginase and other more intensive therapies will usually expedite the response.

Thereafter, treatment is very much along the lines of ALL regimens. Following a three-drug induction with vincristine, steroids and asparaginase, several intensification or consolidation courses are given over the next six months. The number and type of courses needed to produce an optimal response is under active study at present, and one can only say that at least two intensive courses are required and that these can be of short sharp duration or of a more extended type. The drugs used in these courses include an epipodophyllotoxin, anthracyclines, cytarabine, vincristine and steroids. CNS-directed therapy is controversial, and there are proponents of several different modalities and no direct evidence for a superior method. In Britain at present, high-dose methotrexate is used along with continuing intrathecal methotrexate, but radiation therapy to the brain is included in some schedules. The final phase is continuation therapy, to complete a total of 2 years' treatment, with an identical mercaptopurine, methotrexate and pulsed vincristine plus steroid regimen as is used for ALL.

The debate about how to treat localized lymphoblastic lymphoma continues and is somewhat bedevilled by the small numbers and an inability to accurately define prognostic groupings. What we know is that patients who present with a solid lump of pre-B or 'common' (pre-pre-B) ALL, for instance in skin or bone, should be treated on the usual ALL schedules as their liquid counterparts, otherwise they will relapse with leukaemia.

Why these patients have solid lumps of NHL that are very similar to their liquid counterparts remains a mystery in several situations. It is also known that the patients with localized disease who did badly in the past usually turned out to have diffuse high-grade T-cell lymphoblastic disease, and these patients also need to be treated on the ALL-type schedules. The current consensus is also that the small residuum of patients with peripheral T-cell lymphomas should similarly be treated on leukaemia-like regimens. The risk of second malignancies and other toxicities is very low and the risk of relapse otherwise unnecessarily high. Localized diffuse high-grade B-lymphoblastic and Ki-1 lymphomas will be discussed below.

B-cell lymphoblastic lymphoma

The points made above about urate nephropathy apply here to an even greater degree. The tumour growth fraction is extremely high and a high proportion of patients with stage III and IV tumours and those with mature B-ALL develop problems – so much so, that some authorities advise the initial use of a vas-cath for haemodialysis in all patients, changing later to the more usual Hickman type of right atrial catheter. The additional problematic feature of this disease is the occasional occurrence of gut perforation, usually through affected Peyer's patches. Such patients are at high risk of a fatal outcome, and great medical and surgical skill and intensive care are required in order to save them.

The debate continues as to how little therapy one can get away with and still cure children with low-stage B-NHL. Most previous regimens have given about five months of treatment and in recent years have put the patient at small but significant risk of cardiotoxicity and infertility. Current randomized trials are looking at the feasibility of very short intensive regimens lasting as little as 2–3 months and using combinations such as COPAD-M (see Table 14.5). The problem with such trials is that there are few eligible patients and very few events, and this has encouragingly been addressed by international cooperative efforts. The best approach should be known soon.

A similar problem arises with stage III abdominal disease, where it is known from historical results of the 1980s that about three-quarters can be cured with intermediate-intensity protocols. However, the other quarter are very difficult to define in advance, and the best prognostic indicators remain failure to respond (with proven residual viable tumour) after three courses of therapy, and CNS disease from the outset. The results of treating B-NHL are now excellent, with overall survival rates of $94 \pm 8\%$ for stage I and II, $91 \pm 4\%$ for stage III, $89 \pm 11\%$ for stage IV and $90 \pm 6\%$ for B-ALL.

Patients with initial CNS disease do worse, with an event-free survival rate of 81%. These are truly remarkable results when one remembers that 20 years ago the median survival for the high-stage patients was about 6 weeks and that this has been achieved without the need to resort to the damaging effects of allogeneic BMT (allo-BMT). In fact, the only patients receiving radiation are those with CNS disease at diagnosis, and the latest trials have dropped even that approach. So, these patients should survive in good shape, and the ultimate goal of 100% cure is not far away when one thinks that an overall survival of $93 \pm 2\%$ has already been reached.

Patients with primarily resistant disease as defined above, and those who relapse, make up a very small group of children who do very poorly. Very few patients in this situation have been cured, and stem cell rescue from high-dose chemotherapy protocols such as busulphan/cyclophosphamide or busul-

phan/melphalan, or melphalan alone, may be an option when there is no marrow disease. Allo-BMT from related and unrelated donors is also an option for patients who relapse and achieve a stable remission, but the preliminary results have not been overly encouraging.

Anaplastic large cell lymphomas (ALCL)

These are what used to be called the Ki-1 lymphomas and are usually of T-cell type with occasional B-cell variants. Since this is a relatively newly reclassified disease, it is doubtful what are the best prognostic features (although skin disease, lung and mediastinal involvement are good candidates) and the best types of therapy. Efforts have begun to develop collaborative international trials, and there may soon be some answers, but at present the literature is very confusing and the results of therapy are less good than they should be. Part of the problem is that in American trials these lymphomas have been included with other large cell lymphomas, making interpretations of results exceedingly difficult. In addition, there have been champions of a B-cell protocol approach, while others believe that a T-cell-type approach is best. Looking at it dispassionately, the results appear similar, with 70–80% overall survival rates and lower event-free survival outcomes suggesting a significant salvage from relapse. We also know that the histology can be confusingly like Hodgkin's disease and that many patients have 'B'-type symptoms. Also, some relapsed patients have responded very well, albeit temporarily, to Hodgkin's-type regimens such as ChlVPP (chlorambucil, vincristine, procarbazine and prednisolone). Thus we need to investigate more intensive chemotherapy regimens that could be hybrid in nature, and drop the usual oncological prejudice that says that there are such-and-such types of protocols absolutely specific for certain diseases. We must also not forget the low-stage ALCL cases, which are currently usually being treated on B-NHL low-stage protocols. The results of such an approach must be monitored, and this is another instance where a fairly intensive and very short-duration regimen may be curative. Certainly, the current NHL staging systems are of no real value in managing ALCL cases, and it is likely although not certain that skin, mediastinal and lung cases, will be shown to be predictors of a bad outcome.

Late effects of therapy
(see Chapter 17)

The incidence of second tumours following modern chemotherapy regimens is probably going to be low, but all patients should be followed up permanently (as with all childhood malignancy) so that the true risk of this and other very late effects, for example infertility and cardiotoxicity, can be ascertained. The risk of cardiotoxicity is small in this group of patients now that they do not receive mediastinal irradiation as part of primary therapy and receive relatively low doses of anthracyclines. However, the current recommendation is that all patients who have received anthracyclines should be followed up with at least 5-yearly echocardiograms to measure fractional shortening and left ventricular ejection fraction. More frequent tests and cardiological review are required when abnormal test results are found. The ovary is less sensitive than the testes to the effects of cyclophosphamide and cytarabine, and although girls may have raised follicle stimulating hormone (FSH), and oligomenorrhoea has been reported, their prospects for fertility are better than those of men. It is not yet known for sure what dose of these agents is safe, but the total dosage has been reduced, particularly for low-stage B-cell patients, and at the same time in many regimens it has been possible to omit anthracyclines altogether and consequently reduce the cardiotoxicity risk. Males who have received cyclophosphamide and cytarabine may demonstrate abnormalities of spermatogenesis but not steroidogenesis. The secretion of testosterone is not affected, and they experience normal puberty, sexual maturation and libido. They have normal luteinizing hormone (LH) levels but raised FSH, and are thus at risk of developing gynaecomastia. Boys and girls should be followed up with growth charting and semen analysis when appropriate.

CONCLUDING COMMENTS
(see Fig. 14.1)

We are a mere 7% away from curing all children with B-NHL, and what is more the great majority of these patients will not be seriously damaged in any way by the treatment that they have received. Current efforts are aimed at reducing toxicity even further in low-stage patients and in defining risk factors in the small group of patients with a poor outcome, for instance those with ALCL with skin and lung/mediastinal involvement, those with CNS disease at diagnosis and those with primarily resistant disease. Patients with T-NHL fare rather worse if they have stage III and IV disease, and, although the 80% cure rates have been maintained in the face of reduced toxicity, about a fifth of patients still fail to respond to treatment or relapse and have a very poor ultimate outcome with relatively low salvage rates. The challenge, as with T-ALL, is very much to achieve a greater anti-leukaemia/lymphoma effect through the use of more intensive regimens, new drugs and possibly allo-BMT. The best therapy for ALCL is at present undetermined but will probably be low-stage B-cell-like regimens for localized disease and hybrid Hodgkin's/NHL protocols for those with higher stage. In the end, we all hope for more specific treatments such as gene therapy, but for the present we will have to rely on our usual standby of chemotherapy.

FURTHER READING

Atra A, Imeson JD, Hobson R, Gerrard M, Hann I, Eden OB. (2000) Improved outcome in children with advanced stage B-NHL. UKCCSG 9002 protocol. *Br J Cancer* **82:** 1396–402.

Carter RL, McCarthy KP. (1995) Some recent developments in the pathology of acute lymphoblastic leukaemia and non-Hodgkin's lymphomas in childhood. *Baillière's Clin Paediatr* **3:** 659–82.

Eden OB. (1999) Lymphomas. In: Lilleyman JS, Hann I, Blanchette V, eds. *Paediatric Haematology.* Edinburgh: Churchill Livingstone: 565–84.

Hann IM, Eden OB, Barnes J, Pinkerton CR. (1990) MACHO chemotherapy for stage IV B-cell lymphoma and B-cell acute leukaemia of childhood. *Br J Haematol* **76:** 359–64.

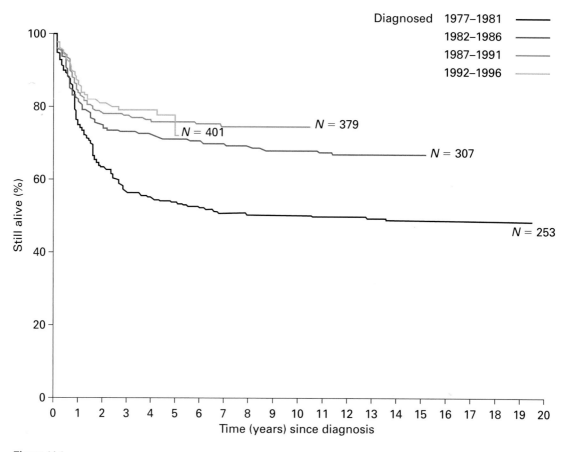

Figure 14.1

Survival with NHL in UKCCSG studies overall approaches 80%, and has improved over two decades despite reduced toxicity of therapy. N = number of patients. With thanks to Dr Gerald Draper and the Children's Cancer Research Group, Oxford, UK.

Patte C. (1995) Management of paediatric lymphomas. *Baillière's Clin Paediatr* **3**: 799–810.

Robison LL, Ross JA. (1995) Epidemiology of leukaemia and lymphomas in childhood. In: Chessels JM, Hann IM, eds. *Leukaemia and Lymphoma*. Philadelphia: WB Saunders: 639–58.

Saha V, Eden OB, Hann IM et al. (1995) Primary extrathoracic T-cell non-Hodgkin's lymphoma of childhood. *Leukaemia* **9**: 40–3.

15 Histiocyte disorders

David KH Webb

INTRODUCTION

Histiocyte disorders are characterized by infiltration of affected tissues with cells of monocyte/macrophage lineage, often mixed with other inflammatory cells, and are divided into two broad categories: reactive disorders, believed to represent a disordered response to immune activation; and neoplastic conditions. However, the boundaries between classes may be blurred, and more than one class of disorder may be present in the same child. To aid study, a classification subdividing the histiocyte disorders into three classes has been proposed (Table 15.1). Abnormal responses to antigen stimulation mediated by inflammatory cytokines have been proposed as mechanisms for the two most common disorders – Langerhans cell histiocytosis (LCH) and haemophagocytic lymphohistiocytosis (HLH) – and it remains unclear whether the histiocytes themselves or other immune active cells are the defective cell population.

The clinical manifestations and prognoses of these diseases are dissimilar: LCH is associated with a low mortality rate but is a cause of considerable acute and chronic morbidity, whereas HLH is often fatal. Understanding of the pathophysiology of these disorders is limited.

AETIOLOGY, EPIDEMIOLOGY AND CLINICAL FEATURES

Most histiocytes are derived from blood monocytes, although local proliferation in the tissues may occur following contact with antigen, and in disease states. Growth and differentiation are controlled by haemopoietic growth factors produced by stromal cells, macrophages and lymphocytes. Differentiation in the tissues occurs under the influence of growth factors and physical stimuli, including contact with antigen. Histiocytes are widely spread throughout the tissues, and include Kupffer cells in the liver, microglia in the central nervous system, Langerhans cells in skin and osteoclasts in bone, and these cells play a key role in host defence, acting as antigen-presenting cells, phagocytes, and generators of inflammation through enzyme release and the production of inflammatory cytokines and cellular growth factors.

Normal histiocytes are divided into two subgroups: dendritic cells (e.g. Langerhans cells, dendritic reticulum cells and interdigitating reticulum cells) and macrophages. Langerhans cells (LCs) are normally found in the epidermis, the mucosa of the bronchial tree, and lymph nodes and the thymus. They are thought to undergo differentiation in the tissues under the influence of the cytokines interleukin-3 (IL-3), granulocyte–macrophage colony stimulating factor (GM-CSF) and tumour necrosis factor α (TNF-α) and physical stimuli, which, in the skin, include low temperature. Characteristic features of LCs include the expression of the CD1a surface antigen, and the presence of specific cytoplasmic organelles (Birbeck granules), which arise either by invagination of the surface membrane during endocytosis of antigen, or as secretory organelles derived from the Golgi apparatus. Birbeck granules may be demonstrated on electron microscopy as rod-shaped structures, often with an expanded end ('tennis racket' appearance). CD1a has considerable homology with HLA class I molecules, and is generally specific for LCs, being expressed otherwise only by cortical thymo-

Table 15.1 Classifications of the histiocytosis syndromes
Class I   Disorders of dendritic cells • Langerhans cell histiocytosis (LCH) • Juvenile xanthogranuloma • Solitary dendritic cell histiocytomas

Class II Disorders of macrophages
• Haemophagocytic lymphohistiocytosis (HLH)
   (i) primary(genetic)
   (ii) sporadic
• Sinus histiocytosis with massive lymphadenopathy (SHML)
• Solitary macrophage histiocytomas

Class III Malignant histiocyte disorders
• (i) Acute monocytic leukaemias
   (AML FAB[a] types M4/M5)
   (ii) Extramedullary monocytic tumours
• Malignant histiocytosis
• Disseminated or localized malignancies with dendritic cell phenotype
• Disseminated or localized malignancies with macrophage phenotype

[a] FAB, French–American–British classification.

cytes. The function of this antigen is unknown, but a role in the immune response, perhaps in antigen presentation to T cells, is possible. Following stimulation by antigen, LCs migrate to lymph nodes, where they present antigen to T cells. Dendritic and interdigitating reticulum cells are localized to lymph nodes, where they present antigen to B and T cells respectively. The location of these cells within the lymph nodes varies, with interdigitating reticulum cells primarily located in the paracortex, and dendritic cells in the lymph node follicle.

CLASS I: DISORDERS OF DENDRITIC CELLS

Langerhans cell histiocytosis (LCH)

The term 'Langerhans cell histiocytosis' has been widely adopted to replace the diagnosis 'histiocytosis X' suggested by Lichtenstein in 1953, following the recognition by Nezelof in 1973 that the presence of LCs is characteristic of lesions in the disorder. LCH is rare, affecting 4 per million children each year, with a peak incidence between 1 and 3 years of age, and is slightly more common in boys. Clinical presentation is variable, and despite the restricted distribution of LCs in health, lesions comprising LCs and other inflammatory cells occur in a wide range of organs, including skin (Fig. 15.1), bone, lymph nodes, liver, spleen, bone marrow, the lungs, central nervous system (CNS) and gut. The proportion of LCs in lesions varies widely, and they may be few in number, or even absent, particularly in lesions of the CNS. Morphologically, LCs in disease are indistinguishable from normal ones, and studies of surface antigen expression show a similar pattern to that of activated LCs in healthy individuals. Later, lesions become characterized by reduced numbers of LCs, and accumulation of lipid-laden macrophages, and ultimate resolution is accompanied by residual fibrosis.

The aetiology is unknown, but LCH is

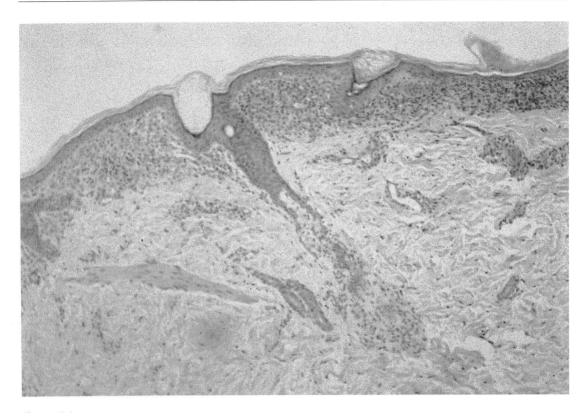

Figure 15.1

Biopsy of skin, showing involvement in Langerhans cell histiocytosis (LCH).

generally considered a reactive disorder resulting from immune activation. Searches for potential triggers have been unsuccessful, and there is no evidence for a viral aetiology. High levels of cytokines (GM-CSF, IL-1, -3, -4 and -8, TNF-α and leukaemia inhibitory factor (LIF)) have been demonstrated in lesions, with GM-CSF and LIF being detected in the serum of children with multisystem disease. Two studies of X-linked DNA polymorphisms have demonstrated clonality in lesional cells. Willman et al used a HUMARA assay to assess clonality in lesional tissues from ten females with various forms of the disease, and demonstrated clonality in nine cases (extreme constitutional lyonization precluded study of the tenth case). The percentage of clonal cells closely approximated the

percentage of CD1a$^+$ cells in the lesions, and there was no evidence of lymphoid clonality by analysis of the immunoglobulin and T-cell receptor genes. Yu et al studied three females with active multisystem disease, again by HUMARA assay, and demonstrated clonality in CD1a$^+$ but not other lesional cells. However, these data are not able to define whether LCH is a neoplastic or reactive disorder, as clonality has been demonstrated in a variety of non-neoplastic disorders.

Skin disease

The skin rash of LCH comprises red or yellow-brown papules on the trunk, erythema in skin folds and behind the ears, and scaling, particularly affecting the scalp

(Fig. 15.2). Rarely, young infants manifest a vesicular rash (Fig. 15.3), similar to varicella, which may be present at birth, and which is generally self-limiting, although a minority of these children subsequently suffer recurrences or develop bone lesions. Ear discharge is a classic sign, and may be due either to skin involvement in the external auditory canal, or bone destruction around and in the middle ear, with polyp formation. Such destructive lesions may result in hearing loss, and formal ENT assessment is essential.

Bone disease

Bone lesions may be occult, but present clinically with pain and soft tissue swelling, and are best seen on plain radiographs as irregular lytic areas, sometimes with marked periosteal reaction, most commonly affecting the skull (Fig. 15.4) and long bones, although any bone may be involved, and there may be pathological fractures. Involvement of the axial skeleton may result in vertebral collapse and vertebral plana, although spinal cord compression is rare. Orbital disease may cause proptosis, another 'classical' feature, but visual impairment is unusual.

Diabetes insipidus

Diabetes insipidus (DI) due to involvement of the hypothalamus and pituitary stalk may occur in both single-system and multisystem

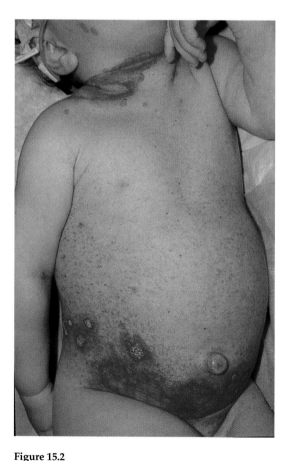

Figure 15.2

Skin rash in Langerhans cell histiocytosis (LCH).

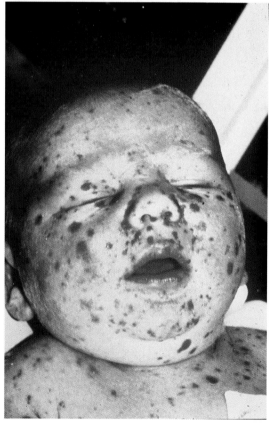

Figure 15.3

Vesicular rash in Langerhans cell histiocytosis (LCH).

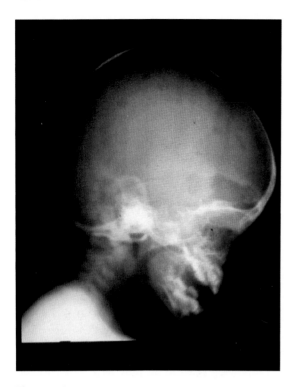 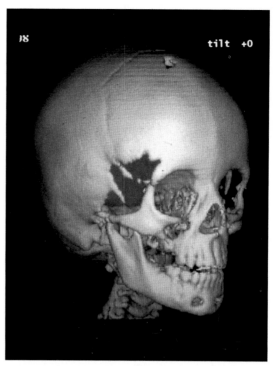

Figure 15.4

Plain radiograph and three-dimensional computed tomography scan of skull, showing lesions in Langerhans cell histio-cytosis (LCH).

disease, although this is far more common in the latter, reaching 40% in some series. Besides multisystem disease, other risk factors for DI include skull lesions and prop-tosis. Because of this risk, study of paired early-morning plasma and urinary osmolali-ties is a standard part of initial assessment, and children with suggestive symptoms require a formal water deprivation test, with measurement of urinary arginine vasopressin (AVP). In children with DI, magnetic reson-ance imaging may demonstrate thickening of the pituitary stalk, a suprasellar mass and/or loss of the posterior pituitary bright signal on T2-weighted images due to the absence of AVP. Some children demonstrate a transient phase of partial DI, but once true DI is estab-lished it is irreversible.

Multisystem disease

Around 40% of children have multisystem disease, and although this group may include individuals with skin and bone disease, it is visceral involvement that carries particular significance with regard to prognosis. In particular, 30% of this group develop organ dysfunction and it is these children who are most likely to die, with a mortality rate reaching 50%. Age is a significant risk factor, and these more severely affected children are predominantly under 2 years of age at diagnosis.

Lung disease

Lung disease occurs in one-third of children with multisystem disease but is very rare as a single site, and is characterized by cough and tachypnoea, with diffuse micronodular shadowing on chest radiograph. Progression to cyst formation and a honeycomb lung appearance occurs, and hypoxia, pleural effusions and pneumothorax may occur in advanced disease. Among adults, tobacco smoking is a risk factor for pulmonary disease. However, lung involvement per se is not a prognostic factor. Histology of affected lung shows peribronchiolar inflammatory infiltrates leading to fibrosis and cyst formation. On occasion, there may be doubt as to the cause of pulmonary signs, and the diagnosis can be confirmed, and infection excluded, by bronchoalveolar lavage or lung biopsy. As LCs are normally present in the bronchial tree, the presence of LCs in lavage fluid is not necessarily diagnostic of lung disease – one study indicated that over 5% $CD1a^+$ cells should be present to support the diagnosis.

Liver disease

Hepatomegaly is common, but documentation of liver dysfunction requires the demonstration of hypoalbuminaemia (<30 g/dl), cholestatic jaundice or prolonged coagulation tests, and hepatomegaly and elevated transaminases (aminotransferases) may occur without evidence of liver infiltration on biopsy. Jaundice may also result from obstruction of the biliary tract by enlarged portal nodes and therefore is not necessarily diagnostic of liver dysfunction. These provisos emphasize the need for careful assessment of mechanisms for clinical findings and investigation results in the initial evaluation. Severe liver disease may result in fibrosis, biliary cirrhosis and hepatic failure, and hepatic failure due to LCH has been successfully treated by orthotopic liver transplantation – 14 out of 17 children reported in the literature were alive at a median follow-up of 3 years. The combination of liver disease with involvement of the lungs or bone marrow has been identified with a poor prognosis in several studies.

Bone marrow disease

A low haemoglobin level is a common finding in active disease, which most often reflects anaemia of chronic disease, and iron deficiency should be excluded in children with microcytosis and hypochromia. Pancytopenia with bone marrow infiltration by macrophages, haemophagocytosis and marrow hypocellularity may occur. These changes often occur with associated splenomegaly in infants, and these children have a poor prognosis. There have been few studies of these changes, but one study found evidence of bone marrow disease in only 3 out of 10 children with haemoglobin <10 g/dl, and in 3 out of 5 with platelets <175 × 10^9/l.

Gut disease

Gut involvement, with failure to thrive, vomiting, diarrhoea, malabsorption and protein-losing enteropathy, occurs in under 5% of children, and requires full investigation, including adequate biopsy for confirmation. Although infiltrates may be seen in the mucosa and submucosa, biopsy of the muscle wall may be required. Barium studies may reveal alternate dilated and stenotic segments throughout the intestine. Mandibular and maxillary disease may result in floating teeth, and there may be gingivitis and buccal ulceration.

CNS disease

Disease in the CNS, excluding diabetes insipidus, occurs in around 4% of cases, and typically affects the cerebellar and cerebral white matter, with ataxia, dysarthria, nystagmus, and cranial nerve palsies. CNS disease usually develops around 5 years from original presentation, and is rarely a feature at diagnosis. Most cases occur in children with multisystem disease, but also in the setting of single-system bone disease (especially of the skull) and in children with diabetes insipidus. On imaging, several patterns are seen:

- Poorly defined changes in the white matter of the cerebellum, cerebrum and basal ganglia. Biopsy in these cases shows perivascular and parenchymal infiltrates of macrophages and lymphocytes with sparse LCs, associated with oedema and demyelination.

- Well-defined lesions in white and grey matter.
- Extra parenchymal masses, generally not in continuity with skull lesions, which on biopsy comprise xanthomatous histiocytes, diffusely infiltrating lymphocytes and Touton giant cells similar to those found in juvenile xanthogranuloma.

Lymphatic system

Lymphadenopathy occurs in both single- and multisystem disease, and cervical nodes in particular may be grossly enlarged. Local pressure effects may cause symptoms and signs due to obstruction of the airway, vasculature or biliary tree, and discharging sinuses may form to the overlying skin. Involvement of the thymus may be detected on chest x-ray, and may be present on tissue examination even without enlargement of the organ.

Juvenile xanthogranuloma

Juvenile xanthogranuloma usually presents with single or multiple yellow-red skin lesions in newborns and infants – in one series, the median age at presentation in 36 children was 0.3 years (range birth to 12 years). Histology shows a cutaneous accumulation of lipid-filled macrophages, Touton giant cells and fibroblasts. Extracutaneous disease may occur in around 10% of patients, involving the CNS, liver, spleen, lung, eye, oropharynx and muscle.

CLASS II: DISORDERS OF MACROPHAGES

Haemophagocytic lymphohistiocytosis (HLH)

Haemophagocytic lymphohistiocytosis is a rare disorder with typical histology showing tissue infiltration by morphologically benign histiocytes, some manifesting haemophagocytosis, and mature lymphocytes. The disorder occurs in primary and secondary forms, with an incidence for primary HLH of between 1 and 2 cases per million children each year in the UK and Sweden.

Primary HLH is a genetic disorder with autosomal recessive inheritance, but the nature of the gene defect is unknown. In a proportion of cases, there is a history of previously affected siblings indicating familial predisposition (familial HLH), and parental consanguinity or onset in early infancy are further supportive features. It appears likely that HLH is due to dysregulated function of T lymphocytes, with tissue infiltrates and haemophagocytosis generated by dysregulated secretion of cytokines, rather than a primary disorder of macrophages. Most children with primary HLH are young – in one series, 16 out of 23 children presented before their first birthday. Cases with no evidence of familial predisposition are termed sporadic, although it remains possible that in some of these cases the index child is the first affected member of a family with genetic predisposition.

Secondary HLH is at least as common as primary disease, and precipitants include viral, bacterial, fungal or protozoan infections, often in an immunocompromised host (infection-associated haemophagocytic syndrome, IAHS). Other precipitants include malignancy, particularly T-cell lymphoproliferative states, and lipid infusions.

Clinical manifestations include fever (84% of cases), splenomegaly (80%), hepatomegaly (88%), lymphadenopathy (50%), pancytopenia (88%), abnormal liver function (86%), coagulopathy (70%), and signs and symptoms referable to the CNS (40%). Occasionally, CNS involvement has been the only evidence of disease at presentation. Initial blood changes may show anaemia or thrombocytopenia, with the development of pancytopenia as the disease progresses. Other features include a high fasting level of triglycerides, low fibrinogen, mononuclear pleocytosis and increased protein in the cerebrospinal fluid, high serum ferritin, and reduced or absent natural killer cell function. Many of these changes result from immune activation with cytokine production, and high levels of circulating IL-1, IL-2 receptor, GM-CSF and TNF-α have been reported. In particular, disturbances in lipid metabolism, with high triglycerides, low levels of high-density lipoproteins and raised very low-density lipoproteins, reflect reduced activity of lipoprotein lipase reductase consequent on cytokinaemia. Involvement of the CNS varies from asymptomatic cerebrospinal fluid pleocytosis (usually to moderate levels and predominantly comprising lymphocytes with occasional macrophages, Fig. 15.5) to symptomatic disease with encephalitis, abnormal head movements, fits, cranial nerve palsies, ataxia, regression of developmental milestones and coma. High levels of neopterins in cerebrospinal fluid are consistent with activation of macrophages, which may return to normal with adequate therapy, resulting in resolution of disease. In children who have died with CNS disease, histology of the brain shows oedema, softening and destruction of tissue, and perivascular, parenchymal and leptomeningeal infiltrates, with necrosis and destruction, especially of white matter.

The Histiocyte Society has established criteria for the diagnosis of HLH (Table 15.2), although not all features are present in every case, and repeated investigation or presumptive diagnosis may be necessary. The tissues that are most frequently sampled to substantiate the diagnosis are bone marrow, lymph node and liver, although fine-needle aspiration of the spleen is reported to have a high diagnostic yield. Diagnostic changes may be difficult to demonstrate, and the bone marrow in particular is hypercellular and reactive in the early stages of the disease, with hypocellularity and haemophagocytosis by histiocytes (Fig. 15.6) later features. Haemophagocytosis may not be a feature on liver biopsy, but there may be prominent sinusoidal Kupffer cells and lymphoid portal infiltrates similar to those seen in chronic persistent hepatitis.

Sinus histiocytosis with massive lymphadenopathy (SHML)

Sinus histiocytosis with massive lymphadenopathy (Rosai–Dorfman syndrome) was described in 1969 by Rosai and Dorfman as a syndrome of cervical lymphadenopathy with typical histology showing preserved lymph node structure, dilated lymph node sinuses containing mixed inflammatory cells, with vacuolated macrophages manifesting haemophagocytosis and emperipolesis of lymphocytes (Fig. 15.7). Fibrosis may be

---

Table 15.2 Diagnostic guidelines for haemophagocytic lymphohistiocytosis (HLH)

Clinical criteria
- Fever
- Splenomegaly

Laboratory criteria
- Cytopenias (affecting >2 of 3 lineages in the peripheral blood):
  Haemoglobin (<9 g/dl)
  Platelets (<100 × 10⁹/l)
  Neutrophils (<1.0 × 10⁹/l)
- Hypertriglyceridaemia and/or hypofibrinogenaemia: fasting triglycerides >2.00 mmol/l; fibrinogen <1.5 g/l

Histopathological criteria
- Haemophagocytosis in bone marrow, spleen or lymph nodes
- No evidence of malignancy

- All criteria are required for the diagnosis of HLH. In addition, the diagnosis of familial HLH is justified by a positive family history, and parental consanguinity is suggestive.
- The following findings may provide strong supportive evidence for the diagnosis: spinal fluid pleocytosis (mononuclear cells); histological picture in the liver resembling chronic persistent hepatitis; low natural killer cell activity; high serum ferritin.

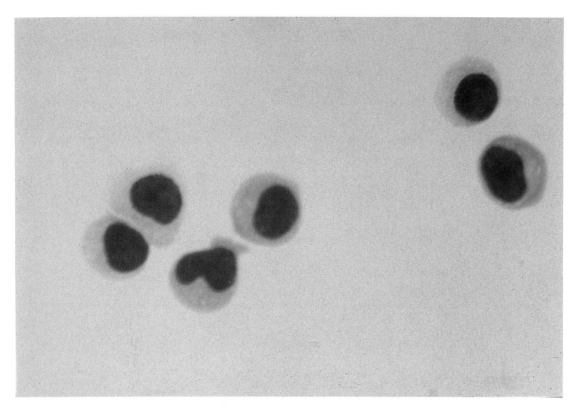

Figure 15.5

Cytospin of cerebrospinal fluid, showing lymphocytes and monocytes in haemophagocytic lymphohistiocytosis (HLH).

marked. Histological features in other tissues are similar, but with increased fibrosis, and less haemophagocytosis. Other features of SHML include systemic ill health with fever and weight loss, destructive infiltrates in skin, bone and other extranodal sites, hypergammaglobulinaemia, elevated erythrocyte sedimentation rate (ESR), reactive leukocytosis, and immune dysfunction including autoimmune anaemia and neutropenia. Although most cases are isolated, SHML has occurred in individuals with malignancy, autoimmune diseases or other histiocyte disorders, especially LCH. Involvement of cervical lymph nodes is present in most cases, but other groups are affected, either jointly or alone. The lymphadenopathy may be gross, and is often painless, and may wax and wane with time. Extranodal disease of the head and neck or a variety of other sites is present in almost half of cases, either alone or in association with lymphoid masses. As with other histiocyte disorders, a possible role for Epstein–Barr virus (EBV) in pathogenesis has been postulated.

CLASS III: MALIGNANCIES

Acute myelomonocytic and acute monocytic leukaemia (AML M4 and M5 respectively according to the French–American–British classification) account for 30% of AML cases in children, and have a standard or, in cases of M4 AML with cytogenetics showing inversion of chromosome 16, favourable prognosis following modern combination chemotherapy. Considerable controversy exists regarding other malignancies of the monocyte/macrophage system, due to difficulties in

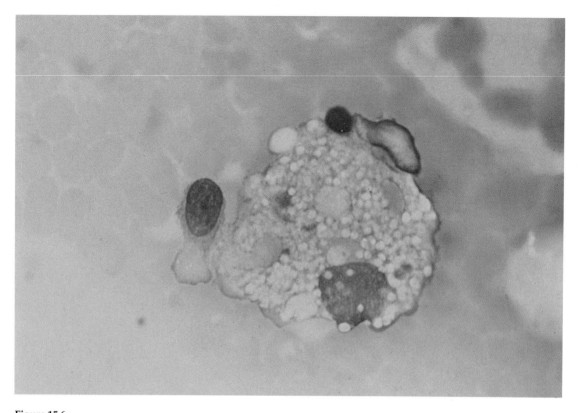

Figure 15.6

Bone marrow macrophage, showing erythrophagocytosis in haemophagocytic lymphohistiocytosis (HLH).

nosology. Malignant histiocytosis was described as a clinical picture of lymphadenopathy, hepatosplenomegaly, fever, wasting and pancytopenia, with histology showing tissue infiltration by large cells with copious cytoplasm and irregular nuclei. However, recent studies of cell lineage in such cases by monoclonal antibodies and immunoglobulin or T-cell receptor gene rearrangements indicate that the majority of these tumours are in fact of lymphoid origin, and reclassifiable as anaplastic large cell (Ki-1[+]) lymphomas. In one overview of experience at the University of Minnesota combined with a literature review, only 19 out of 164 cases originally diagnosed as malignant histiocytosis were confirmed as negative for B- and T-cell markers and positive for monocytic-lineage surface antigens. Accordingly, true 'malig-

nant histiocytosis' is an extremely rare entity, requiring careful pathological assessment to substantiate the diagnosis. Both localized and disseminated malignancies of dendritic cells occur, although these are extremely rare.

MANAGEMENT OF HISTIOCYTE DISORDERS

Langerhans cell histiocytosis (LCH)

Initial workup for a suspected case requires confirmatory biopsy and an accurate assessment of the extent of disease. An exception to this rule regarding the need for tissue biopsy may be made for asymptomatic children with typical lesions, for example isolated lytic lesions of bone, where no specific therapy is

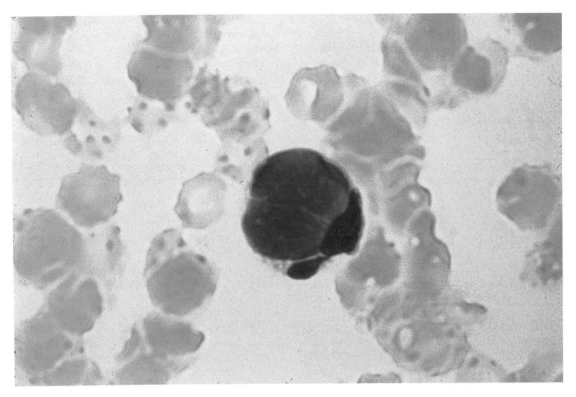

Figure 15.7

Emperipolesis in sinus histiocytosis with massive lymphadenopathy (SHML, Rosai–Dorfman syndrome).

intended. Identification of Langerhans cells within the lesional inflammatory cell infiltrate with demonstration of either the CD1a surface antigen on immunohistochemistry or the presence of Birbeck granules on electron microscopy (Fig. 15.8) is recommended. Disease may be categorized as single- or multisystem, and children with single-system disease may have isolated or multiple sites of involvement. It is important to carefully assess the function of affected organs, as dysfunction carries prognostic significance (see below). Thorough physical examination and investigations are required to determine the extent of disease, and investigations must include a full blood count, liver function tests, serum proteins, a coagulation screen, and skeletal survey by plain radiographs. Further investigations should be guided by

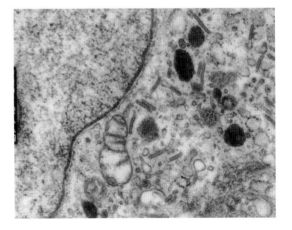

Figure 15.8

Electron micrograph showing Birbeck granules in Langerhans cell histiocytosis (LCH).

the need to explain specific symptoms and signs.

As the majority of cases of LCH eventually resolve spontaneously, and no therapy is uniformly effective, approaches to treatment have varied, with particular controversy regarding the role of intensive chemotherapy for children with multisystem disease. Deaths occur in 10–15% of cases, and are largely restricted to children with organ dysfunction, and for most cases the primary objectives are control of symptoms and limitation of long-term disability, which affects up to 50% of those with extensive disease. Accordingly, observation alone may be appropriate, but for children with skin disease requiring therapy, topical application of corticosteroids may prove beneficial. For those with more severe skin involvement, topical mustine (chlormethine) has proved highly effective – in one study, rapid improvement within 10 days occurred in each of 16 children, with complete healing in 14. The median duration of treatment was 3.5 months, and the only side-effect was contact sensitivity in one child. However, some children require systemic therapy, and oral corticosteroids result in improvement in over half of cases.

Bone lesions may resolve following diagnostic biopsy, but further local therapies include curettage, injected steroids or radiotherapy, although the latter is now uncommon due to concerns over late effects – in particular, secondary malignancies have been described within the radiation field. For children with multifocal bone disease (30% of all children with bone disease), or single, symptomatic lesions unsuitable for local therapy, systemic therapy is indicated. However, further lesions and reactivations of initially responding lesions develop in up to one-third of patients.

Even children with multisystem disease may be managed conservatively, with systemic therapy reserved for those who have organ dysfunction, pain, systemic upset or failure to thrive. For children who require systemic treatment, the most commonly used agents are corticosteroids, vinblastine and etoposide, but a wide range of cytotoxic drugs have been used, including antimetabolites, alkylating agents and anthracyclines. The paucity of randomized trials makes the determination of relative efficacy for these approaches difficult, and the possibility of late effects from some of these agents argues against their use. In particular, secondary malignancy has been described in 1–5% of long-term survivors, and treatments including etoposide, alkylating agents, or radiotherapy carry particular risk.

There is a recognized association between LCH and malignancy, and in one registry-based study 13 children developed acute leukaemia (5 acute lymphoblastic (ALL) and 8 acute myeloid (AML)), 4 lymphomas, and 10 developed other solid tumours. Four cases of ALL predated the LCH, whilst 7 cases of AML developed more than 2 years after diagnosis and treatment with chemotherapy and/or radiotherapy. In another study, a literature review revealed details of 87 LCH-associated malignancies: 39 lymphomas, 62% of which occurred during the course of LCH, 22 acute leukaemias, mostly AML diagnosed after the LCH, and the remainder solid tumours, including secondary tumours arising within fields of previous irradiation. Among 341 children registered in two international treatment trials (LCH I and DAL-HX 83), however, the incidence of secondary malignancy was 1%. Accordingly, only a proportion of cases represent malignancy secondary to therapy for LCH, but this occurrence raises disquiet regarding the use of oncogenic drugs or radiotherapy in those children with little or no risk of a fatal outcome.

Against this background, the outcome for children treated in the UK Children's Cancer Study Group (UKCCSG) centres and registered with the UK Children's Cancer Research Group are of interest. Between 1977 and 1994, 370 children were registered, 191 with single-system disease. When outcomes were compared for three time periods (1977–1984, 1985–1990, 1991–1994), there was no change in prognosis for those with multisystem disease (Fig. 15.9). The great majority of deaths occurred in children with multisystem disease, with the poorest prognosis (60% survival) being for children under 2 years of age at diagnosis (Fig. 15.10).

McLelland et al reported 44 children with extensive disease managed conservatively. Thirty-six required systemic therapy, 17

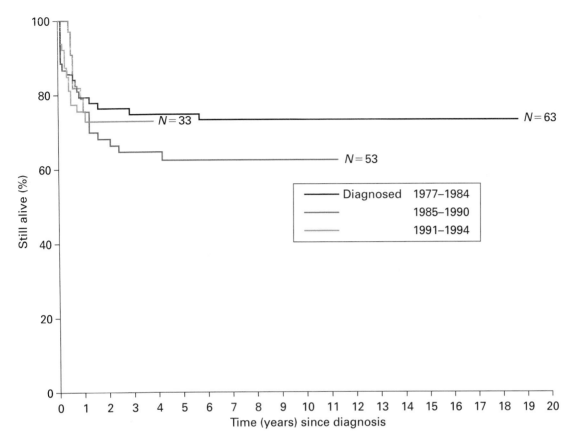

Figure 15.9

Survival of United Kingdom Children's Cancer Study Group (UKCCSG) patients, 1977–1994, according to period of diagnosis.

responded to prednisolone and 19 required further treatment with vinblastine or etoposide. The overall survival rate was 82% (64% amongst those with organ dysfunction), 60% of survivors had late effects and 36% had diabetes insipidus. In an Italian series, 84 children were stratified into good- and poor-risk groups, depending on whether organ dysfunction was present. Good-risk children received vinblastine, doxorubicin and etoposide for a total of 9 months, whereas the poor-risk group were given 9 courses of cyclophosphamide, vincristine, doxorubicin and prednisolone. The overall survival rate at 4 years was 92%, but there was a low complete-response rate in the poor-risk group (2 out of 11 cases), with 6 deaths, and the sur-

vivors had chronic disease. Overall, disease-related sequelae were noted in 45% and diabetes insipidus in 20%. A Dutch study described the results of treatment with cytarabine, vincristine and prednisolone: 8 out of 10 children without organ dysfunction and 5 out of 8 with organ dysfunction had a complete response, with an incidence of diabetes insipidus of 20%. Until recently, there was little evidence that aggressive treatment is beneficial, but Gadner et al, suggested improved disease control and fewer late effects in children with multifocal bone or multisystem disease who were treated with 12 months of combined therapy including prednisolone, vinblastine, etoposide and mercaptopurine, plus methotrexate in children

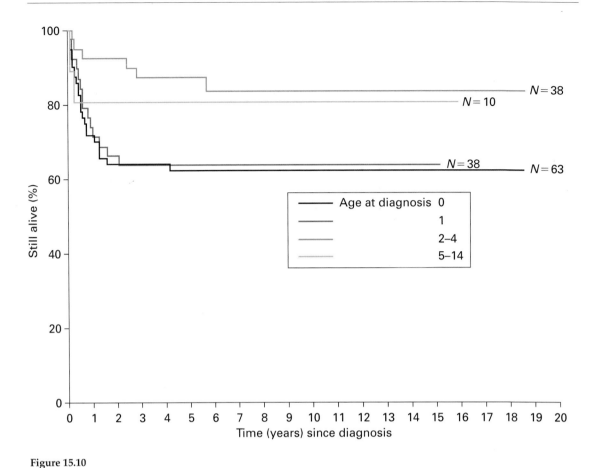

Figure 15.10

Survival of United Kingdom Children's Cancer Study Group (UKCCSG) patients, 1977–1994, according to age at diagnosis.

with organ dysfunction. In these studies (DAL-HX83 and 90), 138 children were stratified and treated with risk-directed therapy. After 6 weeks' treatment, 79% responded, 14% were worse, 19% died, 89% of deaths occurring in children with progressive disease at 6 weeks, and reactivations occurring in 24%, with a cumulative risk of 36% at 2 years.

The uncertainty regarding the most effective and least toxic approach to treatment, together with the rarity of LCH, emphasizes the need for international collaborative randomized studies, and the Histiocyte Society has recently coordinated a trial (LCH I) of vinblastine versus etoposide, both combined with initial prednisolone, in children with multisystem disease. Among 136 children

randomized between etoposide and vinblastine, there were no differences in outcome: 71% responded to therapy and 16% had progressive disease. The mortality rate was 18%, and 9 out of 18 children who died had had progressive disease after the initial 6 weeks of treatment. Reactivations occurred in 19%, with a cumulative probability of 68% at 2 years. These results were considered inferior to the DAL series in both event-free and disease-free survival, which forms the basis of LCH II, although these were not randomized comparisons.

For children who fail first-line treatment, further options are limited. There is little evidence that immune modulation, with cyclosporin A or antilymphocyte globulin, or bone marrow transplantation are effective for most children. Initial reports of responses to 2-chlorodeoxyadenosine (cladribine) are to be assessed in a new phase II trial coordinated by the Histiocyte Society.

LCH is associated with a wide range of potential late effects, particularly skeletal deformity and dysfunction, diabetes insipidus, growth hormone deficiency, ataxia, intellectual impairment, and lung and liver fibrosis. A study in Sweden found at least 1 late effect in 31 out of 58 individuals diagnosed during childhood at a median of 15 years from diagnosis. Among these patients, 10 had diabetes insipidus, 9 had other endocrine disorders, 7 had orthopaedic problems, 6 had CNS abnormalities, and 3 had a later malignancy. These data stress the need for therapeutic trials to include standardized assessments for late effects that can be compared between treatments.

Juvenile xanthogranuloma

In children with juvenile xanthogranuloma, spontaneous resolution is usual, and no treatment has been proven without doubt to be beneficial. For lesions resulting in complications, excision may be indicated.

Haemophagocytic lymphohistiocytosis (HLH)

Careful assessment is required to distinguish those children with true secondary disease (whose disorder will resolve with reversal of any immune suppression, and treatment for or removal of the precipitant) from those individuals with evidence of viral infection but underlying primary HLH. In one series of children and adults diagnosed with IAHS due to viruses (termed virus-associated haemophagocytic syndrome, VAHS), 14 out of 19 patients were receiving immune suppression. Supportive care with withdrawal of immunosupression led to resolution in 13 cases, but amongst the 5 children with no prior immunosuppression, 2 died and 3 improved with steroids and/or azathioprine. However, not all reports show a favourable outcome; for instance, Kikuta et al described 6 children aged 1–12 years with fatal VAHS

related to EBV. Furthermore, Henter et al reported evidence of viral infection in 10 out of 32 children with primary HLH, implicating EBV, cytomegalovirus (CMV) and parvovirus. Among 93 children with HLH reported to the Histiocyte Society registry, there was no difference in outcome between 40 children with and 53 children without evidence of viral infection. These data emphasize the overlap between these disorders and the need for circumspection in determining the best approach to therapy in each case.

There are two standard approaches to treatment for primary HLH: one using etoposide and corticosteroids, and the other using antithymocyte globulin, corticosteroids and cyclosporin A, suggesting that disordered T cells are central to the pathogenesis. Around 80% of patients respond, but eventual disease recurrence is usual in primary HLH unless the child receives an allogeneic bone marrow transplant (BMT): in one study, disease recurrence occurred in 8 out of 10 children treated by etoposide, prednisolone and intrathecal methotrexate, at a median of 5 months from diagnosis. Age is an important determinant of prognosis: in a combined series of 23 cases treated in two London centres, survival was significantly higher in children aged over 2 years at presentation than in younger children. Inadequate disease control or reactivation may also occur in some secondary cases, and these children should then be treated in line with strategies for primary disease. Adequate control of CNS involvement is very important, but the role of routine intrathecal methotrexate in the control of CNS disease is controversial, and cranial irradiation is no longer recommended. The development or progression of CNS disease has been reported to be a feature in children receiving either treatment strategy unless these children receive a BMT, but there is now evidence that changes on imaging and neurodevelopmental performance may improve following a successful BMT. Experience with BMT is greatest using matched sibling donors, with around 70% of children remaining disease-free, but increasing use of alternative donors, including matched and mismatched unrelated donors, and haploidentical grafts from a parent, has demonstrated that similar results may be achieved with this approach. Full engraftment following transplantation is not a pre-requisite for cure, as low levels of donor T cells may provide adequate disease control. Clinical condition at the time of transplant affects outcome, and this emphasizes the importance of initial treatment to establish disease control. A particular worry regarding the use of a sibling donor is that in familial disease there is a 25% risk that the donor will also develop HLH, and continued improvement in the results of alternative donor procedures may make these the treatment of choice. It must also be remembered that some children, usually sporadic cases aged over 2 years at diagnosis, remain well following initial therapy and that BMT is not indicated for this group. The Histiocyte Society has approved an international study for HLH (HLH 94) to provide a uniform approach to assessment, therapy and biological studies. In children with a complete response to initial therapy with etoposide and dexamethasone, and no evidence of familial disease, treatment is discontinued and only recommended if there is reactivation. All children who require continued therapy receive cyclosporin A and intermittent etoposide and dexamethasone, and are eligible for BMT. One particular aspect under investigation is the approach to CNS involvement, as it is possible that better systemic therapy, including dexamethasone (which has good penetration to the cerebrospinal fluid), may obviate the need for methotrexate in some cases.

Sinus histiocytosis with massive lymphadenopathy (SHML)

The natural history of the disorder is chronic, with spontaneous resolution over months or years in many cases, although approximately 5% of patients have died due to immune-mediated organ dysfunction, amyloidosis or infection. Few individuals have died directly as a result of lymphohistiocytic infiltrates. Therapy with steroids, cytotoxic drugs (particularly vincristine and alkylating agents), or radiotherapy has been variably effective, and is unnecessary in most cases.

Management of class III disorders

The uncertainty over the pathology of reported cases of malignant histiocytosis clouds issues regarding therapy. It appears appropriate to treat malignancies of macrophages with AML chemotherapy. The outlook for children with monocytic variants of AML has improved considerably over recent years, with around 50% survival at 5 years from diagnosis following standard chemotherapy regimens. Due to the rarity of dendritic cell malignancies, treatment recommendations are anecdotal, but based on excision with or without adjuvant therapy.

FURTHER READING

Favara BE, Feller AC, Pauli M et al. (1977) Contemporary classification of histiocytic disorders. The WHO Committee on Histiocytic/Reticulum Cell Proliferations. Reclassification Working Group of the Histiocyte Society. *Med Pediatr Oncol* **29**: 157–66.

Gadner H, Heitger A, Ritter J, Gobel U, Janka GE, Kuhl J, Bode U, Spaar HJ. (1987) Langerhans cell histiocytosis in childhood – results of the DAL-HX 83 study. *Klin Pediatr* **199**: 173–82.

Henter J-I, Elinder G, Ost A. (1991) Diagnostic guidelines for haemophagocytic lymphohistiocytosis. *Semin Oncol* **18**: 29–33.

Henter J-I, Soder O, Ost A, Elinder G. (1991) Incidence and clinical features of familial hemophagocytic lymphohistiocytosis. *Acta Pediatr Scand* **80**: 428–35.

Ladisch S, Gadner H (1994) Treatment of Langerhans cell histiocytosis – evolution and current approaches. *Br J Cancer* **70** (Suppl xxiii): S41–6.

McClain K, Ramsay NK, Robison L, Sundberg RD, Nesbit M Jr. (1983) Bone marrow involvement in histiocytosis X. *Med Pediatr Oncol* **11**: 167–71.

McLelland J, Broadbent V, Yeomans E, Malone M, Pritchard J. (1990) Langerhans cell histiocytosis: the case for conservative treatment. *Arch Dis Child* **65**: 301–3.

Schmidt D (1994) Monocyte/macrophage system and malignancies. *Med Pediatr Oncol* **23**: 444–51.

Willman CL, Busque L, Griffith BB, Favara BE, McClain KL, Duncan MH, Gilliland DG. (1994) Langerhans cell histiocytosis (histiocytosis X) – a clonal proliferative disease. *N Engl J Med* **331**: 154–60.

Yu RC, Chu C, Buluwela L, Chu AC. (1994) Clonal proliferation of Langerhans cells in Langerhans cell histiocytosis. *Lancet* **343**: 767–8.

16 Haematological changes in non-haematological disorders

Michael M Reid

INTRODUCTION

The function of the bone marrow and the coagulation system may be affected directly or indirectly by a multitude of pathological processes, many of which are not primarily haematological diseases. The range is enormous. This chapter will focus on some of the more common or particularly striking aspects and will also strongly reflect the author's personal experience. Some topics will get more attention than their rarity might suggest they deserve; this simply reflects the enthusiasm of a morphologist and the inevitable selection bias that accompanies rare disorders! Details of the full diagnostic criteria for or management of the wide variety of disease processes mentioned are not included, nor are the extraordinarily long lists of haematological complications of drugs. The several short tables of information for quick reference are not comprehensive – absence of a particular haematological abnormality or disease from either a tabulated list or the main body of the text should not be assumed to mean that it has not been observed and reported by others.

A valuable source of more detailed information and primary source references can be found in at least one major paediatric haematology text (Stockman and Ezekowitz 1998). Excellent illustrations of haematological abnormalities in many of the conditions mentioned in this chapter may be found in various atlases of paediatric haematology (Hann et al 1996, Smith 1996). Those particularly interested in tropical diseases will also find much more of interest in another well-referenced review (Weatherall and Kwiatkowski 1998).

The anaemia of chronic disease will be discussed first, followed by diseases affecting a variety of organ systems. It should be appreciated that there are considerable overlaps between aspects of the anaemia of chronic disease and more specific causes of anaemia or other haematological abnormalities in many of the diseases covered in this chapter and that comorbidity, such as nutritional iron deficiency or thalassaemia traits (reflecting the local population's ethnic diversity), may contribute to the picture.

ANAEMIA OF CHRONIC DISEASE

This is common and non-specific. The typical pattern is of a normochromic, normocytic (or sometimes microcytic) anaemia with a poor reticulocyte response, often associated with a raised erythrocyte sedimentation rate (ESR), a normal or raised ferritin level, and elevation of other acute-phase proteins. The anaemia is usually modest, but on occasions may be severe enough to cause real clinical worries. Rouleaux may often be seen on the blood film, and there may be some increase in background staining due to hypergammaglobulinaemia or elevated acute-phase proteins. The platelet count is usually normal or raised. Normal or raised ferritin levels may make it difficult to exclude concomitant iron deficiency in microcytic cases. The aetiology of the anaemia is probably multifactorial and related to the interplay of a number of cytokines and to deficiency of or lack of responsiveness to erythropoietin. It is important always to compare red cell indices with age-related normal ranges.

Any list of diseases associated with this form of anaemia will include chronic infections (such as tuberculosis and chronic osteomyelitis), collagen vascular disorders (such as systemic lupus erythmatosus and polyarteritis nodosa), juvenile chronic arthritis and cancer, among others. The most strikingly microcytic examples of anaemia of chronic disease that the present author has seen have been in children with Hodgkin's disease, Wilms' tumour and hepatoblastoma, all of which are relatively rare disorders. Finally, it is unsafe to assume that microcytosis in neonates is ever due to anaemia of chronic disorder or iron deficiency – thalassaemia syndromes are more likely explanations.

In the collagen vascular disorders, immune-mediated neutropenia, haemolytic anaemia and thrombocytopenia may complicate the picture. Lupus inhibitors may cause prolongation of the accelerated partial thromboplastin time but, rather than resulting in a bleeding tendency, are associated with a predisposition to thrombotic events. Many of these complications, together with degrees of marrow hypoplasia, haemorrhage or microangiopathic haemolysis, can occur in many of the conditions that cause anaemia of chronic disorder; it is therefore unwise simply to assume that anaemia is due to no more than the chronic disorder, particularly if other cytopenias or a raised reticulocyte count are present. Table 16.1 summarizes the characteristic features of anaemia of chronic disease.

HEART DISEASE

Fragmentation haemolysis from turbulence induced by heart valves, congenital anomalies or patches can be sufficient to cause clin-ical haemolytic anaemia. Schistocytes, helmet cells and spherocytes may be present on the blood film, and haemosiderin is usually detectable in a spun deposit of the urine. Children with cyanotic congenital heart disease often have erythrocytosis. The mean cell volume (MCV) may be raised – a common finding in patients with an erythropoietin-driven increased red cell mass. The most significant derangements in coagulation usually take place during cardiopulmonary bypass surgery, rather than in the steady state, but both disseminated intravascular coagulation (DIC) and thrombotic complications, exacerbated by erythrocytosis may occur. Both thrombocytopenia and defective platelet aggregation may occur, but it is unusual for these to cause significant clinical problems except during or after surgery. Congestive heart failure and pulmonary oedema may both cause sufficient hypoxia to result in a marked flurry of nucleated red cells in the peripheral blood. Together with the presence of Howell–Jolly bodies (nuclear remnants within erythrocytes), the appearances may suggest, erroneously, asplenia. Table 16.2 shows a list of some common abnormalities.

GUT DISEASE

Problems with atrophic gastritis are usually restricted to adults. However, coeliac disease and other malabsorption syndromes commonly lead to either or both iron and folate deficiency, and surgical removal of the terminal ileum will result, eventually, in vitamin B_{12} deficiency and megaloblastic anaemia. Within neonates, in particular, necrotising enterocolitis is a common cause of microangiopathic haemolysis and DIC.

LIVER DISEASE

Coagulation factor deficiencies, especially of the vitamin K-dependent factors, occur with prematurity and are made worse by infections, hepatitis and liver failure. Again reference to appropriate normal ranges is important in the interpretation of clotting times and factor levels. A wide range of mor-

---

Table 16.1 Typical features of anaemia of chronic disease

- Normochromic, normocytic anaemia; occasionally microcytic
- Poor reticulocyte response
- Normal or raised platelets
- Normal or raised ferritin
- Raised erythrocyte sedimentation rate (ESR), raised acute-phase proteins

Table 16.2 Abnormalities in heart disease

Abnormality	Cause
Fragmented red cells Haemosiderinuria	Turbulence: valves, etc.
Erythrocytosis	Cyanotic heart disease
Clotting factor depletion Platelet dysfunction	Cardiopulmonary bypass
Nucleated red cells, fragmentation Howell–Jolly bodies	Heart failure, hypoxia

phological abnormalities may occur, including macrocytosis, target cells, acanthocytes and spur cells, because of altered lipid metabolism. Viral hepatitis (non-A, non-B, non-C) is one of the few known factors that precipitate severe aplastic anaemia.

LUNG DISEASE

Apart from erythrocytosis due to chronic hypoxia (except that children with cystic fibrosis do not seem to respond with increased erythropoiesis), a wide range of pulmonary pathology may cause significant haematological abnormalities. Among the more prominent are asthma/atopy, sarcoidosis, Löffler's syndrome and various collagen vascular disorders, all of which can all cause eosinophilia. Exacerbations of bronchitis or bronchiectasis may result in the expected neutrophil leukocytosis of infection. Idiopathic pulmonary haemosiderosis may be dramatic in its behaviour, with pulmonary haemorrhage, fever and breathlessness, but the most important cause of anaemia is no more than iron deficiency.

RENAL DISEASE

This has been extensively studied. By far the most important and common haematological abnormality is anaemia due to chronic renal failure. While once thought to be no more than 'anaemia of chronic disease', it is now clear that there is a marked reduction in the kidney's ability to secrete erythropoietin. The advent of recombinant human erythropoietin has transformed the lives of many previously transfusion-dependent children with chronic renal failure. Failure to obtain an appropriate response in haemoglobin to administered erythropoietin is usually due to concomitant iron deficiency or rapid exhaustion of iron stores. Other contributing causes include shortened red cell survival, nutritional deficiencies and some degree of anaemia of chronic disease.

Erythrocytosis is known to accompany hydronephrosis, may occur in other conditions including glomerulonephritis and pyelonephritis, and is sometimes seen after renal transplantation. It is tempting to speculate that, in this last situation, erythropoiesis is more sensitive to the now restored normal erythropoietin drive.

Neutropenia often occurs in patients receiving regular haemodialysis. Mild or modest thrombocytopenia is probably caused by impaired production rather than increased destruction of platelets. Platelets of patients with chronic renal failure also function poorly, but function is improved by dialysis, suggesting that dialysable molecules rather than intrinsic platelet malfunction lie behind this abnormality. There is no doubt that haemorrhagic problems are strikingly more problematic in untreated than regularly dialysed patients with chronic renal failure.

Deficiencies in coagulation factors are usually mild in chronic renal failure (and fibrinogen is often elevated because it is an acute-phase protein). In the nephrotic syndrome, however, only factors IX and XII seem regularly to be depleted, being passed into the urine, but without clinically important consequences. Table 16.3 shows a list of some common abnormalities.

REACTIONS TO ACUTE INSULTS OR STRESS

Neonates

The acutely or chronically stressed neonate (hypoxia, shock, sepsis, haemolytic disease of the newborn) can produce a bewildering array of peripheral blood abnormalities. These include the presence of nucleated red cells, Howell–Jolly bodies, myelocytes and even blast-like cells. It is speculated that oxidative damage may result in mis-shapen red cells, some spherocytes, haemolysis and jaundice; the syndrome is sometimes called infantile pyknocytosis, but is poorly defined and may not be a single, true entity. Some cases may even require phototherapy for this otherwise unexplained jaundice, and the present author has seen two infants who

needed top-up transfusions. It has always resolved without specific therapy (often with no therapy at all) in the author's experience. Sepsis (and some severe viral infections) can also cause DIC with hypofibrinogenaemia and prolonged prothrombin and activated partial thromboplastin times (PT, APTT), fragmented red cells (microangiopathic haemolysis) and profound neutropenia. Again it is important to relate these findings to what is known about the wide range of 'normality'; the mere presence of a nucleated red cell, or an erythrocyte with a Howell–Jolly body, does not by itself imply that the baby is sick! Few, if any, easily found lists of normal ranges of such morphological abnormalities exist, so consultation with experienced haematologists is important in order to interpret the film appearances. Table 16.4 shows a list of some typical 'stress' appearances.

Older infants and children

All the features in neonates described above may also occur in older infants and children, but they are less striking. Thrombocytosis, on the other hand, sometimes reaching levels of >1000 × 10^9/l, often follows surgery of almost any kind, or in a rebound after some courses of cytotoxic chemotherapy or after splenectomy, or as an accompaniment of some infections (e.g. chickenpox) or in rarer conditions

Table 16.3 Abnormalities in renal disease	
Abnormality	**Cause**
Anaemia	Erythropoietin deficiency Anaemia of chronic disease
Erythrocytosis	Hydronephrosis Pyelonephritis
Neutropenia	Haemodialysis
Platelet dysfunction	Chronic renal failure
Prolonged activated partial thromboplastin time (APTT)	Loss of factors IX and XII in nephrotic syndrome

---

Table 16.4 Typical abnormalities in stressed or infected infants

- Nucleated red cells and Howell–Jolly bodies in blood
- Irregular, mis-shapen, spherocytic red cells (pyknocytosis)
- Myelocytes in blood
- Disseminated intravascular coagulation (DIC)
- Thrombocytosis or thrombocytopenia
- Pancytopenia or neutropenia

---

such as Kawasaki disease. It is striking how frequently marked thrombocytosis is seen after even simple operations such as those for pyloric stenosis in infants.

INFECTIONS

Neonates

In addition to those more general features mentioned above, congenital infections with toxoplasma, rubella, cytomegalovirus (CMV), other herpes viruses, syphilis and human immunodeficiency virus (HIV) may all cause varying degrees and combinations of cytopenias, hepatosplenomegaly, jaundice and DIC. Human parvovirus B19 can cause prolonged red cell aplasia and result in stillbirth or hydropic fetuses and newborns.

Older infants and children

The lists here are truly enormous. Only a few examples will be highlighted. The most fulminating pictures with DIC and microangiopathic haemolysis occur in bacterial septicaemias – pneumococcal and meningococcal being particularly prominent. Verotoxin-secreting *Escherichia coli* may cause haemolytic uraemic syndrome. Temporary red cell aplasia has been seen – and confirmed on bone marrow examination – that appeared to have been caused by *Pseudomonas* septicaemia.

Viral infections also cause some striking haematological pictures. Infectious mononu-

cleosis is caused by Epstein–Barr virus (EBV) and, on occasions, with superficially similar appearances, by CMV. Although the presence of atypical mononuclear cells is by far the most common haematological manifestation of EBV infection, neutropenia, red cell aplasia, thrombocytopenia, immune haemolysis and even acute cold haemagglutinin disease with haemoglobinuria may occur. The immunological changes following infection with EBV have been extensively studied, but most are relatively unimportant to practising paediatricians and haematologists. Heterophile antibodies produced during infectious mononucleosis can be detected by a variety of commercial kits, but positive tests are not specific for EBV infection. Demonstration of IgM anti-EBV antibodies is more specific. Rather more clinically demanding are the problems caused by EBV in malarious areas of Africa (Burkitt's lymphoma), the increasing number of lymphomatous or abnormal lymphoproliferative diseases precipitated by this virus in immune-suppressed transplant recipients, the much rarer X-linked lymphoproliferative disease and infection-associated haemophagocytic conditions (see below under 'Histiocytoses'). Purpura fulminans can be precipitated by chickenpox, especially in children with protein C deficiency. Red cell aplasia, and accompanying neutropenia and thrombocytopenia, is one result of human parvovirus B19 infection (especially noticeable in any child with a short red cell survival, such as with spherocytosis, sickle cell disease or other haemolytic anaemia). Thrombocytopenia and low CD4$^+$ T-cell numbers may precede the hallmark infections of AIDS caused by HIV infection. Finally, there is a curiosity that is becoming more familiar: the development of a lupus-like anticoagulant with anti-prothrombin antibody resulting in prolongation of both the PT and APTT may be found as a temporary disturbance after a range of acute viral infections. In most cases, there is nothing else to raise the possibility of lupus, nor is it more likely to develop subsequently in such children (as far as is known). These are but a few of the well-known infection-associated abnormalities caused by diseases endemic to the UK.

Tropical infections are becoming ever more common. The old classic is malaria. Here, the full blood count is less important, apart from noting those cases with severe anaemia or with thrombocytopenia. More important is the detection and accurate identification of the plasmodium involved. It should be remembered that haematologists will only look for malarial parasites if prompted in some way to do so; clinical details will help, and a history of travel abroad (and exactly where, too) is useful and may help in the consideration of other non-malarial tropical diseases. Falciparum malaria may progress rapidly to death with cerebral malaria; rapid, accurate diagnosis and prompt appropriate treatment is crucial. The percentage of red cells infested with *Plasmodium falciparum* is important, and high levels should make one consider exchange transfusion, for example. In such cases, the haematology laboratory will be drawing attention to dangerous levels of parasitaemia.

Somewhat more exotic infections (but they are by no means particularly exotic in the countries in which they are contracted) are becoming more common as a result of the increasing number of people returning or newly arriving from countries that only 20 years or so ago might have been considered exotic themselves. Leishmaniasis may be contracted after sandfly bites from most tropical regions of the world, but also, closer to home, from Mediterranean countries. Fever, hepatosplenomegaly and pancytopenia in advanced cases may mimic cancer. Finding bone marrow macrophages containing Leishman–Donovan bodies provides a simple way of making the diagnosis. Dengue viruses are widespread throughout the world. Apart from the severe aches, bone pains and fever associated with dengue viruses, haematological disturbances are prominent; marked temporary neutropenia is a classical feature and may cause considerable alarm if discovered in a febrile child recently returned from a holiday in Thailand! Southeast Asian dengue may cause the fulminating dengue haemorrhagic fever/shock syndrome. At least as severe are the other viral haemorrhagic fevers and similar infections. Profound coagulopathy arising from DIC is a prominent feature. Guidance from an expert in tropical medicine is essential whenever such infections are suspected. Table 16.5 shows a very brief list of some important tropical diseases. More comprehensive lists with, in particular, discussion about the dengue haemorrhagic shock syndrome, can be found elsewhere.

NON-HAEMOPOIETIC TUMOURS

Most peripheral blood abnormalities (other than those caused by treatment) are either due to the anaemia of chronic disease, with or without reactive thrombocytosis, or to the effects of bone marrow infiltration. In those with leukoerythroblastic features (myelocytes and nucleated red cells in the blood film), the possibility of marrow infiltration should be seriously considered. Protocols for initial investigations in several types of childhood cancer require bone marrow examination irrespective of the peripheral blood findings. In some tumours, the initial presentation may be precipitated by bone marrow failure: anaemia and/or neutropenia and/or symptomatic thrombocytopenia.

The small round cell tumours (Table 16.6) often invade bone marrow, but only exceptionally rarely is it suggested that the malignant cells can be seen, by standard light microscopy, circulating in the blood stream. The term 'small' may be misleading; in cytological preparations (such as aspirated bone marrow), they may vary in size from a lymphoblast to a small megakaryocyte. The

Table 16.5 Tropical infections	
Infection	**Important features**
Malaria	Identify parasites in red cells Level of parasitaemia
Leishmaniasis	Hepatosplenomegaly Leishman–Donovan bodies in macrophages
Dengue	Neutropenia, haemorrhagic shock
Viral haemorrhagic fevers	Fulminating DIC

Table 16.6 Small round cell tumours	
Tumour type	**Appearance in infiltrated marrow**
Neuroblastoma Ewing's sarcoma	Clumping of 'blasts'. Reactive fibrosis Often patchy distribution
Rhabdomyosarcoma	Vacuolated large 'blasts', little clumping Often mistaken for leukaemia, lymphoma Little fibrosis, alveolar pattern in biopsy, often extensive distribution
Non-Hodgkin's lymphoma[a]	Similar to leukaemia appearances, no clumping Often diffuse, rather than localized, infiltrate
[a] NHL cells are positive for, and non-haemopoietic tumours negative for, haemopoietic cell markers.	

importance of detecting infiltration of the marrow lies in accurate staging (to guide treatment intensity and accuracy of prognosis) and, in those rare cases where no primary tumour can be found or it cannot safely be biopsied, in helping to make the diagnosis. On the whole, non-haemopoietic tumours tend to form clumps in aspirated bone marrow, while leukaemias and lymphomas do not. Other specialized immunocytochemical, cytogenetic and molecular biological tests may also distinguish between various small round cell tumours and provide conclusive evidence of their non-haemopoietic origin, but it is not always as simple to make a precise diagnosis. Such tests tend to be restricted to specialized centres. The role of detecting minimal levels of infiltration, or submicroscopic levels of circulating tumour cells, by molecular or immunological tests remains unclear. Bone marrow trephine biopsy is an important adjunct to aspiration because infiltration with non-haemopoietic tumour tends to be patchy, unlike the widely diffuse infiltration found in leukaemia. Some lymphomas, notably Hodgkin's disease and some more 'adult' forms of lymphoma, can also have a very patchy distribution within the marrow. In such circumstances, aspirated bone marrow often fails to reveal the presence of an infiltrate. Similar caveats apply to investigation of other non-malignant conditions that may infiltrate the marrow: tuberculosis, other granulomatous conditions, histiocytoses (see below) and others.

HISTIOCYTOSES

These are now classified into three groups (Table 16.7). They are covered in more detail in Chapter 15. In Langerhans cell histiocytosis (LCH, class I), important haematological abnormalities are rare. The marrow may be infiltrated in disseminated disease. The present author has only seen this, and been convinced by it, twice in the past 17 years, but routine staging bone marrows have not been demanded by many management protocols.

Opinions vary about the clinical importance of detecting marrow infiltration. This is hardly surprising in view of the lack of standardization of investigation required by different protocols. In the two cases mentioned above, the children had extensive infiltration detectable in aspirated marrow. The cells were histiocytes, but did not look like normal marrow macrophages or monocytes, nor did they look 'malignant'. Haemophagocytosis by the infiltrating cells was not a prominent feature in either case, in sharp contrast to haemophagocytic lymphohistiocytosis (HLH, see below). Occasional macrophages with some ingested cellular material could be found, but they were no more striking than similar reactive changes in a host of other conditions. The trephine biopsies showed extensive though patchy replacement of areas of marrow, interspersed with patches of morphologically normal haemopoietic tissue. Both children had neutropenia, which first, and unexpectedly, developed during the course of treatment. Neither has succumbed but follow-up was still, at the time of writing, less than 5 years in both.

Within the HLH syndromes (class II), it may be difficult or impossible to distinguish between the sporadic, presumably infection-associated, syndrome and the familial form. The clinical features (apart from a strong associations of the sporadic form with viral infections, of which EBV is the most prominent) of both types may overlap or even be identical; both types may have cytopenias, fever, malaise, hepatosplenomegaly, prolonged clotting times, hypofibrinogenaemia, hyperlipidaemia and other evidence of liver dysfunction, together with the striking presence of macrophages ingesting both nucleated and non-nucleated red cells, granulocytes and platelets in the bone marrow, lymph nodes, spleen or liver. Although central nervous system (CNS) involvement may occur, it is less common to find large numbers of such characteristic macrophages in cerebrospinal fluid (CSF); more usually, the CSF contains increased neutrophils and macrophages, without gross haemophagocytosis. It is worth re-emphasizing the point made in several atlases that haemophagocytosis by macrophages is not a diagnosis, merely a microscopic appearance. Decisions about

Table 16.7 Histiocytoses		
Histiocytosis class	**Cell of origin**	**Infiltrating cells in bone marrow**
Class I: e.g. Langerhans cell histiocytosis (LCH)	Dendritic cell	Morphologically non-malignant histiocytes. Little haemophagocytosis
Class II: e.g. haemophagocytic lymphohistiocytosis (HLH)	Tissue macrophage	Macrophages with numerous ingested haemopoietic cells
Class III: Malignant, e.g. acute monocytic leukaemia	Monocyte	Monocytoid blasts

Table 16.8 Storage diseases	
Disease	**Haematological abnormality**
Sphingolipidoses	
Gaucher's disease	Gaucher cells: macrophages with 'crumpled tissue paper'
Niemann–Pick disease	Foamy macrophages, occasional sea blue histiocyte
Mucopolysaccharidoses	
Hurler's, Hunter's syndromes, etc.	Alder–Reilly bodies in neutrophils, vacuoles with inclusions in lymphocytes, foam cells in marrow
Mucolipidoses	
Mannosidosis, fucosidosis	Vacuoles in lymphocytes
Others	
Glycogen storage disease (Pompe's)	Periodic acid Schiff reagent (PAS)-positive vacuoles in lymphocytes
Batten's disease	Vacuoles in lymphocytes
Wolman's disease	Foamy macrophages, Oil Red O positive for lipid

treatment may be difficult, and options include withdrawal of immunosuppression (in those being so treated for other reasons), high-dose intravenous immunoglobulin, interferon, chemotherapy regimens containing etoposide, and bone marrow transplantation. A number of other rare forms of histiocytosis have also been included within class II, but will not be considered here.

The malignant histiocytoses (class III) comprise acute monocytic leukaemia, 'granulocytic sarcoma' of monocytic origin and true 'histiocytic' lymphoma – a contradiction in terms! Overlap in their clinical and pathological features exists. They will not be considered further in this chapter (see Chapter 15).

STORAGE DISEASES

The haemopoietic cells that are sought in order to help make morphological diagnoses of storage diseases are often macrophages (in bone marrow) or other peripheral blood cells. They contain excessive amounts of material – sphingolipids, mucopolysaccharides or oligosaccharides. Various forms of 'storage cells', such as foamy macrophages, Gaucher cells or sea blue histiocytes, can be found in bone marrow aspirates. None is pathognomonic of a particular disease; all these various 'storage cells' may occur in other conditions. Peripheral blood cell vacuolation, especially of lymphocytes, may help raise the suspicion of various other storage diseases. Table 16.8 shows a brief list of some of these conditions and the characteristic storage cells. Other haematological abnormalities (e.g. bone marrow failure and hypersplenism) may develop. Complete diagnostic criteria comprise a complex mixture of clinical features and specific enzyme deficiencies; they, and the potential benefits of any interventions, such as specific enzyme replacement or bone marrow transplantation, are beyond the scope of this chapter.

FURTHER READING

Hann IM, Lake BD, Lilleyman J, Pritchard J. (1996) *Colour Atlas of Paediatric Haematology.* Oxford: Oxford University Press.

Smith H. (1996) *Diagnosis in Paediatric Haematology*. New York: Churchill Livingstone.

Stockman JA, Ezekowitz RAB. (1998) Hematologic manifestations of systemic disease. In: Nathan DJ, Orkin SH, eds. *Hematology of Infancy and Childhood*, 5th edn. Philadelphia: WB Saunders: 1841–91.

Weatherall D, Kwiatkowski D. (1998) Hematologic manifestations of systemic disease in children of the developing world. In: Nathan DJ, Orkin SH, eds. *Hematology of Infancy and Childhood*, 5th edn. Philadelphia: WB Saunders: 1893–914.

17 Late effects of therapy

Meriel EM Jenney

INTRODUCTION

It is because the survival rates for children with both acute lymphoblastic leukaemia (ALL) and acute myeloid leukaemia (AML) have improved so dramatically over the past 20 years that the issue of the late effects of therapy has assumed increasing importance in paediatric haematology. The number of children surviving continues to rise and their life expectancy is likely to be good (although this will not be truly known until current cohorts are followed for several decades). Any adverse treatment effects acquired will therefore have a very long-term impact. Before exploring these effects in detail, it is important to understand a number of issues relating to the interpretation of investigations of children and adolescents following therapy, to put findings in context and to appreciate the limitations of many current studies.

The treatment regimens for childhood haematological malignancies are changing continually – the late effects apparent in survivors treated 10 years ago may not be present in the current cohort. (An example of this would be the ubiquitous use of cranial irradiation throughout the 1980s for children with ALL, now only used for children designated 'high-risk' or with disease within the central nervous system (CNS).) There has been a steady increase in the intensity of systemic chemotherapy used, which, with improved supportive care, has led to improved survival rates for the children. Whether this leads, for example, to an increase in the number of infertile survivors or an increase in the rate of second cancers remains to be seen, but when counselling families at the time of therapy, many details are unknown for an individual's risk of specific late effects of therapy.

Children, although more tolerant of intensive chemotherapy than adults, are more sensitive to many of the late effects of treatment. Growth and maturation are not complete and some complications may not become apparent until the child enters puberty, when an accelerated rate of growth or maturation may not occur or may be subnormal. Organ dysfunction (e.g. cardiac or pulmonary) may also become apparent at that time. Late effects of therapy are more directly related to the therapy received than to the diagnosis. They are more frequent and severe for children who have relapsed and have had additional intensive therapy or a bone marrow transplant (BMT) than for children with the same diagnosis who have received standard therapy. The late effects of therapy can be physical, emotional and/or social, and, for some survivors, can have a major impact on the individual's quality of life.

Identification of the late effects of therapy is important, as intervention may be required (e.g. growth hormone replacement or psychological support), and delay in diagnosis and intervention may lead to further problems for the child or adolescent. As future treatment strategies are planned, an understanding of the long-term impact of therapy is important so that adverse effects of therapy can, if possible, be minimized without compromising cure.

As the data relating to the late effects of childhood cancer is now reviewed, these issues should be kept in mind. The causes of many of the late sequelae are often multifactorial (cytotoxic chemotherapy, intercurrent infection, age at therapy, gender, etc.), although particular aspects of therapy may be primarily responsible. Current research continues to explore the relative impact of different therapeutic modalities. Many of the cohorts examined are not population-based (research has centred around those on active follow-up); therefore there may be an overestimate of the frequency of some of the late effects seen, assuming that those not attending routine clinics are well! The details of sequelae after therapy will be described, with their likely causes; where specific agents or modalities of therapy are known to be associated with particular late effects, this will be clarified.

HISTORICAL PERSPECTIVE

In the early 1960s, the outlook for children with leukaemia was bleak, with only an occasional survivor, the majority of children suffering CNS relapse and progression of their disease. The introduction of CNS-directed therapy in the form of craniospinal irradiation for children with ALL dramatically reduced the relapse rates and in turn improved overall survival. The subsequent modifications of CNS-directed therapy demonstrate the importance of the recognition of late effects and how therapy can be modified to minimize toxicity without compromising cure. Studies of the long-term survivors of the 1960s demonstrated an adverse effect on educational achievement (fall in intelligence quotient, IQ) and growth impairment in children who received craniospinal radiotherapy, and in the early 1970s, the Medical Research Council (UK) ALL trials addressed some of these issues. Cranial irradiation only was used in UKALL II (1972) and UKALL III (1973), to minimize the effect on spinal growth (and the acute myelosuppressive effect), and the dose was reduced in 1980–84 (UKALL VIII) from 24 Gy to 18 Gy in an attempt to further reduce toxicity. More recently, alternative CNS-directed therapy for children with standard-risk disease has been introduced (high-dose systemic methotrexate with intrathecal methotrexate or intrathecal methotrexate alone). As the CNS-directed therapy has been reduced, so the use of systemic cytotoxic chemotherapy has been significantly increased. (An example is the introduction of anthracyclines, which, despite

concerns of acute and long-term cardiotoxicity, have enhanced survival overall.) Survival rates have been maintained with reduced CNS toxicity, although much of the long-term toxicity of the newer CNS-directed therapy and more intensive systemic therapy has yet to be defined.

The prognosis for children with AML remained poor until recently. Through national and international randomized trials, progress has now been made with the use of intensive cycles of chemotherapy, including high-dose anthracyclines, alkylating agents and a number of patients undergoing BMT. Long-term toxicity is therefore greater for these survivors, and for some patients with 'good prognostic indicators', modifications of therapy aiming to reduce toxicity are now being made.

ENDOCRINE EFFECTS

The endocrine effects following treatment for childhood haematological malignancies are perhaps the most important, since early diagnosis and intervention, particularly with respect to growth, can dramatically improve outcome. Many of the effects described result from the use of cranial irradiation in ALL and the dose-dependent effect that this has on the pituitary gland. As the treatment regimens for childhood leukaemia have changed, particularly with the reduction of the use of irradiation and substitution by more intensive chemotherapeutic regimens, one might expect a change in the pattern of the early and late toxicity seen.

Growth

The commonest cause of growth impairment following treatment for ALL is growth hormone deficiency (GHD) following cranial irradiation. Growth hormone (GH) is the most sensitive of the pituitary hormones to radiotherapy, and abnormalities of production are seen to occur at doses of 18 Gy and above. The higher the dose, the greater the incidence of GHD in the cohort and the more rapid the onset from the time of irradiation. Children younger at the time of irradiation also appear to be more susceptible. Despite a normal response to provocation tests, GH production may be impaired (e.g. disturbances of the periodicity of growth hormone secretion) and GHD may therefore be difficult to diagnose. All children who have received cranial irradiation as part of their therapy for leukaemia should therefore have regular, accurate assessment of their growth until they have completed puberty.

One important clinical point is that the pubertal growth spurt can occur early in some children who have received cranial irradiation, particularly girls. In these children, the onset of GHD may be masked by the pubertal growth spurt. If GH production is impaired, the growth spurt will be inadequate and the epiphyses will fuse early, limiting the growth potential of the child. It is therefore essential that pubertal staging is also monitored closely – puberty can then be delayed, GH given and the height potential of the child improved.

The spinal component of craniospinal irradiation has a direct effect on spinal growth. The younger the child at the time of irradiation, the greater the effect. It has been estimated that for a child aged 5 years at the time of therapy, the expected spinal loss would be 7 cm, and for one aged 10 years, approximately 5.5 cm.

Chemotherapy has also been shown to have an adverse effect on growth. Although catch-up growth can occur, there is some evidence in survivors of childhood ALL that the intensity of cytotoxic chemotherapy (dose and duration) is related to long-term impairment of growth, although the effect is less profound than that following radiotherapy. Nutritional and emotional effects of therapy also impair growth during therapy; whether there is long-term impairment is less clear.

Sexual development and fertility

Males and females differ in their sensitivity to chemotherapy and radiotherapy used in the treatment of leukaemia and other haematological malignant disorders. The testis is more sensitive than the ovary and has less capacity to recover.

Chemotherapy in girls

The ovulatory and secretory functions of the ovary are closely associated. Therefore, normal progression through puberty with the onset of menarche and regular menses is likely to be associated with ovulatory cycles and normal sex hormone levels. The vast majority of survivors of childhood ALL will have received low-dose multi-agent chemotherapy (vincristine, prednisolone, daunorubicin, asparaginase, methotrexate and 6-mercaptopurine). This results in little significant impairment of ovarian function (hormonal output or fertility potential), although some evidence of structural damage has been demonstrated. In a large study of 97 survivors of ALL who had not received radiotherapy to the abdomen or spine, only 9% had raised gonadotrophin levels. Those patients who do have impairment of ovarian function after chemotherapy for ALL are likely to have relapsed and to have required additional chemotherapy, in particular alkylating agents (e.g. cyclophosphamide) and cytarabine together with radiotherapy. There is little evidence of significant long-term ovarian toxicity with standard chemotherapy alone. Fewer studies of survivors of childhood AML have been undertaken to date, although many of these children undergo BMT and therefore may have long-term problems (see below).

Radiotherapy in girls

Some girls surviving ALL will have received radiotherapy to a region with possible scatter to the ovary (e.g. craniospinal radiotherapy) and are thereby at increased risk of significant dysfunction. Many patients who have received such therapy have a period of normal ovulatory cycles but may go on to have premature ovarian failure. However, among girls who have received total body irradiation (direct radiation to ovary) prior to BMT (usually in combination with high-dose cyclophosphamide), almost all experience primary ovarian failure and develop symptoms of early menopause. In a large series (Sanders and Sullivan 1989), a small proportion did experience recovery of ovarian function, although this was only transient. In addition to the impact of radiotherapy on the ovary, there may also be direct radiation effects to the uterus and the vasculature of the uterus, limiting its ability to expand normally during pregnancy, with the result of a high frequency of miscarriage or mid-trimester abortion.

Premature puberty has been recognized as a complication of the treatment of ALL, particularly following cranial irradiation. Those patients who are youngest at the time of cranial radiotherapy are most likely to have significant disturbance of pubertal timing.

In summary, for the majority of girls who receive standard treatment for ALL, there will be no significant long-term fertility problems, with the exception of three groups: (i) patients who relapse and receive further intensive chemotherapy including alkylating agents; (ii) girls receiving BMT (total body irradiation and high-dose alkylating agents); (iii) girls receiving radiation with significant scatter to the ovaries.

Chemotherapy in boys

A normal progression through puberty in boys is not predictive of normal fertility. The testis is more sensitive to chemotherapy than the ovary. The Leydig cells (responsible for steroidogenesis) are more robust than the Sertoli cells (spermatogenesis), although both will be affected by significant doses of irradiation.

Alkylating agents are the main group of drugs that cause testicular damage, although the cumulative doses of cyclophosphamide used in the treatment of ALL are usually below gonadotoxic doses. Some patients with AML will have received high doses of alkylating agents and may demonstrate abnormalities of spermatogenesis but not steroidogenesis. The boys are likely to experience normal puberty, sexual maturation and libido. They will have normal luteinizing hormone levels, but their follicle-stimulating hormone levels may be raised. If the gonadotoxicity is significant, the testicles may be smaller than normal (approximately 12 ml or less). Recovery of spermatogenesis can occur but is unpredictable.

Radiotherapy in boys

The majority of boys receiving testicular irradiation will have had ALL and will receive a dose (24 Gy) that will render the child sterile. The majority will also require androgen replacement therapy to allow normal pubertal development. For boys with AML, although the dose of total body irradiation used as conditioning for transplantation is lower than that for testicular relapse, usually 12–14 Gy, these patients will also receive high-dose cyclophosphamide, rendering the majority sterile and requiring androgen replacement therapy for normal progression through puberty. There is also a risk of gonadal damage after spinal irradiation with scatter to the testis, although this is smaller.

All peripubertal boys who receive gonadotoxic treatment should have the opportunity to store seminal fluid prior to cancer therapy. Some may not have achieved spermatogenesis at the time of presentation – new techniques of sperm and spermatid retrieval are currently under evaluation.

Effects on offspring

For both males and females, there is currently no evidence that there is an increased risk of congenital abnormalities in the offspring of survivors who have received cytotoxic chemotherapy or radiotherapy and have retained their fertility.

Obesity

A progressive increase in body mass index (BMI) has recently been demonstrated in survivors of childhood ALL following completion of therapy. A further observation is that survivors undertake less aerobic activity than their peers, and when undertaking exercise in a controlled environment, their maximal oxygen uptake ($\dot{V}O_2$ max – a measure of exercise potential) is significantly less than that of control subjects. What is less clear is whether the obesity occurs primarily as a result of physiological changes following therapy and this in turn leads to lower motivation towards exercise (and in turn a lower exercise capacity), or whether there are psychological or other reasons that lead to the survivors undertaking less exercise on a daily basis leading to the lower $\dot{V}O_2$ max and obesity. Does the decrease in activity lead to obesity or vice versa? Obesity is associated with an increase in morbidity and mortality in later life and has adverse socioeconomic implications – it will be important to understand the underlying mechanisms and use preventative interventions wherever possible for these survivors.

Changes in bone mineral density

Osteoporosis has long been recognized as a complication of acute leukaemia at the time of presentation and in patients receiving therapy with high-dose steroids. More recently, a fall in bone mineral density has been identified in patients who have completed therapy for acute leukaemia in childhood, raising concerns that these patients may be at risk of significant osteoporosis in later life, particularly if there are other factors present (e.g. inactivity or sex hormone imbalance) that may compound the problem. There are several reasons why this cohort may be at risk of osteopenia – the disease itself, nutritional factors, growth hormone insufficiency or prior radiotherapy – and there is now evidence suggesting that chemotherapeutic agents may also have an adverse effect on bone turnover. Identification of patients at particular risk is again important, as intervention may result in a significant improvement in outcome.

Thyroid function

Although resistant to chemotherapeutic damage, the thyroid is sensitive to the effects of irradiation, and patients receiving total body or craniospinal irradiation with significant scatter to the thyroid will be at risk of long-term dysfunction. The latency period between the time of radiotherapy and the onset of clinical problems can be several years. There may be abnormalities of structure with the development of nodules that occasionally can become malignant, or of secretory function. A fall in thyroxine production with a raised thyroid-stimulating hormone (TSH) level clearly indicates a need for replacement therapy. An isolated elevation of TSH (with normal serum thyroxine) can also occur, and patients with this secretory pattern should also receive replacement therapy because of concern that a persistently raised TSH can further increase the risk of the development of malignant nodules.

Patients who have received a significant radiation dose or scatter to the thyroid should have regular, life-long biochemical monitoring of thyroid function and clinical palpation of the thyroid gland. Ultrasound scans may also be of value, but are not generally performed on a regular basis.

SECOND MALIGNANCIES

Children surviving ALL and AML are known to be at an increased risk of developing a second cancer when compared with the cancer risk of the general population. For children with ALL, this has been estimated at 2.5–8% at 15 years. The risk for all survivors of haematological malignancies is related to three main factors:

- *Cytotoxic agents:* (i) topoisomerase II inhibitors, for example etoposide (scheduling and cumulative dose); (ii) alkylating agents, for example cyclophosphamide (cumulative dose); (iii) anthracyclines.
- *Radiotherapy:* dose- and site-related.
- *Genetic risk:* there are familial germline mutations now recognized (e.g. abnormalities of the *p53* gene) in which an increased number of family members may be susceptible to early cancer. Although uncommon, this or similar genetic risk may contribute to the increased number of second cancers seen in survivors.

As therapeutic regimens change (intensify) and greater numbers of children survive and are followed up into adult life, the incidence of second cancers seen in this population is likely to increase.

CARDIAC SEQUELAE

The anthracycline antibiotics (e.g. daunorubicin, doxorubicin and mitoxantrone) are important agents used in the treatment of childhood leukaemia, particularly AML. Since the late 1970s, early and late cardiotoxicity associated with these agents has been recognized. The risk of toxicity is dose-related and exacerbated by irradiation (direct or scatter) to the heart (e.g. craniospinal or total body irradiation). Although children receiving chemotherapy doses as low as 45 mg/m^2 have been reported to have minor abnormalities of cardiac function, significant toxicity is unlikely for children receiving under 200 mg/m^2, although there are individual differences in sensitivity. Some survivors of childhood leukaemia, however, are at a particular risk: (i) children with AML, who will receive at least 300 mg/m^2 of anthracyclines as standard therapy and some of whom will go on to have a BMT; (ii) children with ALL who have relapsed and require additional therapy with anthracyclines; many of these also undergo BMT.

For many children, long-term cardiac dysfunction is subclinical. The implications of this are poorly understood, and prospective studies of these survivors are currently underway to identify whether children in whom dysfunction is identified during therapy are those who go on to have later significant cardiac dysfunction. There is a gender difference in that girls appear to be more sensitive than boys to cardiac dysfunction following a given dose of anthracyclines at a given age. For some previously asymptomatic individuals, cardiac function may apparently worsen during or following puberty. The mechanism of this is not fully understood but may be related to a failure of adequate cardiac adaptation during the physiological growth spurt.

It is now recommended that all children who have received anthracyclines as part of therapy be followed throughout therapy and afterwards. All patients should at the very least have an electrocardiogram (ECG) and resting echocardiography at the start of therapy, after alternate courses of anthracyclines and within 3 months of completion of therapy. If the end-of-treatment studies show abnormality, further evaluations should be undertaken at least annually; if normal, then evaluation should be at 3-yearly intervals. Holter monitoring (24-hour ECG monitoring) is also recommended at 5-yearly intervals. For patients in whom cardiac abnormalities are demonstrated, many are seen to worsen with time, and long-term follow-up into adulthood is essential.

RESPIRATORY FUNCTION

The majority of patients surviving acute leukaemia will not have significant respiratory dysfunction in the long term. However, a number of patients will have subclinical evidence of lung damage, usually a restrictive defect. Patients at particular risk are those who have received radiotherapy to an area involving, or with scatter to, the lung fields (spinal radiotherapy or total body irradiation). Other agents used in the treatment of leukaemia that can predispose to long-term pulmonary dysfunction are cyclophosphamide, busulphan and methotrexate. During therapy, a number of patients will also have experienced a significant lower respiratory tract infection (bacterial, *Pneumocystis carinii*, viral or fungal). This may predispose to long-term pulmonary dysfunction, particularly fibrosis.

Exercise tolerance is known to be lower in survivors of leukaemia when compared with a peer group. How much of this is related to prior lung damage (rather than obesity, lack of activity or cardiac dysfunction) remains to be seen – its aetiology is clearly multifactorial.

NEUROPSYCHOLOGICAL SEQUELAE

There has been considerable interest in the neuropsychological outcome for children after treatment for leukaemia. Research has focused on the effects of CNS-directed therapy in ALL, which have become increasingly important as survival rates have improved. Following the introduction of cranial radiotherapy in the early 1960s, a number of adverse effects were reported (e.g. memory impairment or fall in IQ). These effects appear to be dose-related, and the younger the child is at the time of therapy, the greater the effect. Girls appear to be more sensitive than boys, particularly with respect to fall in IQ, and problems may be exacerbated by the use of intrathecal drugs (e.g. methotrexate). Structural abnormalities of the brain can be identified in patients who have received high doses of radiation, for example, cortical atrophy, vascular damage (mineralizing microangiopathy) or leukoencephalopathy. Calcification of the basal ganglia and/or grey or white matter junctions has been associated with poor intellectual and memory functioning in survivors of leukaemia during infancy. Early recognition of adverse cognitive function is important, as additional help with schooling may be of value and improve the long-term outcome for the child.

TRANSFUSION-RELATED COMPLICATIONS

Many children with malignant and non-malignant haematological disorders will be exposed to multiple transfusions of blood products. Transmission of infections (usually viral) has been dramatically reduced through screening and heat treatment of pooled blood products; however, it continues to occur, and all patients receiving blood products are at some risk. In the UK, there is now a national retrospective study ('Lookback study') underway, screening those patients who have received blood products over a particular time period from donors subsequently identified as testing positive for hepatitis C. The screening of patients who received blood products prior to this period is now being undertaken by some centres, although the role of intervention (interferon-α) has yet to be fully evaluated. Survivors of childhood leukaemia are not routinely screened for HIV, although occasional patients are now presenting with evidence of HIV infection. This is a well-recognized complication in recent years in patients with coagulation disorders (e.g. haemophilia) who have received regular transfusions of pooled blood products.

Patients with non-malignant disorders who require repeated red cell transfusions are at particular risk of iron overload in the long term. This is discussed in detail in Chapter 5.

CONCLUSION

The outlook for children surviving haematological malignancies during childhood is good. There are significant physical late effects of treatment that are now recognized, particularly following bone marrow transplantation. The majority of children, however, receive lower-intensity chemotherapy with minimal toxic effects. The long-term social and psychological effects of treatment are less well understood, and systematic evaluation is necessary to determine patients at risk and where psychological intervention may be appropriate and beneficial. Whilst it is important to focus on the late effects of treatment, it is of greater importance to maintain survival rates and to modify therapy to reduce toxicity only where this will not compromise cure.

FURTHER READING

Cousens P, Waters B, Said J, Stevens M. (1988) Cognitive effects of cranial irradiation in leukaemia: a survey and meta-analysis *J Child Psychol Psychiatry* **29:** 839–52.

Liesner RJ, Leiper AD, Hann IM, Chessells JM. (1994) Late effects of intensive treatment for acute myeloid leukaemia and myeloidysplasia in childhood. *J Clin Oncol* **12:** 916–24.

Lipshultz SE, Colan SD, Gelber RD et al. (1991) Late cardiac effects of doxorubicin therapy for acute lymphoblastic leukaemia in childhood. *N Engl J Med* **324:** 808–15.

Neglia JP, Meadows AT, Robison L et al. (1991) Second neoplasms after acute lymphoblastic leukaemia in childhood. *N Engl J Med* **325:** 1330–6.

Sanders J, Sullivan K. (1989) Long term effects and quality of life in children and adults after bone marrow transplantation. *Bone Marrow Transplant* **4:** 27–9.

Schwartz CL, Hobbie WL, Constine LS, Ruccione KS, eds. (1994) *Survivors of Childhood Cancer. Assessment and Management.* St Louis, MO: Mosby.

Wallace WHB. (1997) Growth and endocrine function following treatment of childhood malignant disease. In: Pinkerton CR, Plowman PN, eds. *Paediatric Oncology. Clinical Practice and Controversies*, 2nd edn. London: Chapman & Hall: 706–31.

Index

Ferguson